Handbook of Family Planning and Reproductive Healthcare

Fifth Edition

Edited by

Anna Glasier BSc MD DSc FRCOG FFFP OBE

Lead Clinician for Sexual Health in NHS Lothian; Honorary
Professor at the University of Edinburgh School of Clinical Science
and at the Community Health and University of London School of
Hygiene and Tropical Medicine, UK

Ailsa E Gebbie MB ChB DCH FRCOG FFFP

Consultant in Community Gynaecology, NHS Lothian; Honorary
Senior Lecturer, University of Edinburgh, Edinburgh, UK

Foreword by

John Guillebaud MA FRCSE FRCOG FFFP HON FCOG (SA)

Emeritus Professor of Family Planning and Reproductive Health
University College London, UK
Trustee of the Margaret Pyke Memorial Trust
Formerly Medical Director of the Margaret Pyke Family Planning
Centre, London, UK

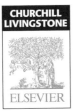

CHURCHILL
LIVINGSTONE

ELSEVIER

Edinburgh   London   New York   Oxford   Philadelphia   St Louis   Sydney   Toronto   2008

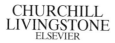
CHURCHILL
LIVINGSTONE
ELSEVIER

An imprint of Elsevier Limited

© 2008, Elsevier Limited. All rights reserved.

© Harcourt Publishers Limited 2000

The right of Anna Glasier and Ailsa Gebbie to be identified as authors of this work has been asserted by them in accordance with the Copyright, Designs and Patents Act 1988.

Fourth edition 2000

Third edition 1995

Second edition 1991

First published 1985

ISBN: 9780443068874

British Library Cataloguing in Publication Data
A catalogue record for this book is available from the British Library

Library of Congress Cataloging in Publication Data
A catalog record for this book is available from the Library of Congress

Note

Knowledge and best practice in this field are constantly changing. As new research and experience broaden our knowledge, changes in practice, treatment and drug therapy may become necessary or appropriate. Readers are advised to check the most current information provided (i) on procedures featured or (ii) by the manufacturer of each product to be administered, to verify the recommended dose or formula, the method and duration of administration, and contraindications. It is the responsibility of the practitioner, relying on their own experience and knowledge of the patient, to make diagnoses, to determine dosages and the best treatment for each individual patient, and to take all appropriate safety precautions. To the fullest extent of the law, neither the Publisher nor the Editors assume any liability for any injury and/or damage to persons or property arising out or related to any use of the material contained in this book.

The Publisher

Foreword

The foreword to the last edition by Dr Nancy Loudon OBE, whose 'baby' (first born in 1985) this Handbook was, started with the words: 'Family planning has been one of the success stories of the 20th century'. Yet, she also pointed out, world population had at the start of that year (2000) just passed six billion and more than 120 million women in developing countries had no modern way of preventing pregnancy. So it was maybe a success story but also undoubtedly a could-do-better story – due to not receiving the priority, especially the funding priority it merits, whether worldwide or in the UK.

In the same year, 189 governments committed themselves to achieving eight highly estimable Millennium Development Goals (MDGs) to improve the welfare of the people of developing countries by 2015. But by 2007 the UK All-Party Parliamentary Group on Population Development and Reproductive Health issued its Report on Hearings at Westminster and concluded that 'at current rates of progress . . . we will not meet these goals' and specifically that 'the MDGs are difficult or impossible to achieve with the current levels of population growth'.

What do the following have in common? Controlling climate change, saving the wild mountain gorillas of Rwanda, reducing the carnage of about 550,000 women dying annually through unsafe abortion, pregnancy and childbirth, and improving the long-term life prospects for many UK teenagers? What these highly disparate problems share is the major contribution to their solution that could come from improved availability and uptake of family planning (for humans). Potentially this would mean: fewer climate changes; the conservation of more habitats in the wild; about 30–40 percent fewer women in Africa dying through pregnancies they have no desire to have; and fewer teenage mothers who are everywhere 'more likely to drop out of school, to have no or low qualifications, to be unemployed or low-paid, to live in poor housing conditions, to suffer from depression, and to live on welfare'.

In the light of these and even more potential benefits to all life on the planet, James Grant of UNICEF in 1992 declared that *'family-planning could bring more benefits to more people at less cost than any other single technology now available to the human race.'*

Why then, in almost all countries, is there such a tragic mismatch between the value of this 'technology' and its perceived priority on the ground, in competition with the many concerns of civil society? UK readers of this book will not need reminding how clinicians battle endlessly to maintain staff morale and face the often difficult choice between the training of doctors in long-acting reversible contraception (ironically a government priority) and keeping their services open, free and accessible. As Richard Ma, a London GP, wrote in the BMJ in 2006, contraceptive services are 'about sex, but not sexy enough' – meaning that in the decisions by primary care organizations they are 'not as worthy of attention as information technology, management consultants, cancer and children's services'. The title of another article by Meera Kishen, President of the UK Faculty of Family Planning and Reproductive Health Care said it all: *Contraception in Crisis*. She wrote in the Faculty journal at the end of 2006, 'Though political commitment to contraception has been expressed in all national policy documents the reality on the ground, being experienced by clients and clinicians, seems very different. . . . If current trends in contraceptive provision in the UK are not addressed as a matter of urgency then single mothers, teenagers, migrants, refugees, sex workers and other marginalised groups . . . will face barriers to obtaining the more effective methods of fertility control'.

Teenage pregnancy is a major unresolved problem in the UK yet it could also be said to be THE problem, everywhere. The Earth faces the largest generation of young people in its history – a 'youthquake' of some 1200 million people between the ages of 10 and 19, or three billion under the age of 25. The 'demographic momentum' they generate means global population will continue to grow for decades, even if replacement fertility is achieved. How many youngsters thronging the slums of the world's mega-cities will be able, as they pass puberty and 'come into the sexual market-place', to access the sex and relationships education and the contraceptive services they need and deserve?

Nancy Loudon's 2000 Foreword made another point which remains – and for all the same reasons – unquestionably true for this edition: that although improvements in many methods appear throughout the Handbook, and new ones are predicted in the final chapter, 'no major breakthrough appears on the horizon'. But be that as it may, we are far better off with what we do have than our grandparents were. Much of great value will result if the words of this Handbook are read, inwardly digested and can then be fully implemented by its expected many readers.

John Guillebaud

Preface

This is the fifth edition of the Handbook and the third one to include the broader aspects of reproductive healthcare. Since the last edition was published in 2000, the specialty of family planning and reproductive health has become much more closely linked with genito-urinary (GU) medicine. Reflecting this, the specialty has become known as Sexual and Reproductive Healthcare as many family planning services are providing integrated care with GU medicine.

While the last seven years have seen little in the way of new contraceptive methods – only the combined contraceptive patch and a new type of progestogen-only pill have become available in the UK – there has been a profusion of strategies and guidelines relating to our specialty. Northern Ireland, Wales, England and Scotland have all published strategies for improving sexual health. While these strategies and their implementation have brought family planning and genito-urinary medicine services into greater prominence within the National Health Service (NHS), this plethora of interest threatens to be short lived. Inevitable financial overspends in the NHS have led within the last few years to closure of many family planning services in parts of England. It is ironic that this is happening just as the specialty of family planning has a flourishing professional organisation and integrated approach to healthcare delivery.

The thriving professional interest in this specialty is illustrated by the abundance of evidence-based clinical guidance for family planning providers. By the middle of 2008 the Clinical Effectiveness Unit of the Faculty of Family Planning will have produced a complete set of guidance documents for all available methods of contraception in the UK together with guidance on the needs of special groups and on managing common conditions related to contraceptive use. Additionally, two international clinical guidelines developed under the auspices of the World Health Organization have been adapted for use in the UK – the Medical Eligibility Criteria and the Selected Practice Recommendations. These guidelines are now widely available to all family planning professionals and should result in much improved clinical practice. Many of the chapters in this edition of the Handbook refer directly to these evidence-based guidelines. Even the National Institute for Health and Clinical Excellence (NICE) in the UK has been active in the area of contraception; producing in November 2005 the very welcome guideline on long-acting reversible methods of contraception.

Guidelines are only meant as a guide to clinical practice; to be a good clinician you need to have an understanding of how contraceptive methods work, the biological basis for their side effects, risks and benefits and how to provide contraception effectively. We hope that this new edition of the Handbook provides a useful and readable source for health professionals to acquire a better understanding of the theory underlying modern family planning and reproductive healthcare.

We have made several changes to this new edition of the Handbook and have involved a number of new authors who are all either respected authorities in their field or have very longstanding practical expertise. Dr Charlotte Ellertson who wrote the chapter on 'Contraceptive Choice' in the last edition of the Handbook tragically died in 2004. We highly valued Charlotte's old chapter so have updated it and kept it for one more edition. We are honoured that Professor John Guillebaud has written the foreword for this edition. John, who is now retired from clinical practice, contributed to all the previous editions of the Handbook. The author of the very first Handbook was Dr Nancy Loudon and it has been a great privilege to have continued editing the book which she first conceived and guided into print in 1985. Finally, Dr Lulu Stader was an extremely efficient editor for Elsevier. We appreciated her patience and skill in keeping the book on track.

It has become traditional for authors of medical textbooks to acknowledge the tolerance of their families whilst they slaved away with the writing, editing and final proof checking of their emerging textbook, in addition to carrying on with existing medical day jobs. This book of course has been no exception and we gratefully acknowledge the support of our families who only occasionally objected to the contemporaneous lack of domestic endeavour. This book is dedicated to them in the hope that they will feel the final result was worth it.

Contributors

Richard A Anderson MD PhD MRCOG
Professor of Clinical Reproductive Science, The University of Edinburgh; Consultant in Reproductive Medicine, Royal Infirmary of Edinburgh, Edinburgh, UK
Vasectomy

Paula Baraitser MBBS MFFP MD MFPH
Clinical Champion, Lambeth and Southwark Sexual Health Modernisation Programme, London, UK
Sexual health services for young people

Alison Bigrigg FRCOG MFFP FRCS (Ed) FRCP (Gla) DM MBA
Director and Lead Clinician Sexual Health, The Sandyford Initiative, Glasgow, UK
Service provision in the UK

Susan Brechin MRCOG MFFP MD ILTM DIPM
Senior Clinical Lecturer in Sexual and Reproductive Health, Aberdeen University, Aberdeen, UK
Emergency contraception

Audrey H Brown MBChB MRCOG
Consultant in Sexual and Reproductive Healthcare, Sandyford Initiative, Glasgow, UK
Abortion

Sharon Cameron MD MRCOG
Consultant Gynaecologist, Dean Terrace Centre and Royal Infirmary of Edinburgh, Edinburgh, UK
Gynaecological problems in the family planning consultation

Susan V Carr MB ChB FFFP DRCOG MPhil
Consultant in Sexual and Reproductive Healthcare, Sandyford Initiative, Glasgow, UK
Sexuality and family planning

Charlotte Ellertson MPA PhD (deceased)
Former Director of Reproductive Health for Latin America and the Caribbean, Population Council, Mexico City, Mexico and in 2002, founder of IBIS Reproductive Health, Boston, USA
Contraceptive choice

Marian P Everett MB ChB FFFP
Consultant in Sexual and Reproductive Health and Clinical Lead for Family Planning, Hull and East Yorkshire, UK
Progestogen-only pill

Ailsa E Gebbie MB ChB DCH FRCOG FFFP
Consultant in Community Gynaecology, NHS Lothian; Honorary Senior Lecturer, University of Edinburgh, Edinburgh, UK
Intra-uterine systems; Menopause

Anna Glasier BSc MD DSc FRCOG FFFP OBE
Lead Clinician for Sexual Health in NHS Lothian; Honorary Professor at the University of Edinburgh School of Clinical Science and Community Health and University of London School of Hygiene and Tropical Medicine, UK
Contraceptive choice; Combined hormonal contraception

Michael J K Harper PhD ScD MBA FIBiol
Professor of Obstetrics and Gynecology; Director Consortium for Industrial Collaboration in Contraceptive Research at CONRAD, a project of the Department of Obstetrics and Gynecology, Eastern Virginia Medical School, Arlington, Virginia, USA
Contraceptives of the future

Martha Hickey FRANZCOG MD
Professor of Obstetrics and Gynaecology, School of Women's and Infants' Health, University of Western Australia, Subiaco, Australia
Progestogen-only implants

Sally Hope MA [Oxon] FRCGP DRCOG
GP at the Woodstock Surgery, Oxfordshire; Hon Research Fellow in Women's Health, Dept of Primary Health Care, University of Oxford, Oxford, UK
Screening and health promotion

Susan Jones MA LLB MBBS FFFLM MRCGP DRCOG
Senior Medicolegal Adviser, Medical Protection Society, Leeds, UK
Legal aspects of family planning

Meera Kishen MD Dip GUM FFFP
Consultant in Contraception and Reproductive Healthcare, Abacus Clinics, Liverpool PCT, UK
Intrauterine devices

Diana Mansour MB BCh
Head of Contraception and Sexual Health Services, Medical Director, Community Services, Newcastle Primary Care Trust, Graingerville Clinic, Newcastle General Hospital, Newcastle upon Tyne, UK
Progestogen-only injectables

P M Shaughn O'Brien MD FRCOG
Professor of Obstetrics and Gynaecology, Keele University; Consultant Obstetrician and Gynaecologist, University Hospital North Staffordshire, Stoke-on-Trent, UK
Premenstrual syndrome

Mary W Rodger MBChB MRCOG MD
Consultant Obstetrician and Gynaecologist, Glasgow Royal Infirmary and The Princess Royal Maternity, Glasgow, UK
Female sterilization

Jane Smith BSc MB ChB FFFP
Associate Specialist, Family Planning and Sexual Health in NHS Lothian, Edinburgh, UK
Fertility awareness methods and postpartum contraception

Madelaine Ward RGN RNT ENB FFFP
Clinical Nurse Specialist Contraception and Reproductive Health Care, West Side Contraceptive Services, London, UK
Barrier methods

Christopher Wilkinson MBBS FFFP
Consultant in Sexual and Reproductive Health, Margaret Pyke and Mortimer Market Centres, Camden PCT, London, UK
Sexually transmitted infections

Contents

1 Contraceptive choice

Charlotte Ellertson and Anna Glasier

FERTILITY REGULATION STRATEGIES VERSUS METHODS

• Methods as building blocks

Family planning handbooks have traditionally presented the options for women or couples seeking to limit their fertility as a list of methods, each with its advantages and disadvantages. As the menu of contraceptive choices grows longer and more intertwined, however, and as the needs of couples who use contraception grow more complex, it may be more useful to think in terms of fertility control strategies rather than methods. A woman who perceives herself to be at risk of sexually transmitted infections (STIs) might choose condoms, even though these have a relatively high contraceptive failure rate, but might opt to back them up with emergency contraception to create a contraceptive strategy that is reasonably effective and also protective against STIs. Another woman who does not consider herself at risk of STIs might choose a method with higher contraceptive efficacy such as oral contraception, but which offers no protection against STIs. A woman who has intercourse infrequently but with a mutually monogamous partner, and who does not wish to use a method that requires daily action on her part, might prefer a combination of a diaphragm and spermicide, aware that if her contraception fails she has the back up of abortion (three methods combined, creating a highly effective and acceptable strategy), while another woman who would not like to rely on abortion might prefer the intrauterine device (IUD) in such a situation (a strategy involving just one method).

This chapter presents a brief overview of the various methods of family planning, but with the idea that they are building blocks that women or couples might use singly or in combination to construct a strategy that meets their needs.

• The lifecycle approach

Since methods of contraception which men can use are limited to withdrawal, condoms and vasectomy we can think of the 'typical' family planning client as a woman. Over the course of her life, a woman's needs will vary greatly. If she is from an industrialized country, as an adolescent, she is likely to have intercourse sporadically and at unpredictable times, but with partners that place her at risk of STIs. She may feel that her protection must be kept private from parents or friends, and her family planning goal may be to protect herself against pregnancy in a way that preserves her options for future fertility, preferably using methods that also offer STI protection. Later, as she enters a more stable relationship, and her sexual activity is more socially sanctioned, she may feel better able to negotiate condom use, or more willing to use a method that requires daily activity on her part. If she wants children, her needs during the next stage may be for methods that help her to space the births appropriately. Finally, she may reach a point where she no longer wants the option of childbearing, and she or her partner may choose a permanent method. A woman who has a large array of family planning options available to her throughout the course of her reproductive life will have an easier time meeting the needs she faces at each one of these stages.

• UK and international patterns of family planning

Two demographic trends in the UK currently influence the method mix in this country. First, the proportion of couples who opt not to have children at all is rising, and is currently around 25%. Second, the average age of women having their first baby is climbing, and is now nearly 30 years. Thus women today spend more years requiring contraceptives that preserve their fertility and fewer years needing permanent contraception, such as sterilization. Indeed the number of women being sterilized in Scotland has fallen dramatically over the last few years. In the calendar year 1998 in Scotland 7339 women were sterilized (a rate of 67.5/10 000), in 2005 the number had fallen to 2334 (22.1/10 000). While changes in the availability of the procedure and the willingness of health professionals to recommend and provide it may account for some of this decline, it does seem as though at least in Scotland, female sterilization may have become unfashionable.

Figures 1.1–1.3 show the patterns of contraceptive use found in a nationally representative survey of women aged 16 to 49, carried out in Britain in 2005/06.[1] Respondents were asked which methods (if any) 'you (and your partner) usually use at present'. A total of 74% of women under 50 years of age were using contraception and over 90% of those who believed themselves to be fertile and were not pregnant or trying to get pregnant were using contraception. Use of contraception was related to educational status with the least-well-educated women being less likely to use any method. The data shown come from female respondents and are presented by age group, since the method mix varies dramatically by this variable. Fifty-three percent of women were using a reversible method of contraception. Younger women (those under 29) favour the oral contraceptive pill and barrier methods and in

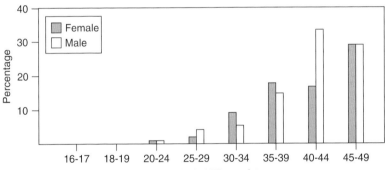

Figure 1.1 Use of male and female sterilization in the UK in 2005/06

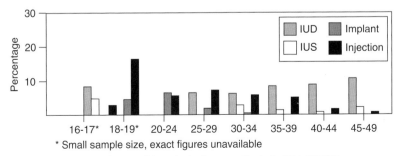

Figure 1.2 Use of long-acting reversible methods of contraception in the UK in 2005/06

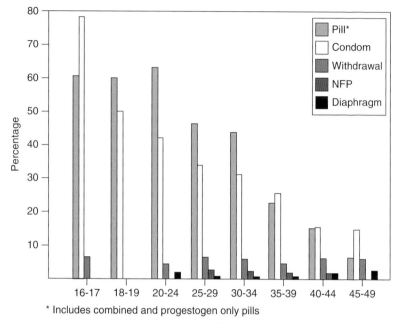

* Includes combined and progestogen only pills

Figure 1.3 Use of oral contraceptives, barrier methods, NFP and withdrawal in the UK in 2005/06

2005/06 compared with previous years, an increase was seen in young women using contraceptive implants and injections. In the next age category (30–39), the IUD and sterilization start to grow in popularity, as couples complete their families, and move toward longer-acting methods. Finally, in the older age groups (40 and over), oral contraceptive use falls to a fraction of its popularity with younger women, and sterilization (most commonly vasectomy) moves into the lead as the most widely used method. Interestingly female but not male sterilization was related to education with the least-well-educated women being most likely to have been sterilized. A disappointingly large proportion of women still rely on rather ineffective methods of contraception. Withdrawal is used more commonly than the LNG-IUS and natural family planning methods are used by more women than are diaphragms.

In the USA, nationally representative data are available from a large government survey, the National Survey of Family Growth (NSFG), that is repeated every few years (and seems to take forever to be reported). Data from 1995 show that, female sterilization, the pill and the male condom were the most widely used methods.[2] Between 1988 and 1995, however, pill use dropped from 31% to 27% of respondents, while condom use rose from 15% to 20%, with growth in condom use most marked among younger unmarried women. Clearly, in the late 20th century concerns about HIV and other STIs changed family planning strategies dramatically in the USA.

Worldwide, sterilization is by far the most widely used method. Nearly half of all sterilized men and women of reproductive age live in China (37%) or India (22%). In Canada, South Korea and the territory of Puerto Rico, over 40% of the population of reproductive age are sterilized. Except in the UK, India and Nepal, where the proportions are roughly equal, far more women than men are sterilized. IUDs are the second most popular method worldwide, driven largely by the popularity of the method in China, where a third of all couples using contraception employ it. Hormonal contraceptives as a group rank third in world usage. The bulk of this use is oral contraception. Some countries, however, may rely heavily on one particular method. For example, the South African national programme relies overwhelmingly on injectables. Condoms are used relatively little in developing countries, although they have grown in popularity as concerns about HIV spread. Japan, where oral contraceptives were approved only in the late 1990s leads the list, with 44% of contraceptive-users relying on the condom. Singapore and the Nordic countries (Denmark, Finland and Sweden) have rates of around 20% condom use.

EFFECTIVENESS

When guiding a new user through the array of contraceptive methods, undoubtedly the single most important question to ask about a method is 'how well does it work?' Unfortunately, the answer is sometimes quite complicated. The following brief guide to interpreting the efficacy literature may be helpful for those readers who do not simply want to trust the authors of handbooks!

• Measuring effectiveness

There are several pitfalls to notice when considering the effectiveness of contraceptive methods. First, not all of the women who use a given method would become pregnant even if the method were completely useless (such as crossed fingers). A certain percentage (perhaps 15%) of couples will not conceive within a year of trying, and for this fraction, 'using' even a useless method would still appear to provide 100% effective contraceptive protection. Second, many users participating in effectiveness studies of various methods do not use the method correctly and consistently every time they have intercourse. Third, some user characteristics of the participants in the study can have an enormous impact on the failure rates. Studies filled with younger women will tend to have higher failure rates (because younger women are more fecund), as will studies in which the participants have sex very frequently.

With most data taken from clinical studies, contraceptive effectiveness is typically presented in terms of failure rates rather than success rates. Failure rates are often subdivided into two categories: perfect-use failure rates and typical-use failure rates. A perfect-use failure rate refers to the number of pregnancies observed during cycles when the method was used consistently and correctly at every act of intercourse. Typical-use failure rates, by contrast, are derived from a mixture of perfect- and imperfect-use failure rates. Pregnancies counted during imperfect use include those that occurred when the user actually did not 'use' the method at all, leaving the diaphragm in the drawer, for instance, or missing her pills for several days in a row. The difference between typical- and perfect-use failure rates reflects how easy the method is to use.

As shown in **Figure 1.4** many methods have no or virtually no difference between their perfect- and typical-use failure rates. For instance, sterilization or an IUD requires almost nothing of the user once the method is started. By contrast, some methods have a tremendous gap between perfect- and typical-use failure rates. Abstinence, as one example, has a theoretical failure rate of 0%, but in practice, the method is prone to misuse (couples fail to abstain!), and has a typical-use failure rate of about 25%. Importantly both the combined pill and the condom (the two most commonly used methods in the UK) have much higher failure rates during typical use than during perfect use – and of course, by definition, most people use the methods 'typically'.

By contrast, effectiveness statistics based on community or population surveys, such as the Oxford Family Planning Association study in the 1970s or the NSFG in the USA, tend to reflect actual use experiences (typical use). These

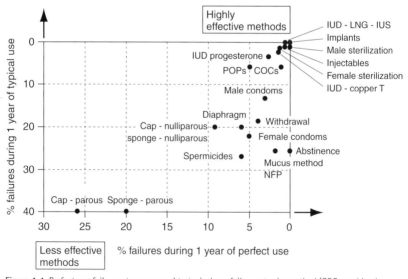

Figure 1.4 Perfect use failure rates compared to typical use failure rates by method (COC, combined oral contraceptive pill; IUD intrauterine device; NFP, natural family planning; POP, progestogen only pill)

types of studies, however, tend to suffer from under-reporting of abortion (and therefore artificially low failure rates of contraceptive methods) and also over-reporting the number of women using any contraceptive method.

There are two exceptions in the family planning literature concerning the way that effectiveness is measured: abortion and emergency contraception. In measuring the effectiveness of various abortion methods, researchers can use standard probabilities analogous to the cure rates used in other areas of medicine. This intuitively more straightforward method is possible since, in each case, 100% of the women who use the method start out pregnant and only a few remain pregnant following use of the method. Emergency contraception researchers typically present two effectiveness statistics. The first is a straightforward and easily interpretable failure rate. This percentage reflects the number of women who use emergency contraception in the trial and end up pregnant anyway. Unfortunately, the failure rate is only partially a reflection of how well the method works. It also reflects the underlying pregnancy risks of the women in the trial. For instance, an emergency contraception trial of extremely cautious women who all took emergency contraception because they had unprotected sex during menses would be expected to have a far lower failure rate than a trial of women who all had unprotected sex during their mid-cycle peak fertility days and took emergency contraception. For this reason, good emergency contraception researchers also present the results that estimate the number of expected pregnancies (added up by assessing the theoretical risk of pregnancy the study participants were facing) that were averted by the use of the method.

Over the past decades, family planning researchers have made great strides in measuring the effectiveness of contraceptives. In many older studies, effectiveness is described in terms of the somewhat misleading Pearl index. Developed by physician Raymond Pearl early in the last century, the Pearl index represents the number of pregnancies observed in a cohort of women using a given method divided by the total number of cycles in which the method was used by all the women put together. It is then usually multiplied by 1300 to standardize the results to reflect the experience of 100 woman-years with each woman contributing 13 cycles per year. The main flaw with the Pearl index is that it is not stable over time, and so researchers can ensure a low Pearl index for whatever method they are studying by running the study for a longer time. For example, in a hypothetical study of the male condom (based on actual data from the 1973 NSFG), the Pearl index would be 7.5 for the first 12 months, but only 4.4 if 60 months of data were analysed.[3] The reason is that the most fecund women will become pregnant first, and for at least a few months, they will not be at risk of falling pregnant again. The remaining women staying in the study will be the less fecund ones. Modern contraceptive researchers rely on life-table techniques that correctly reflect the exposure to pregnancy that each woman contributes starting from the time she joins the trial.[4] The results are presented as the number of pregnancies experienced during 100 woman-years of use of the method (a woman-year is

Table 1.1 Effectiveness of contraceptive methods: percentage of US women experiencing an unintended pregnancy during the first year of use (failure rates)

Method	% pregnant	
	Typical use	Perfect use
No method	85	85
Spermicides	29	18
Withdrawal	27	4
Periodic abstinence	25	
Calendar	9	
Ovulation method	3	
Sympto-thermal	2	
Cap		
parous women	32	26
nulliparous women	16	9
Diaphragm	16	6
Condom		
female	21	5
male	15	2
Combined pill and minipill	8	0.3
Combined hormonal patch (Evra)	8	0.3
Combined hormonal ring (NuvaRing)	8	0.3
DMPA (Depo-Provera)	3	0.3
IUD		
copper T	0.8	0.6
LNG-IUS (Mirena)	0.1	0.1
Implant	0.05	0.05
Female sterilization	0.5	0.5
Male sterilization	0.15	0.10

From Ref. 4

defined as 13 cycles), and are standardized by 1-year, 2-year, 5-year (or much shorter or longer) cut-off points.

One difficulty that remains is extrapolating effectiveness rates from the literature to the typical clinic population. On the one hand, failure rates might be expected to be higher in 'real life' than in a clinical trial because the users are perhaps less motivated than they would need to be to endure the extra burden of participating in a trial. In addition, perhaps they receive less counselling and special attention than they might in a trial. On the other hand, participants in clinical trials are sometimes selected because of their uniquely high risk. Focusing on a high-risk population can dramatically reduce the number of users needed in a trial, but it will also result in the trial showing a higher failure rate than would be true in real life. Table 1.1 shows summary estimates of the 1-year life-table perfect-use and typical-use failure rates for currently available methods. These are derived from a combination of population-based studies (wherever possible) and clinical trials judged to be of good quality. The failure probabilities for the various methods of early abortion and for emergency contraception appear in Chapters 8 and 11.

SAFETY

• Measuring safety

The second most common question about a method is likely to concern its safety. Measuring and comparing the safety of family planning methods is also difficult, but the reason in this case is that most methods are so safe that serious adverse events are extremely rare. Less serious ones are often quite subjective. Moreover, it is difficult to extrapolate side-effect profiles from clinical trial populations to real-life clients, in part because the users who join clinical trials often do so because they are not satisfied with any of the existing methods. These 'fussy customers' may be especially sensitive to side effects, and study staff prompt them to report side effects that would typically go unreported or unnoticed in a cohort of general users. It is these 'side effects' that make it into the patient information leaflet produced by the manufacturers and they often make the method seem much more likely to cause side effects than it actually is. Finally, safety events often affect only a subset of the users of a given method. For such users, the risks may be too high to justify the benefits, but for the rest of users the risks may be negligible.

• Safety of various methods of family planning

Safety may be divided into several categories: the most common side effects (including the medically trivial), any serious dangers that the method might entail (even if rare), and the risks of death. Table 1.2 summarizes safety considerations for each of the methods of fertility regulation currently available. In choosing methods it is important to bear in mind that pregnancy, particularly unwanted pregnancy, is not without health effects and risks of its own. Fully 100% of pregnant women experience 'side effects' and the risk of death from carrying a pregnancy to term is approximately 1/10000 in the developed world.

• Contraindications

Most contraceptive users are young and medically fit and can use any available method safely. A few medical conditions, however, are associated

Table 1.2 Chief side effects and dangers, and risks of death of selected family planning methods

Method	Side effects	Serious dangers	Risk of death
Spermicides	Reproductive and urinary tract infections, allergy (causes itching)	None	None measurable
Cervical cap, diaphragm, sponge	Reproductive and urinary tract infections	Toxic shock syndrome	None measurable
Condoms (male latex)	None	Anaphylactic reaction	None measurable
Oral contraceptives (combined)	Nausea, weight gain, dizziness, spotting, breast tenderness, chloasma, decreased libido	Cardiovascular complications, hepatic adenomas, possible increased risk of breast and cervical cancers	Non-smokers aged <35: 1/200 000; non-smokers aged 35+: 1/28 600; heavy smokers <35: 1/5300; heavy smokers 35+: 1/700
Oral contraceptives (progestogen-only)	Headaches, irregular bleeding, androgenic effects		None measurable
Emergency contraception (Hormonal)	Nausea, headaches, breast tenderness	None	None measurable
Abortion (mifepristone-PG in first 9 weeks LMP)	Bleeding, pain, gastrointestinal side effects	Haemorrhage, retained tissue	None measurable
Abortion (surgical)	Pain, bleeding	Anaesthesia complications, uterine perforation, cervical/uterine trauma, infection	<9 weeks: 1/262 800; 9–12 weeks: 1/100 000; 13–15 weeks: 1/34 000; 15+ weeks: 1/10 200
Injectables	Cycle changes, weight gain, headaches, changes in lipid profile, breast tenderness	Allergic reaction, bone density loss	None measurable

Table 1.2 (Continued)

Method	Side effects	Serious dangers	Risk of death
IUD (copper)	Increased menstrual cramping, spotting and bleeding	PID following insertion, uterine perforation, iron deficiency anaemia	1:10 000 000
Implants	Tenderness at implant site, cycle changes, alopecia, breast tenderness	Infection at implant site, removal complications	None measurable
Female sterilization	Pain at incision site, possible regret that method is permanent	Infection at surgical site, anaesthesia complications, ectopic pregnancy	Laparoscopic tubal ligation: 1/38 500; hysterectomy: 1/1600
Male sterilization	Pain at incision site, possible regret that method is permanent	Infection at surgical site, anaesthesia complications	Vasectomy: 1/1 000 000

LMP, Last menstrual period; PID, pelvic inflammatory disease.
Sources: Medical Economics Company 1999; World Health Organization 1996; other chapters in this book.

with theoretical increased health risks with certain contraceptives, either because the method adversely affects the condition or because the condition, or its treatment, affects the contraceptive. The combined pill for example may increase the risk of a woman with diabetes developing cardiovascular complications; some anti-convulsants interfere with the efficacy of the combined pill. Since most trials of new contraceptive methods deliberately exclude subjects with serious medical conditions, there is little direct evidence on which to base sound prescribing advice. In an attempt to produce a set of international norms for providing contraception to women and men with a range of medical conditions which may contraindicate one or more contraceptive methods, the World Health Organization (WHO) developed a system addressing medical eligibility criteria (MEC) for contraceptive use.[5] Using evidence-based systematic reviews, conditions are classified into one of four categories (Table 1.3). Category 1 includes conditions for which there is no restriction for the use of the method, while category 4 includes conditions that represent an unacceptable health risk if the contraceptive method is used (absolutely contraindicated). Classification of a condition as category 2 indicates that the method may generally be used but that more careful follow-up is required. Category 3 conditions are those for which risks of the COC generally outweigh the benefits (relatively contraindicated). Provision

---

Table 1.3 WHO Medical Eligibility Criteria Classification categories

The suitability of different contraceptive methods was categorized in the presence of specific illnesses or conditions. The categorization was achieved by weighing the health risks and benefits of using a particular contraceptive method when any of these conditions are present:

1. A condition for which there is no restriction for the use of the contraceptive method.
2. A condition where the advantages of using the method generally outweigh the theoretical or proven risks.
3. A condition where the theoretical or proven risks usually outweigh the advantages of using the method.
4. A condition which represents an unacceptable health risk if the contraceptive method is used.

The classification also includes the medical criteria for the initiation and continuation of use for all methods. Only those instances where the criteria for continuation of a method differed from criteria for initiating the method are included.

---

of a method to a woman with a category 3 condition requires careful clinical judgement since use of that method is not recommended unless there is no acceptable alternative. It may be sensible in these circumstances for the provider to seek advice from someone with expertise in contraception. For some conditions the MEC distinguish between a method being started for the first time (initiation) and continuation of a method (continuation). If for example a women has a stroke while she is using the progestogen-only pill, continuation of the method is a category 3 (the theoretcial risks of using the POP outweigh the benfits). If a woman who has had a stroke wants to start using the progestogen-only pill it is a category 2 condition and the benefits of using the method outweigh the theoretical risks. The document is available on the web and a system is in place to incorporate new data into the guideline as they become available. The Faculty of Family Planning and Reproductive Healthcare (FFPRHC) has produced a UK version of the WHOMEC. The UK medical eligibility criteria will be presented for each contraceptive method in the appropriate chapters in this textbook.

NON-CONTRACEPTIVE BENEFITS

Modern users of contraceptives want more from their methods than just safe and effective contraceptive protection. In one recent study from the USA,[6] for instance, male users, describing the factors important to them in choosing a method of family planning, rated protection from STIs as highly as they did contraceptive protection. Other contraceptive users may be attracted to the benefits for acne, or the reduction in dysmenorrhoea, offered by certain oral contraceptive formulations. For this reason, family planning providers should be familiar with the non-contraceptive benefits associated with several of the family planning methods. Although these are covered in detail in the chapters relevant to each individual method, the few most important are covered briefly here.

• Protection against sexually transmitted infections

As described more fully in Chapter 18, protection from STIs in the context of family planning is chiefly a function of physical barriers. The male and female condoms, designed to prevent the greatest amount of skin-to-skin contact, offer the best protection. Partial barriers, including the diaphragm and cervical cap, may confer some protection, particularly for the cervical infections chlamydia and gonorrhoea and for cervical neoplasia. Chemical barriers of the future (often called 'microbicides') have such protection as an overt goal, and several possibilities are now entering advanced clinical testing. The important point to stress is that while the risk of pregnancy is concentrated during certain times of the menstrual cycle, the risk of transmitting or acquiring an STI is present at all times. In addition, depending on the pathogen, the likelihood of transmission during a single act of unprotected intercourse can far exceed the likelihood of pregnancy during a single act, even at a time in the cycle when the woman is most at risk of pregnancy.

• Menstrual disorders and bleeding control

Some hormonal contraceptives can reduce menstrual bleeding, and can help to alleviate the discomfort and inconvenience of irregular or painful periods. For women on honeymoon, women who travel frequently, women who compete in athletic competitions, or women who want, for any other reason, to time their bleeds precisely, combined oral contraceptives can be used continuously (discarding the placebos from everyday (ED) packets). Amenorrhoea is becoming increasingly acceptable in the Western world and methods which are likely to confer amenorrhoea (Depo Provera and the LNG-IUS) are getting more popular.

• Other non-contraceptive benefits

Several family planning methods offer non-contraceptive benefits, ranging from delays in premature ejaculation (male condoms) to protection against pelvic inflammatory disease (PID) and even certain cancers (several of the hormonal methods) to improvements in acne (oral contraceptives).

USER CONSIDERATIONS

Family planning has advanced farther than perhaps any branch of medicine in user autonomy and responsibility for decision-making. Methods of contraception are relatively safe and effective and the users are typically healthy and expected to use contraception for decades. Information is needed to allow the user to choose a method and is typically straightforward. The law and policy governing access to contraception is well developed in the UK. Family planning healthcare providers are able to act as a resource for information, and to offer counselling, where welcomed, to help the user reach an informed choice. In the equality of this partnership, family planning is a model area of medicine.

• Measuring user attitudes

Discontinuation rates

One indirect measure of user's satisfaction with a contraceptive method is the discontinuation rate. This measure shows the number of users, from a standardized starting cohort of 100, who have stopped using a method at a certain period in time, typically after 1 year of use. Methods that demand a great deal of the users, or impose a lot on them in terms of the side effects that must be tolerated, tend to have higher discontinuation rates than methods that require little, all other things being equal. Table 1.4 shows the 1-year discontinuation rates associated with the main reversible methods of family planning. The data come from the US. Data from the UK are hard to find and most come from clinical trials which, as discussed earlier, are not representative of normal use. Discontinuation rates for all methods are disappointingly high. Methods which require removal by a health professional (IUD/IUS and implants) tend to have higher continuation rates than those which the user can simply stop.

One criticism of the discontinuation rate as a measure is that it fails to reflect that people often choose specific methods for short periods of time and use them happily during this time, but with no plans for long-term use. For instance, users might opt for condoms in the first 3 months of a new relationship, but then switch to oral contraceptives if the relationship appears to stabilize into a mutually monogamous one.

Other measures of user satisfaction

At least in the clinical trial literature, several measures of user satisfaction are common. These include a user's willingness to use the method again and willingness to recommend the method to others. Many studies also inquire directly about satisfaction, asking users to rate the method overall (either numerically or qualitatively) and to rate their satisfaction with specific features of the method (e.g. interference with sexual pleasure, partner's reaction).

Continuation rates and willingness to use a method again are only indirect measures of acceptability. To avoid pregnancy contraception must be used, many women do so with some reluctance and their chosen method may represent 'the best of a bad lot'.

Helping a woman to determine her contraceptive needs and then to find a contraceptive strategy that meets them will make her feel in control

Table 1.4 1–year method–related discontinuation rates of selected family planning methods (reproduced with permission from Ref. 3)

Method	% of users discontinuing use at 1 year[a]
Spermicides	60
Periodic abstinence	37
Calendar	
Ovulation method	
Symptothermal	
Post-ovulation	
Cap	
Parous women	58
Nulliparous women	44
Sponge	
Parous women	58
Nulliparous women	44
Diaphragm	44
Condoms	
Female (Reality)	44
Male	39
Oral contraceptives	29
IUD	
Progesterone T	19
Copper T 380A	22
LNG-IUS	19
Injectable (depot medroxyprogesterone acetate)	30
Implants (Norplant and Norplant-2)	12
Female sterilization	0
Male sterilization	0

[a] Among users attempting to avoid pregnancy.

of her sexuality and reproductive health generally. As discussed earlier, in family planning, relative to nearly every other area of medicine, the role and responsibility of the user is uniquely important. It is critical that women and men who seek contraceptive advice and assistance feel that the family planning choices they have made are their own.

In working through a family planning counselling session, Box 1.1 may be helpful. It presents a summary checklist of factors to discuss. There are many factors to consider. These may be grouped into factors related to back-up options the woman is willing to use, factors related to her interaction

Box 1.1 Checklist of user considerations

	Implications
Attitude towards back-up options	
Attitude towards abortion	If willing to consider as a back-up, opens a wider range of choices for creating an effective family planning strategy
Attitude towards emergency contraception	Emergency contraception back-up, even without abortion as a safety net, widens options for creating an effective strategy involving methods with important benefits, such as STI protection
Interaction with the healthcare system	
Regular access to a clinic	Methods that require frequent clinic visits may be inconvenient
Provider's role	Provider's personal concerns can influence method selection
Sexual lifestyle	
Frequency of actions required	Some methods require daily action; others require action at the time of sex; others require initial or intermittent action only
Privacy	For younger users, or others whose sexual activity may not be socially sanctioned, discreet methods may be critical. Methods involving storage or disposal problems, are more vulnerable to discovery
Partner's role	Users may desire or may reject methods that involve a large role for the partner. Many methods can be used in ways that make family planning mutual
Frequency of intercourse	If intercourse is very infrequent, users may prefer methods that they use only at the time of coitus
Future fertility	
Wish for future fertility	Male and female sterilization are only for users who do not wish any pregnancies in future
Desired timing of future fertility	If a woman plans to conceive soon, her planning would differ from a woman who plans to conceive in 10 years or more
Cost	
Out-of-pocket costs	Methods impose different cost structures on the user. Time, travel and item costs are all factors

with the healthcare system, factors related to her sexual lifestyle and factors related to her future fertility plans.

• Back-up options

The strength of a user's desire to avoid pregnancy is a critical factor in determining the methods that are right for her. But if she is open to back-up methods, her choices for creating a highly effective family planning strategy will be greater.

Abortion

Given the length of time that most women in the UK will use contraception, a huge proportion of them will likely experience at least one contraceptive failure. For instance, the woman who starts pill use at age 16, and continues until she is 30, faces a risk of more than 50% that her method will fail (during this 14-year span, if her annual failure rate is 5%, her cumulative risk of pregnancy is $[1.0 \times (1.0 \times 0.05)^{14}]$ or 51.2%). Even perfect users of most contraceptive methods can expect one or more failures during their lifetimes. For example, the 1-year perfect-use failure rate of the diaphragm is 6%. If we assume for the sake of simplicity that for a given user, this rate stays constant over time, then after 12 years of use (say age 17–29), a woman is more likely than not (52.4%) to have experienced a failure. Many women will choose to resolve their unplanned pregnancies by abortion. Modern methods of medical and surgical abortion are exceptionally safe and easy to use, and it is critical that family planning providers do not stigmatize this choice. If a woman is open to using abortion as a back-up, she may also be willing to consider some of the slightly less effective but otherwise very appealing family planning methods available such as diaphragms or condoms offering non-contraceptive benefits, such as protection from HIV, that may be life-saving in a global context.

Emergency contraception

Even for those women who would not consider using abortion as a back-up method, but who are otherwise highly motivated to prevent pregnancy, emergency contraception (see Ch. 11) can reduce the risk of pregnancy after certain types of contraceptive accidents. If a woman is willing to use emergency contraception as part of her family planning strategy, her choices about a primary method may be wider than if she would not consider this back-up option and still is highly motivated to avoid pregnancy.

• Interaction with the healthcare system

Reducing the number of visits made to clinics may improve continuation rates. Supplying 12 months supply of oral contraceptive pills to women who have no contraindications for example, saves both the woman and the health service time and money. A new formulation of the long-acting progestogen-only injectable contraceptive Depo Provera® theoretically allows women to self-administer the method rather than having to attend a clinic every twelve weeks for injection.

• Sexual lifestyle

A user's sexual patterns are an important determinant of the methods that would be suitable for her during a given phase in her reproductive life.

Frequency of actions required

Some users may want a method that requires little or no action on their part. 'Birth control you think about just four times a year' is the slogan for Depo Provera® in the USA. At one extreme are the sterilization methods, the implants and the IUDs. Once action to start use is taken, the user can essentially forget about contraception for at least several years. At the other extreme are the 'coitus-dependent' methods, such as withdrawal, diaphragms, condoms or spermicides, that require action on the user's part with each act of intercourse. Also at this end of the spectrum are the methods that require daily action even in the absence of sexual intercourse, such as oral contraceptive pills or certain forms of fertility awareness that require daily temperature-taking, or cervical mucus evaluation. Some users prefer routine daily actions to those that may be required less often but that can interrupt sexual spontaneity. Other users, particularly if they are sexually active only infrequently, may prefer methods that require action only when needed. A user's daily schedule and ability to stick to a routine are of paramount importance in evaluating her needs along this dimension. If she travels frequently and unexpectedly, has stressful and unpredictable deadlines, or is generally not a creature of habit, then methods requiring strict adherence to a daily regimen might be less desirable.

Partner cooperation

Methods range widely in the role that each member of the couple is required to play. For some methods, such as sterilization, IUD or implants, one of the partners bears the entire responsibility. For others, such as periodic abstinence or withdrawal, both must be willing to cooperate. For some, token responsibility can be shared. For example, a male partner can prepare or insert a diaphragm for a woman, or can even take the placebo pills in her oral contraceptive cycle. A woman can roll the condom onto a man's penis. In choosing a method, the user should consider the role she wants and can reasonably expect her partner to play. If both partners are very committed and cooperative, the range of options is wider than if one partner has strict limitations.

Privacy

Family planning users may attribute the utmost importance to several privacy considerations. In particular, younger women or women who are engaging in sexual relationships that might not be socially sanctioned for them may feel strongly that they need discreet methods. One consideration is storage and disposal of contraceptives. Oral contraceptives, condoms or spermicides kept in a purse or drawer, or thrown in the household rubbish, may be more vulnerable to discovery than injectable methods or IUDs. Another consideration is tell-tale changes in bleeding patterns, although there are so many causes for cycle disturbance that most changes entailed by contraceptive methods would be unlikely to arouse comment or suspicion.

• Plans for future fertility

It is essential to determine whether and when a user plans to become pregnant in future. Many methods are advisable or cost-effective only if the woman does not have immediate plans to become pregnant. For instance, a woman seeking to conceive within the next few months would be a poor candidate for an implant or an IUD. With the exception of the progestogen-only injectable methods (see Ch. 5), however, all other reversible methods are considered to offer an immediate return to fertility once use is halted.

COSTS

The cost of a family planning strategy is properly measured by including the cost of the method itself (Table 1.5), the costs of the woman's and provider's time, as well as all other indirect costs, including travel to the clinic for visits. Such studies are extremely complicated to undertake, and so are rare. Family planning methods also vary tremendously in the ways in which the costs to the user and provider are spread out over time. In the UK, all methods of contraception, except male and female condoms and Persona are free to the user, who can therefore ignore the costs of the method. Male and female condoms are provided free by most family planning clinics (FPCs) but not by general practitioners. The provider, whether general practitioner or FPC, however, is increasingly aware of the cost of contraceptive methods, particularly those like the IUS and implants which have high upfront costs.

Another important aspect to cost, at least from the perspective of the NHS or of society as a whole, is the cost of the unintended pregnancies and side effects that result from contraceptive failure. For instance, a year of contraceptive protection using the cervical cap may seem to cost less (counting only the cost of the method) than a year of contraceptive protection from a hormone-releasing IUD. But if the far higher failure rates of the cap and the subsequent costs of the births or abortions are added in, the picture changes. All things considered, the copper IUD is probably the most cost-effective method available. In 2005 the National Institute for Health and

Table 1.5 Price to the National Health Service for selected contraceptive commodities, September 2006

Method	Months of protection	Price range (£UK)
Combined oral contraceptives	3	1.20–14.70
Combined transdermal contraception	3	16.26
Progestogen-only oral contraceptives	3	2.10–8.85
Progestogen-only injectables	3	3.95–5.01
Implant	36	90.00
LNG-IUS	60	83.16
Framed copper IUD	60–120	8.00–13.50
Frameless copper IUD	60	25.19
Diaphragm	–	5.78–7.23
Condoms	–	Variable
Spermicidal gel	–	2.40
Emergency contraception (LNG)	–	5.11

Clinical Excellence (NICE) in the UK published a guideline on long-acting reversible methods of contraception (LARC). It included a cost-effectiveness analysis. The guideline concluded that all LARC are cost effective and that even the most costly (IUS and implant) are more cost effective than either the pill or condoms even if used for only 1 year – because of their low failure rates.

CONCLUSION

Never in history have so many options for planning and regulating fertility been so widely available. The majority are also safer than ever before, as new and improved methods emerge, and better knowledge about how to reduce risks with older methods accumulates. Family planning is also a model area of medicine in terms of advances in user autonomy and responsibility. The challenge for future years will be to develop still better and more diverse methods, and to help users combine the existing methods to build strategies that meet their needs over the decades of use that characterize modern family planning users. Particularly important in this regard will be to reduce the stigma and bias associated with emergency contraception and abortion, just as cultural obstacles to oral contraceptive use, and indeed the barrier methods, were fought earlier last century.

REFERENCES

1. Taylor T, Keyse L, Bryant A. Contraception and Sexual Health 2005/06. Omnibus Report No. 30. Office for National Statistics. London 2006

2. Piccinino LJ, Mosher WD (1998) Trends in contraceptive use in the United States: 1982–1995. Family Planning Perspectives 30(1): 4–10, 46.

3. Hatcher RA, Trussell J, Stewart F, et al. (1998) Contraceptive Technology, 17th revised edn. Ardent Media, New York.

4. Trussell J, Kost K (1987) Contraceptive failure in the United States: A critical review of the literature. Studies in Family Planning 18(5): 237–283.

5. World Health Organization (1996) Improving access to quality care in family planning: Medical eligibility criteria for contraceptive use. World Health Organization, Geneva.

6. Grady WR, Klepinger DH, Nelson-Wally A (1999) Contraceptive characteristics: The perceptions and priorities of men and women. Family Planning Perspectives 31(4): 168–175.

7. Faculty of Family Planning & Reproductive Health Care. UK medical eligibility criteria for contraceptive use (UKMEC 2005/2006. www.ffprhc.org.uk)

FURTHER READING

Oddens BJ, Visser AP, Vemer HM, Everaerd WTAM, Lehert P (1994) Contraceptive use and attitudes in Great Britain. Contraception 49(1): 73–86.

Pearl R (1932) Contraception and fertility in 2000 women. Human Biology 4: 363–407.

Segal SJ (1993) Trends in population and contraception. Annals of Medicine 25: 51–56.

Shah IH (1994) The advance of the contraceptive revolution. World Health Statistics Quarterly 47(1): 9–15.

Wilcox AJ, Baird DD, Weinberg CR (1999) Time of implantation of the conceptus and loss of pregnancy. New England Journal of Medicine 340 (23): 1796–1799.

2 Service provision in the UK

Alison Bigrigg

Chapter contents

Family planning (FP) is rather an old-fashioned term but remains in common use due to its familiarity to both professionals and users. It is commonly understood to include contraception and related sexual and reproductive health issues. In the UK, FP services are delivered by both general practitioners (GPs) and specialists within the community. Many specialist services are now using more explicit names such as Contraception and Sexual Health (CASH). Others choose a generic name for the service (e.g. Abacus in Liverpool), which the local population knows, through word of mouth and advertising, to be their local contraceptive service.

The professional training programme for consultants preparing to lead FP services is currently known as the sub-specialty of Sexual & Reproductive Health.

HISTORY OF FAMILY PLANNING SERVICES

The first birth control clinic was founded in London in 1921 by Marie Stopes. By 1930, there were five separate birth control societies operating clinics in various parts of the country. These organizations united to become the National Birth Control Council whose main objective was 'to promote the provision of facilities for scientific contraception so that married people may space or limit their families and thus mitigate the evils of ill-health and poverty'. Almost a decade later, the National Birth Control Association became the Family Planning Association (FPA); its new title indicating a concern with the whole issue of fertility including promotion and prevention.

In 1946, the National Health Service Act empowered local health authorities and regional boards to open contraceptive clinics. The FPA led the development of services which were used almost exclusively for married women, the majority of whom had to pay for the service and for contraceptive supplies, although payment could be waived if necessary. At that time, contraceptive methods were limited to abstinence, the rhythm method, coitus interruptus, spermicides, diaphragms, condoms or, unusually, sterilization by tubal ligation following childbirth.

The 1960s was a decade of rapid social and technological progression. In 1960 Helen (later Lady) Brook started an evening session for unmarried women and in 1963 the Board of the Marie Stopes Clinic agreed to sponsor a young people's advisory session. The FPA approved the use of oral contraceptives in its clinics in 1961 and IUDs in 1965. The first vasectomy clinics were opened by the FPA in 1968 and advancements in laparoscopic techniques saw female sterilization become a less-invasive procedure. In 1967 the National Health Service (Family Planning) Act 1967 became law. The Act conferred permissive powers on local health authorities to give birth control advice to people regardless of marital status, and on social as well as medical grounds. In 1967 the Abortion Act was passed, bringing to an end illegal abortion and its tragic sequelae.

The 1970s saw the achievement of the long-term aim of the FPA of having family planning incorporated into the NHS. In 1974, they began a phased handover of 1000 FPA clinics and domiciliary services to Area Health Authorities. In addition, all contraceptive advice provided by the NHS and all supplies were made free of charge. In 1975 GPs joined NHS FP services providing contraception free at the point of delivery.

In 1980 the Department of Health issued guidance to doctors regarding contraceptive advice to young people and the right to prescribe to under-16-year-olds without parental consent was confirmed in 1986 following the House of Lords overturning a ruling of the Court of Appeal (Chapter 15).

In the 1990s widespread concern developed over the number of unplanned pregnancies (particularly in young people) and then over the increasing prevalence of sexually transmitted infection (STI). In 1991 the Royal College of Obstetricians and Gynaecologists (RCOG) recommended that each Health

Table 2.1 Strategic Planning Documents published in the UK between 1999–2006

- Promoting Sexual Health – A Strategy for the Northern and Social Service Board Area 1999[2] (Northern Ireland)
- Teenage Pregnancy Strategy 1999[3] (England)
- A Strategic Framework for Promoting Sexual Health in Wales 2000[4]
- A Strategic Framework for Promoting Sexual Health in Wales – Post-consultation Action Plan 2000[5]
- The National Strategy for Sexual Health & HIV for England 2001[6]
- The National Strategy for Sexual Health & HIV for England Implementation Action Plan 2002[7]
- Effective Commissioning of Sexual Health & HIV Services 2003[8] (England)
- Choosing Health – Making Healthier Choices Easier 2004[9] (England)
- Respect & Responsibility Strategy and Action Plan for Improving Sexual Health in Scotland 2005[10]
- Recommended Standards for Sexual Health Services 2005[11] (England)
- Recommended Service Specification for integrated Sexual Health Services (in Wales) 2005[12]
- Proposed Sexual Health Services Quality Requirement for Wales 2006[13]
- Proposed Sexual Health Standards for Wales 2006[14]

Authority should consider the appointment of a senior specialist to oversee the provision of contraceptive and abortion services. In 1992 England, Wales and Northern Ireland (and later Scotland) published targets to reduce the number of unplanned pregnancies in young people. In 1993, the Faculty of Family Planning and Reproductive Health Care (FFPRHC) of the RCOG was established and in 1994, the first trainee was accredited after completing the training programme in the sub-specialty of community gynaecology, later to be known as sexual and reproductive health.

During the late 1990s and the beginning of the 21st century, a plethora of national strategic planning documents were introduced (Table 2.1). The impact on frontline services has been variable as successive NHS re-organizations have unpredictably supported or impeded their implementation. At present some services in England are flourishing, while others are suffering cutbacks and even closures.[1] In Scotland, funding from the National Scottish Sexual Health Strategy has reached frontline services and there is strong emphasis on integration and coordination with Genitourinary Medicine (GUM) services. The Welsh Assembly has recommended ring-fenced funding for integrated contraceptive and STI services as well as the development of sexual health networks, standards and leadership.

CRITERIA FOR PLANNING CONTRACEPTIVE AND SEXUAL HEALTH SERVICES IN THE UK

During the last 10 years, contraceptive provision, previously a Cinderella service, has been developing into an essential element of the NHS health improvement programme.

Service providers, together with local partners, should consider how their services meet the needs of the population. In other words, as well as ensuring the quality of one-to-one consultations, contraceptive services should also consider the needs of non-users and attempt to provide comprehensive contraceptive, sexual and reproductive health services which are easily accessible in their geographical area. This end is often achieved by forming a local sexual health committee or network where GPs, voluntary organizations, health promotion experts, FP consultants, education and other local authority representatives are all represented. This is not a guarantee of service development or even defence against service closure, but generally does strengthen the position of services within their local NHS structure. The lead clinician from specialist family planning services has a vital leadership role in these groups and should strive to improve the following key service themes.

CHARACTERISTICS OF A FAMILY PLANNING SERVICE

• Access

'Providers must ensure that services are accessible to all members of the community, e.g. through appropriate opening times, and location, and provision of services to vulnerable and socially excluded groups.'[8]

FP clinics have traditionally been exemplary in providing extended opening times in the evening and at weekends and a wide choice of geographical sites. 'Drop-in' or walk-in clinics have always been a key element of most services. Clinic location, range of services and opening times need constant review against the needs of users and complementary service provision from GPs, GUM services and others.

Advertising of services to potential clients is often neglected. At a minimum, contraceptive services should be publicized in local telephone directories, local GP practice leaflets and notice boards and by other sexual health providers. Information for young people should ideally be available in schools. Local authorities may also be amenable to displaying information about specialist clinics in libraries, youth clubs and other public venues.

It is clearly essential that service providers ensure fellow professionals such as NHS Direct/NHS 24, pharmacists, hospital specialists, school nurses, GPs and social workers have easy access to information describing opening times and location of services. This can be done by paper communications but many services are making use of the internet and developing their own websites. These also need to be publicized but have the advantage of being updatable instantly.

If an appointment system is in place, it should be possible to make an appointment at any time during the working day and on any working day, not just when the clinic is open. This remains a challenge to many specialist FP services which attempt to provide clinics as locally as possible through weekly or fortnightly sessions.

Diversification of providers has also improved access to contraception in the UK in recent years. For example, emergency contraception is now provided by pharmacists and STI screening commonly takes place in specialist FP clinics.

• Capacity

'Services need to be adequately resourced to enable sufficient time in consultations to support holistic care.'[11]

Improved capacity can be achieved through process improvement and service modernization, but resources are ultimately finite. In recent years, service capacity has been enhanced in the UK in many different ways such as:

- Increasing the role of nurses, both in GP and specialist clinics.
- 'One-stop shop' approach for sexual and reproductive health.
- Focusing specialist GUM tests on those most in need and undertaking screening in the community setting.
- Reducing routine regular (and unnecessary) follow-up consultations, e.g. providing a 12-month supply of oral contraceptive pills for women in stable medical and social circumstances.

Ultimately, however, if the workload increases exponentially, consultations will become progressively shorter with a resulting focus on minimizing input. Health promotion, holistic care, information giving and informed choice are all likely to suffer.

The FFPRHC has recommended a minimum time for each type of consultation[15] (e.g. practitioner or clinician teams to have 20 minutes for new consultation and 10 minutes for a routine follow-up appointment), but this may be insufficient in certain situations, e.g. when a procedure is required in addition to counselling .[16]

Much of the emphasis on measuring capacity has been on waiting times for appointments (e.g. 48-hour limit for General Practice and GUM) and the number of attendances, but these are not good proxies for quality of service and irrelevant when open-access services are provided.

Service providers should work to demonstrate the efficiency and importance of their services and negotiate improved national and local contracts which will ultimately result in a better deal for patients.

• Choice

'The fundamental principle should be that every person should have a choice when accessing Sexual Health services and be able to self refer to all such services.'[10]

Choice is fundamental to the provision of FP services. An individual *chooses* to attend a FP service and a method of contraception is much more likely to be continued when the user has chosen one that most suits her/ his circumstances. Within services there should be choice of a drop-in or appointment system and choice of gender of clinician. It is also a fundamental principle of FP provision in the UK to give a choice of providers. GPs will continue to provide most contraceptive care, but over 1 million people attend community FP clinics in England every year. The reasons for this are varied; some GPs provide only basic contraceptive services and the alternative provider serves people with complex or particular needs. Sometimes individuals will choose an alternative provider to preserve anonymity or confidentiality. For instance young people may prefer not to see GPs who provide health care to other members of their family, and local surgeries may have members of staff who are known to them in the community.

The alternative provider is usually a community clinic supported by a Primary Care Trust or Health Board, but can be a GP specialist running an open-access service.

• Equity of service provision

'Sexual Health matters to everyone, but we also know that sexual health needs vary from one person to another and from one community to another as well as evolving throughout life.'[11]

Provision of contraceptive services is not currently equitable across the United Kingdom. The variation is remarkable; some areas have virtually no specialist community-based provision while others have comprehensive well-targeted services (see **Fig. 2.1**).[6]

Different geographical areas face different challenges – such as low density of population in rural areas – but it is not these barriers that usually set the extent of provision, but the priority that the local health system places on contraceptive and abortion services. For example the percentage of abortions funded by the NHS varies between 46% and 96% in different health authorities in England and there is no evidence that this relates to variation in need.[6] In Wales a large proportion of women have to travel to England for abortions in the charitable sector. Even though the National Institute of Clinical Effectiveness (NICE) guidelines on Long Acting Reversible Methods of Contraception (LARC)[17] have demonstrated the cost effectiveness of these methods, availability is often patchy. The Scottish Executive has recently developed a set of Key Clinical Indicators to compare

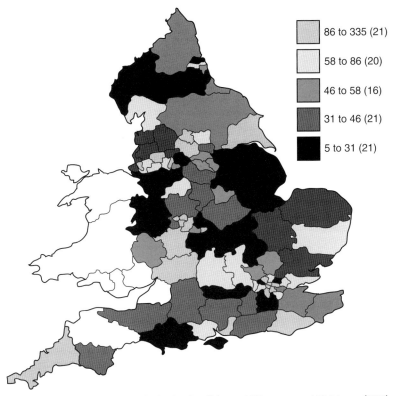

86 to 335 (21)

58 to 86 (20)

46 to 58 (16)

31 to 46 (21)

5 to 31 (21)

Figure 2.1 Rates of first contacts at family planning clinics per 1000 women aged 20–24 years (2000) (From Department of Health, London 2001,[6] Crown Copyright, with permission)

service provision between different Health Board areas in the hope of stimulating debate and investment where required.

In order to ensure equity for the whole local population, it is necessary to address the unequal needs and barriers to access that exist between different groups in local communities. Young persons' sexual health clinics were established as early as the 1980s and are now recognized as a fundamental element of a comprehensive contraceptive service. Also within these specialist clinics, providers should address inequalities by ensuring that the particular needs of sub-groups are being met, e.g. young people who are looked after and accommodated by social services or girls from black minority ethnic populations.

Thirty years ago in FP services, domiciliary visiting was common to try to address the special requirements of the most socially deprived women, those with disabilities or addictions. Today best practice is to facilitate access to mainstream or specially targeted services.

Equity of provision in any geographical area will require regular needs assessment and consultation with local communities and stakeholder groups.

• Coordination of approach

'Joined up action – It is essential to put in place (new) structures that co-ordinate action.'[3]

Over the last 10 years, there has been a gradual realization that a fragmented approach to service provision does not serve the population well. Traditionally contraception has been delivered mainly from GP and community contraceptive services, sexually transmitted infections have been managed in hospitals and some community settings and abortions have been provided both by the hospitals and independent sector organizations. These arrangements can be wasteful of resources, inconvenient for the client and lead to lost opportunities, not least for health improvement.

The National Strategy for Sexual Health and HIV for England (2001)[6] suggested that comprehensive care to a local community could be delivered by commissioners and providers in primary and acute care working together to set up a network providing three different levels of care (Table 2.2).

It was intended that level 1 provision would be available in the majority of general practices, level 2 would be provided by specialist general practitioners or community teams while level 3 clinicians would provide most specialist care and take responsibility for needs assessment, clinical governance and maintaining service quality.

The expert group advising the Scottish Executive on the development of the Scottish Sexual Health Strategy[15] recommended a similar approach but expanded the model to five tiers taking into account sources of advice for self-management and a greater diversity of providers, such as community pharmacies. The strategy also recommended nomination of a lead NHS executive for Sexual Health, lead clinician within each Health Board area and local authority lead officer. These individuals are responsible for the development of a local inter-agency Sexual Health Strategy involving all statutory providers as well as voluntary organizations and local communities.

The Welsh Assembly recommended the establishment of 'Sexual Health Units' that should encompass management of contraception, STIs, HIV, abortion, psychosexual medicine as well as providing training for Primary Care. Sexual Health Units are expected to meet the needs of the local population through working with other partners such as Primary Care and voluntary sector organizations within a managed sexual health network.

In 2005, the Department of Health in England endorsed a similar concept in the Recommended Standards for Sexual Health services published on its behalf by MedFASH,[11] where the establishment of local managed service networks is one of the ten main standards.

The need for co-ordination of care between GUM and FP services is now universally accepted. Few would dispute that care pathways should appear

Table 2.2 National Strategy for Sexual Health and HIV for England – Suggested Model of Working

Level 1
- Sexual history and risk assessment
- STI testing for women
- HIV testing and counselling
- Pregnancy testing and referral
- Contraceptive information and services
- Assessment and referral of men with STI symptoms
- Cervical cytology screening and referral
- Hepatitis B immunization

Level 2
- Intrauterine device (IUD) insertion
- Testing and treating STI
- Vasectomy
- Contraceptive implant insertion
- Partner notification
- Invasive STI testing for men (until non-invasive tests are available)

Level 3
- Outreach for STI prevention
- Outreach contraception services
- Specialized infections management, including co-ordination of partner notification
- Highly specialized contraception
- Specialized HIV treatment and care

(data from Ref. 6)

seamless to clients, but there are currently a range of models of care which are employed to achieve this (see **Fig. 2.2**).

Within GP services, co-ordination of approach between the various practitioners is as important as within a community service. Each practice needs to consider what level of provision across the range of contraceptive and sexual health services it will deliver and how it will signpost users to other providers.

• Quality of care

'Clinical Governance and risk assessment: achieving safe, effective patient-focused care and services.' [19]

National level

The last 10 years have seen the emergence of a robust and extensive framework of guidelines and service standards for contraceptive provision

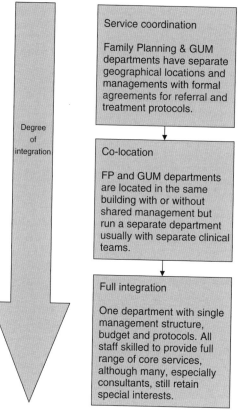

Degree of integration

Service coordination

Family Planning & GUM departments have separate geographical locations and managements with formal agreements for referral and treatment protocols.

Co-location

FP and GUM departments are located in the same building with or without shared management but run a separate department usually with separate clinical teams.

Full integration

One department with single management structure, budget and protocols. All staff skilled to provide full range of core services, although many, especially consultants, still retain special interests.

Figure 2.2 Range of service models

within the UK. The FFPRHC has been the main mover producing several clinical guidelines each year and a series of service standards as well as UK versions of World Health Organization (WHO) guidance relating to contraception. Further details can be found on the various college/society' websites listed at the end of this chapter.

The Clinical Effectiveness Unit (CEU) of the Faculty of Family Planning & Reproductive Health Care provides a clinical enquiry service which responded to over 500 queries in the first 3 years of its operation. CEU clinical guidance documents and evidence-based reviews of new products have become the gold standard underpinning clinical practice in most family planning services throughout the UK.

Local level

The above resources support the production of local guidelines and evidence-based practice in our field. Audit against these standards is of course critical to demonstrate quality of provision and stimulate change as required.

As a minimum, a clinical governance programme report for a FP service should include sections on:

- Department and area wide audits
- Child protection training and monitoring
- Complaints/litigation
- Adverse events and incident reporting
- Staff governance
  - Competencies and qualifications
  - Sickness rates and vacancies
  - Health and safety
- Training provided for in-house staff and other providers
- Public and stakeholder involvement.

RANGE OF SERVICE PROVISION

It is estimated that 6 million women use services throughout the UK per year. The Office for National Statistics Omnibus Survey (2004)[20] reported that 81% of women between 16–50 years had seen their own GP or practice nurse in the last 5 years for contraceptive advice; 32% had been to a community clinic; 3% had seen another GP or nurse; 8% sought advice from a pharmacist and 1% had used a walk-in service.[20] There is some evidence that community clinics offer a greater variety of methods with more emphasis on long-acting methods of contraception and that young people prefer community clinics, particularly dedicated youth sessions.[21]

• The basic consultation for contraceptive advice

Whatever the setting of a FP consultation, it should have a number of components including listening, understanding the individual's needs, taking a comprehensive medical and social history and information provision. Verbal advice should be backed up by written information and both should cover how each method works, how it is used, its efficacy, minor and serious side effects, and non-contraceptive benefits. Once a method is selected, further information on its safe and effective use and a contingency plan if any adverse effects are experienced (e.g. telephone helpline) are required.

The opportunity should not be lost to discuss the need for screening and protection against STI and cervical cancer and the risks associated with different lifestyles (Chapter 17). Other issues such as a risk assessment for child protection and confidentiality policies need to be raised as appropriate.

• Family planning provision in primary care

Family planning services remain free at the point of access in the UK, but funding of providers drives the range of provision.

The general medical service (GMS) Contract (2003) for GPs is aimed at investing in primary care providing a practice-based contract with a quality and outcomes framework. The GMS Contract describes essential, additional and enhanced services. Essential services must be provided by all GPs and include the management of patients who are ill, terminally ill or who have a chronic illness.[22] Additional services cover the provision of cervical screening and a range of basic contraceptive services (Table 2.3). These services are roughly equivalent to those included in level 1 service provision of the National Sexual Health & HIV Strategy for England.[7]

Most GPs deliver these additional services, but they have the right to opt out with the commensurate loss of income. To be funded for basic contraceptive services, GPs therefore only have to provide advice about the full range of methods not deliver them. This does, however, encourage appropriate referral to other services able to provide a full range of contraceptive methods.

Local and national enhanced services are commissioned by Primary Care organizations and local health boards to meet local needs. The two relevant national enhanced services are for 'IUD fittings' and for 'Sexual Health'. For national enhanced services, the Department of Health (DH) in England specifies the minimum service provision and sets the financial reward.

Table 2.3 Contraceptive service provision in the new GMS Contract

1. Provide advice about the full range of contraceptive methods.
2. Where appropriate, examine patients seeking contraceptive advice.
3. Treat patients for contraceptive purposes and prescribe contraceptives or refer for the fitting of intrauterine contraceptive devices or implants.
4. Provide advice about emergency contraception and where appropriate supply or prescribe emergency hormonal contraception. Where the doctor has a conscientious objection to emergency contraception, the patient must be promptly referred to a health professional who has no such objection.
5. Provide advice in cases of unplanned or unwanted pregnancy including advice about the availability of free pregnancy testing in the practice area. Where the doctor has a conscientious objection to termination, the patient must be promptly referred to a doctor who has no such objection.
6. Give initial advice about sexual health promotion and sexually transmitted infections.
7. Refer as necessary for specialist Sexual Health services, including tests for sexually transmitted infections.

(From Department of Health, London December 2003 Delivering Investment in General Practice: Implementing the new GMS Contract, Crown Copyright, with permission)

Enhanced services for IUDs are generally popular, with a proportion of practices within each area usually providing the service. However, few GPs have been offered and accepted a sexual health enhanced service contract as it is generally seen as being overtly proscriptive and too inflexible to meet local needs. Another common enhanced service is for the provision of contraceptive implants. The FFPRHC together with the Royal College of Nursing, the FPA and the Royal College of General Practitioners have developed a recommended framework.

An alternative method of funding for GPs for contraceptive services is through personal medical services (PMS) contracts. Contraceptive services within PMS are remunerated as additional service points.[23]

All funding for enhanced services comes from a Primary Care organization administered budget for GMS/PMS Contracts. This is a ring-fenced allocation with a minimum spend set by the UK Technical Steering Committee for these contracts. Rarely a Primary Care organization may choose to spend more using other funding sources.

• Family planning provision by community services

The number of women attending family planning clinics was around 1.1 million in 1993–1994 rising to 1.2 million in 2003–2004 in England alone. Table 2.4 shows number of attendances per country in the UK family planning clinics.[24]

The number of attendances does not reflect volume of work, as the types of service have expanded over the last decade with increased emphasis on reducing the number of clinic visits and targeting women with more complex, social or medical needs. The peak age of attendance remains 16–19 years with 182 out of 187 NHS contraceptive services in the UK providing clinics especially for young people. In addition, there are 17 contraceptive services run by Brook or Caledonia Youth (in Scotland) for this age group.

The vast majority of services are managed within a primary care trust or health board, but a few remain in acute trusts. The number of attendances per service varied from a few 100 to nearly 100 000 in 2004.[25]

Table 2.4 Attendances in FP clinics in UK 2003/4

Country	No of attendances
England	2.7 million
Northern Ireland	61 000
Scotland	292 000
Wales	56 000

(data from Ref. 24)

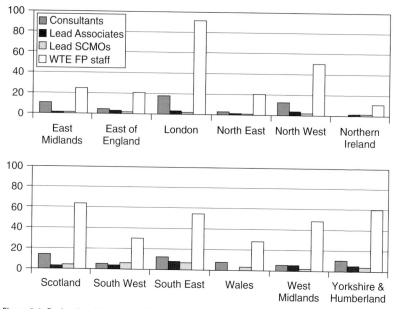

Figure 2.3 Regional variation in workforce in 2005. Data from: Regional Totals 2005 from the FFPRHC Census of Family Planning Workforce in the UK 2005

All FP clinics provide a basic range of services, but an ever-increasing number are expanding their provision to meet the range of sexual and reproductive health needs covered in this Handbook. The number of FP services providing enhanced provision is likely to be increasing year on year in line with the increase in the number of consultants and other specialist staff (see Figs 2.3 and 2.4).

• Health improvement role of the services

As well as providing one-to-one clinical services, many FP services undertake a substantial health improvement or public health role. The extent of this depends on local needs and resources within the department, but may include the following.

Condom provision

This may be limited to distribution during one to one consultations or by virtue of an 'open-access' scheme. In order to improve provision (and contain costs), 'C Card' schemes are becoming increasingly popular. The exact structure of these schemes varies from area to area, but usually involves inviting individuals for a brief interview where the benefits of condoms, types available and how to use them effectively are explained.

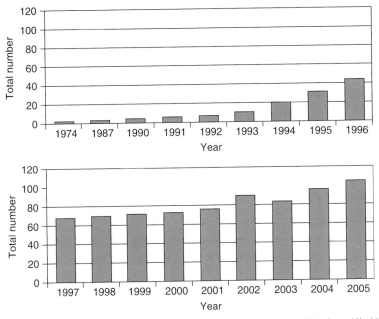

Figure 2.4 Number of consultants in family planning (with permission from J Fam Plan Reprod Health Care 2005: 31(4) and later data; from The Seventh & Eighth Census of the Family Planning Workforce in the United Kingdom 2003 and 2004 Faculty of Family Planning & Reproductive Health Care (FFPRHC))

The individual is then issued with a card which allows him/her to claim a free supply of condoms from the clinics and other outlets within the area which vary from health centres to record shops and youth clubs. Child protection concerns do need to be addressed when structuring these schemes for younger clients.

Emergency contraception availability

As well as providing all forms of emergency contraception, FP services are in an ideal position to lead the area-wide response to ensuring good access. They are often involved in training and quality assurance provision of other providers, such as pharmacies, accident and emergency departments, school nurses, GP out-of-hours services and others.

Screening programmes for STI

See Chapter 17.

Information provision

Information (both written and verbal) is essential to allow individuals to make an informed choice. Core provision needs to cover a full range of contraception, STIs, options for unwanted pregnancy, common gynaecological conditions and local service provision including confidentiality. Extended provision can involve a vast range of literature, for example for use in sex education, psychosexual problems, colposcopy, issues around sexuality, sexual violence, female genital mutilation and so forth.

The role of FP services is to liaise with local health promotion services and be aware of all national and local resources, associated costs and methods of distribution. To ensure the cost-effective use of this important resource, the needs of the local population require careful assessment. If local material is produced, this should be done in liaison with or at least piloted with its intended users.

When financial resources are available, information technology can make a substantial contribution to ensuring the chosen information resource is available at the right time for the right person. Some services enable GPs to download information leaflets from the local specialist health service.

Where possible, information should be available in different languages according to the populations who use the clinic or practice, consideration should be given to using pictorial, recorded or video format for those with poor literacy skills.

Commissioning planning and needs assessment

FP services and GPs with a special interest must play an active role in planning as well as delivery of services in their area. To fulfil this role, it is necessary for lead clinicians to be skilled in research methodology, needs assessment, data handling and interpretation.

Involvement of users and local community

Although it can sometimes be challenging to engage with users and the local community because of the nature of FP services, the techniques listed below can be utilized:

- Written surveys
- Comment cards
- Focus groups
- Stakeholder groups
- Face-to-face or telephone interviews
- Volunteer schemes
- Open days.

• Reducing health inequalities

FP services should be available to all who need them and should empower the users to make decisions that enhance their lives. Services need to be designed to work in partnership with the broad range of individuals – the healthy, the physically or mentally ill, sex workers, those with a learning disability, young people, people from different ethnic groups, homeless and other vulnerable groups, such as those with addictions.

Nearly all community FP services have found it beneficial to have specific services for young people (see Chapter 14). Larger services, or those serving particular communities offer specific outreach, facilitated in-reach or full discreet services to other groups such as sex workers. General practices and small community services are skilled in the provision of tailored services within a generic environment. The ability to do this is however limited if the patient or client does not feel comfortable talking about aspects of their current and past life, such as prostitution or previous abuse. This can be overcome in some circumstances by the ability of the clinician to develop a long-term relationship but is also an important reason to ensure the choice of FP and sexual health service provider is available. Finally, services which cater for specific groups can provide information and research to assist others with their work with these particular individuals.

The homeless

This is a group within our population with numerous complex, medical and social needs. Up to 50% have severe mental health problems and up to two-thirds of young homeless are drug users and all have a reduced life expectancy. Needs assessment has shown much unmet need around sexual and reproductive health issues, such as a high incidence of prostitution, concerns around STIs and unplanned pregnancies. It is difficult for a homeless person to prioritize contraception and sexual health. Not least, access to conventional services may be problematic. Many are not registered with a GP and they may have no way of receiving notification of appointments. Even if they can give a temporary address, they may have been 'moved on' before essential correspondence arrives. Previous negative experiences with conventional services may also make homeless individuals reluctant to attend. To overcome these problems, services with large homeless populations may consider setting up clinics in homeless hostels or other environments more familiar to this group. Ideally these clinics should be combined with fast-track support of the mainstream services. Smaller services should consider forming links with health- and social-work staff with specific remits for the homeless to ensure facilitated access.

FP staff working with this group should be familiar with the challenges of their everyday lives. For example, they may have nowhere secure to keep contraceptive supplies and prolonged bleeding may be difficult if there is inadequate access to toilet facilities or sanitary protection due to costs.

Sex workers

There is an overlap between the homeless population and those involved in prostitution. For both groups, drug use and experience of violence and sexual assault are common. Choice of contraceptive method is complicated by medical problems associated with drug use, such as deep venous thrombosis and by other factors such as women wishing to work but not experience vaginal bleeding.

In a number of large urban services, specific clinics have been developed which offer a range of services to this client group in addition to sexual health including needle exchange, counselling and social support to exit prostitution. Even outwith such specialist provision, FP services can be an important venue where women will reveal their situation perhaps for the first time. This is particularly likely as relevant questions about sexual relationships are asked. This then provides a valuable opportunity to refer to the relevant support agencies.

Ethnic minorities

Black and ethnic minorities like other client groups, include a range of people with many different needs and expectations. Those seeking asylum or recently arrived in this country often have different needs from those who have spent their childhood and adolescence in the UK. FP services need to be aware of, and provide for, these needs which include not only language barriers but religious and cultural issues affecting choice of contraception. For example, examination by a male doctor may be unacceptable to Hindu women and fasting during Ramadan is forbidden to Muslim women who are menstruating, as is entering a mosque.

All FP services should be able to arrange for interpreters to be present when the need is identified in advance. The wishes or beliefs of the individual may be different from that of the immediate community and this can be a problem if services rely only on help from family members or friends of the client.

People with learning disabilities

FP services need to be flexible in order to meet the needs of this group. Establishing an appropriate level of communication is vital and takes time. If a service normally only provides walk-in clinics, alternative arrangements are likely to be required. Building up of trust may necessitate repeated consultations with the same clinician. Provision of appropriate written and possibly audio/video information will greatly assist the process. It is essential the individuals are able to express their own views and not be 'spoken for' by their carer. However, involvement of other workers and supporters with the consent of the individual is beneficial, particularly, for example, when a couple wish to embark on a pregnancy.

TRAINING

Since their incorporation into the NHS, specialist FP services have been recognized as having an important role in training, not only for their own staff, but all other providers of contraceptive and related services. Traditionally FP services provide both theoretical and practical training in contraception for GPs, practice nurses and trainees in obstetrics and gynaecology, as well as GUM. Today with the increasing recognition of the importance of sexual health, this has expanded to include school nurses, pharmacists, addiction nurses, teachers, social workers and other professionals. The training for the latter groups may be provided by FP services alone or in partnership with health promotion and GUM.

• Doctors

The mainstay of training for other medical professionals and the recognized gold standard qualification for basic sexual and reproductive health remains the Diploma of Faculty of Family Planning (DFFP). Details of training which is overseen nationally by the Faculty but delivered locally, are shown in Appendix 2.1.

• Nurses

FP services have traditionally been multidisciplinary. This important characteristic has been retained as the role of the nurse develops within the NHS. Nurses are being encouraged to become fully competent across a range of FP and sexual health services so as well as contraceptive advice and treatment, they are able to provide sexual health screening, TOP services and nurse-led clinics. Mechanisms have been developed which allow nurses to extend their contribution within the specialist services and GP bases include Patient Group Directions (PGD) and Nurse Prescribing. A PGD is a specific written instruction relating to the appropriately trained nurse being able to supply and administer named medicines in an identified clinical situation. Nurse prescribing enables non-physicians to prescribe within their level of competence. In addition, many nurses are now fitting and removing contraceptive implants and a few are fitting IUDs after appropriate training.

As some nurses become highly skilled, individual services need to consider the skill mix within their nurse workforce. Some tasks such as chaperoning, pharmacy stocking, room preparation may be better undertaken by healthcare assistants.

SUPPORTING SERVICE PROVISION

Delivery of the services described above requires adequate premises, equipment and support services.

• Premises

The ideal scenario is to secure dedicated accessible premises, but most FP services have to share all or some of their accommodation. The latter has the advantage of sharing building costs and security, but should not compromise opening hours, good transport links and adequate space. There should be at least one clinical room for each clinician with additional facilities for practical training. The rooms should be co-located to promote team working and wherever possible, close to a dedicated waiting area and reception with facilities storing patient records.

• Equipment

In a modern service, patient safety and quality of experience should not be compromised by less than optimal equipment or support. Resuscitation equipment including oxygen should be easily accessible. Where intrauterine contraception is being fitted, consideration should be given to provision of electronic lithotomy couches and ceiling-mounted lamps. Equipment used in invasive procedures should either be single-use or sterilization procedures regularly monitored according to national and local standards.

• Support services

Modern clinical services cannot work in isolation and require all the usual modern support services. The importance of communication within and outwith the FP organization is worthy of special mention and modern IT systems with good clerical administrative support are essential.

• Important service linkage

Modern FP services should not be working in isolation from the rest of the health services. This should be considered when service configuration is reviewed. If a 'traditional' service of single weekly or fortnightly clinics on any particular site is preferred (and it does have many advantages), extra effort is needed to ensure good communication and relationships with other services.

A list of important service linkages are given below:

- Maternity and gynaecological services
- Pathology and radiology services
- General medicine, paediatrics and dermatology
- GPs, public health nurses, including health visitors, school nurses, pharmacists
- Youth and community services
- Child protection services
- Social care
- Schools and colleges
- Drug agencies and HIV services
- Voluntary organizations active in sexual and reproductive health
- Police
- Public health
- Health promotion.

Partnership working with these agencies ensures the most vulnerable in the population can benefit from specialist FP services, but this does require time over and above that required for direct client contact.

REFERENCES

1. Kishen M, Belfield T (2006) Contraception in crisis. The Journal of Family Planning and Reproductive Health Care 32(4): 211–212.

2. Department of Health and Social Services Northern Ireland (1999) Promoting Sexual Health – A Strategy for the Northern Health and Social Services Board Area. Northern Ireland.

3. Social Exclusion Unit (1999) National Teenage Pregnancy Strategy. London.

4. Health Promotion Division (2000) The National Assembly for Wales. A Strategic Framework for Promoting Sexual Health in Wales. Cardiff.

5. Health Promotion Division (2000) The National Assembly for Wales. A Strategic Framework for Promoting Sexual Health in Wales – Post Consultation Action Plan. Cardiff.

6. Department of Health (2001) The National Strategy for Sexual Health & HIV. London.

7. Department of Health (2002) The National Strategy for Sexual Health & HIV Implementation Action Plan. London.

8. Department of Health (2003) Effective Commissioning of Sexual Health & HIV Services. London.

9. Department of Health (2004) Choosing Health – Making Healthier Choices Easier. (A Public Health White Paper). London.

10. Scottish Executive (2005) Respect & Responsibility – Strategy and Action Plan for Improving Sexual Health. Edinburgh.

11. Medical Foundation for AIDS and Sexual Health (MedFASH) (2005) Recommended Standards for Sexual Health Services produced on behalf of the Department of Health London.

12. Recommended Service Specification for integrated Sexual Health services in Wales, Marion Lyons, National Public Health Service, Welsh Assembly Government, Cardiff (2005).

13. Consultation Document: Proposed Sexual Health Services Quality Requirements for Wales, Department for Health & Social Services, Welsh Assembly Government, Cardiff (2006).

14. Proposed Sexual Health Standards for Wales, National Public Health Services, Welsh Assembly Government, Cardiff (2006).

15. FFPRHC Service Standards for Workload in Contraception (May 2005) Available: www.ffprhc.org.uk

16. George VA, Kishen M (2006) Assessment of workload: intrauterine device/ intrauterine system provision. The Journal of Family Planning and Reproductive Health Care 32(3): 171–172.

17. National Institute for Health and Clinical Excellence (2005) Long-acting reversible contraception Clinical Guideline 30. Available: www.nice.org.uk/CG030.

18. Scottish Executive (2003) Enhancing Sexual Wellbeing in Scotland. Sexual Health & Relationship Strategy supporting paper 5a: An integrated tiered service approach. Edinburgh.

19. NHS Quality Improvement Scotland (2005) Clinical Governance and Risk Management: Achieving safe, effective, patient focused care and services. Edinburgh and Glasgow.

20. Office for National Statistics London on behalf of the Department of Health (2004) Contraception and Sexual Health 2003. A report on research using the ONS Omnibus Survey.

21. Mansour D (2005) Contraception and contraceptive use. Overview of contraceptive methods: a provider's perspective. Glasier A, Wellings K and Critchley H (eds). RCOG Press: London, pp. 44–77.

22. Department of Health (2003) Delivering Investment in General Practice. Implementing the new GMS Contract. London.

23. Department of Health (2004) Sustaining Innovation through the new Personal Medical Services (PMS) Arrangements. London.

24. Horrocks C (2005) Workforce specialty review for Family Planning and Reproductive Health Care 2003/4: England, Wales, Northern Ireland and Scotland. Journal of Family Planning and Reproductive Health Care 31(4): 325–328.

25. FFPRHC (2005) The Seventh and Eighth Census of the Family Planning Workforce in the United Kingdom 2003 and 2004. Available: www.ffprhc.org.uk

USEFUL WEBSITES

- Faculty of Family Planning and Reproductive Health Care (FFPRHC) – www.ffprhc.org.uk
- Royal College of Obstetricians and Gynaecologists (RCOG) – www.rcog.org.uk
- British Association for Sexual Health and HIV (BASHH) – www.bashh.org
- National Institute for Health and Clinical Excellence (NICE) – www.nice.org.uk
- Department of Health (DH) – www.dh.gov.uk
- Scottish Executive (SE) – www.scotland.gov.uk/topics/health

Appendix 2.1

SUMMARY OF PROFESSIONAL TRAINING PROVIDED BY THE FACULTY OF FAMILY PLANNING AND REPRODUCTIVE HEALTHCARE IN THE UK

The Diploma of the Faculty of Family Planning (DFFP) is the 'gold standard' Level 1 qualification in sexual and reproductive health.

Letters of Competence (LOC) in intrauterine techniques, subdermal contraceptive implant techniques and medical education are for those members who wish to achieve and maintain these skills and/or become Registered Trainers for the Faculty.

The Membership of the Faculty of Family Planning (MFFP) examination is a senior postgraduate examination for specialists in sexual and reproductive health.

Special Skills Modules are competency-based, structured training modules on specific topics, open to clinicians working in the broader field of sexual and reproductive health.

Career Grade Training is a 3-year certificated modular training programme for non-consultant clinicians who choose to become specialists in sexual and reproductive health.

Subspecialty Training in Sexual and Reproductive Health is a 3-year training programme entered by open competition for obstetrics and gynaecology specialist registrars who wish to specialize in, and become service leaders in, sexual and reproductive health.

3 Combined hormonal contraception

Anna Glasier

Chapter contents

The combined oral contraceptive pill was first marketed in the US in 1959 and in the UK in 1961. Over 45 years later it is used all around the world and is the most popular method of contraception in most industrialized countries. There can be very few women in the UK over the age of 30 who have never taken the combined oral contraceptive pill. Although 'the pill', as it is known, is widely credited as being the cause of the 'second contraceptive revolution' and of the emancipation of women in the Western world, it is still a controversial drug and is never far from newspaper headlines. Frustratingly for health professionals the media are enthusiastic about reporting any data suggesting a theoretical risk of the pill, but totally disinterested in good news about its real or potential benefits. Many women are influenced by this negative reporting and need to be reassured that combined hormonal contraception is extremely safe and highly effective for the vast majority of them.

In contrast to progestogen-only contraception, until the last few years combined hormonal contraception was available only as an oral preparation. Recently however transdermal and injectable preparations have become available and a vaginal ring delivering a combination of estrogen and progestogen is now marketed in some countries. The patch, ring and combined injectable contraceptives are no different from the pill in terms of safety and efficacy. However, as with all methods which do not require the user to remember to do something every day or with every act of intercourse, there may be advantages in terms of demands on compliance.

ORAL

The combined oral contraceptive pill (COCP) contains estrogen (almost always ethinyl estradiol) and a progestogen, both of which are orally active. Progestogens are synthetic formulations of progesterone which mimic its action, particularly on the endometrium. Since the pill was first introduced in the late 1950s, pharmaceutical companies have gradually reduced the dose of estrogen, and modern pills contain less than 35μg ethinyl estradiol (EE). The drive to lower the dose, in the interests of safety since most of the serious side effects are thought to be due to the estrogen component of the pill, risks compromising efficacy. There is no evidence that a pill containing 20μg EE is less effective than one containing 30μg. However the pill-free interval (PFI, see below) is often shortened, or in the US estrogen alone is included in the PFI, when brands containing 20 or 15μg of EE are marketed.

Pharmaceutical companies have also spent a great deal of effort and money experimenting with the progestogen component of the combined pill. Norethisterone and its pro-drugs (norethisterone acetate and ethynodial diacetate) and levonorgestrel are known as second-generation progestogens. Closely related to testosterone, these drugs when given without estrogen are more androgenic than the so-called third-generation progestogens (desogestrel and gestodene). Much of the marketing material promoting these third-generation progestogen-containing oral contraceptive pills emphasized their reduced androgenicity and their consequent 'lipid-friendly' nature. In reality, when combined with 20 or 30μg of ethinyl estradiol, the progestogens behave very differently than when they are administered alone and the androgenic effects are largely overwhelmed by the presence of estrogen. In the UK the most recently marketed pill contains a new progestogen, drospirenone. This compound is anti-androgenic and also has some anti-mineralocorticoid properties. The manufacturers have been careful to avoid the use of the term fourth-generation progestogen.

Oral contraceptive pills differ not only in the dose of estrogen and the type of progestogen but also in the dose of the combination of the two hormones. Monophasic pills contain the same dose of both progestogen and estrogen throughout the full 21 days of treatment. Biphasic pills contain two different dose formulations through the 21 days and triphasic pills three. The biphasic and triphasic pills were developed in an attempt to improve cycle control by 'mimicking' the normal cycle. There is no evidence that cycle control is improved with these preparations and they make the contraceptive regimen more complicated. There is no advantage to their use over the simpler and cheaper monophasic preparations.

The oral contraceptive pill was developed as a 21-day regimen followed by 7 days without treatment, known as the pill-free interval (PFI). Cessation of steroid treatment results in a withdrawal bleed and thus the 21/7 regimen confers a cycle of 28 days, mimicking the 'normal' cycle. The developers of the pill thought that this would make it more acceptable to women and to the church. In addition to inducing a withdrawal bleed, the pill-free interval frees the ovary from the suppressive effects of steroid hormones and allows the resumption of follicular development. On the last day of the pill-free interval one in five women will have ovarian follicles greater than 10 mm in diameter measurable on ultrasound. Delaying the start of the next packet of pills and thus extending the pill free interval to 8 or 9 days or more, risks follicle growth and subsequent ovulation despite the pill being restarted. Missing a number of pills in the last 7 days of the packet will have the same effect. Shortening the pill free interval (to only 4 days) or giving 10 μg of ethinyl estradiol on 5 of the 7 days are two strategies that have been adopted in recent years by pharmaceutical companies to increase the theoretical effectiveness of very low-dose pills. In some countries packets of pills are marketed with 21 active pills followed by 7 placebo pills (every day, ED preparations) enabling women to take a pill every day thus, in theory, making it easier to remember to take them.

TRANSDERMAL

It was a surprisingly long time after the use of transdermal estrogen replacement therapy for postmenopausal women became commonplace, before a contraceptive patch was developed. Only one preparation is currently marketed and it delivers 20 μg ethinyl estradiol and 150 μg norelgestromin daily. Like the oral contraceptive pill, the patch is designed to be used for 21 days followed by a 7-day patch-free interval. Each patch lasts for 1 week.

COMBINED INJECTABLE

A once/month injectable contraceptive containing 5 mg estradiol cypionate and 25 mg medroxyprogesterone acetate has been in fairly widespread use in Latin America and was marketed in the US recently. Injections are administered intramuscularly every 28 days. Bleeding patterns and efficacy are comparable with the combined oral contraceptive pill. Bleeding episodes can be anticipated 18–22 days after injection and are induced by a fall in estrogen concentrations to 50 pg/ml or less.

Approximately 70% of women experience one bleeding episode per month, with only 4% experiencing amenorrhoea over three treatment cycles.

VAGINAL RING

A combined contraceptive vaginal ring (CCVR) releasing 15 μg ethinyl estradiol and 120 μg etonorgestrel is licensed in the US and in much of Europe. Made of soft ethylene–vinyl–acetate (EVA) copolymer, the ring has an outer diameter of 54 mm and a cross-sectional diameter of 4 mm. Designed to last for 3 weeks, a 7-day ring-free interval is associated with bleeding patterns which appear superior to those associated with the combined pill. Compared with an oral contraceptive containing 30 μg ethinylestradiol and 150 μg levonorgestrel, the incidence of irregular bleeding in the vaginal ring appears to be significantly less (2% versus 39%).

MODE OF ACTION

All combined hormonal contraceptives inhibit ovulation. In addition both estrogen and progestogen have an effect on cervical and vaginal mucus reducing the likelihood of successful transportation of sperm into the upper genital tract. There is good evidence too that endometrial growth is suppressed by combined hormonal contraception; the endometrium is thin and its cellular and biochemical characteristics are altered in such a way that implantation is less likely to take place should ovulation occur. Efficacy of the combined pill depends on perfect use (see below). Missed pills, as with extended pill-free intervals, theoretically risk follicle growth and ovulation. In reality there seems very little chance that missing two or even three pills in the middle of the packet is sufficient to allow ovulation to occur. It seems much more likely that women who conceive while 'taking the pill' are probably taking it very inconsistently or chaotically. The recently revised rules for what to do when pills are missed (see page 63) reflect this fact.

EFFECTIVENESS

Combined hormonal contraceptives, regardless of their route of administration, are highly effective when used perfectly (Chapter 1, Table 1.1). For all methods, fewer than one in 100 women will get pregnant during 1 year of perfect use. Failure rates associated with typical use are of course much higher and an estimated eight per 100 women will get pregnant every year while using the combined oral contraceptive pill. This is because of incorrect and/or inconsistent use. Compliance with pill taking is notoriously poor. In an elegant study undertaken in the US in the late 1990s, new users were given their pills in an electronic dispenser which recorded whether they were removed from the packet (although not whether they were swallowed).[1] The average number of missed pills per cycle was 2.6 and rose to 3.5 in cycle three when half the women missed three or more pills. None of these women got pregnant. As discussed earlier combined hormonal contraceptives with a slightly longer action (1 week for the patch, 4 weeks for the CCVR and injectable method) may be associated with better compliance than the pill and so typical-use failure rates may be lower.

INDICATIONS

The pill is licensed for contraception. However it is often prescribed for its additional health benefits, usually to women who also need contraception but not infrequently to women who are not sexually active or who have been sterilized. If it is not being used for contraception, then the COCP (and other combined hormonal contraceptives) is being prescribed outside the terms of the product licence and the prescriber needs to make this clear to the user (and document that she/he has done so).[2] That said, it is extremely common practice to prescribe the COCP for the relief of menstrual dysfunction such as dysmenorrhoea, premenstrual symptoms and menorrhagia. It is also of benefit to women with acne (see page 68).

CONTRAINDICATIONS

While the majority of women who use contraception are young and healthy and have no contraindications to combined hormonal contraception certain conditions, including chronic disease such as diabetes, do theoretically interfere with the relative safety of the pill. As discussed in Chapter 1, the World Health Organization Medical Eligibility Criteria distinguish between category 4 conditions when the pill should not be used and category 3 conditions when the pill can be used but only if other methods of contraception are unavailable, unacceptable or inappropriate. Table 3.1a and b list the category 3 and category 4 conditions as laid out in the UK Medical Eligibility Criteria.

ADVANTAGES

Combined hormonal contraception is simple to use, highly effective when used perfectly, reasonably effective when used typically, and relatively inexpensive. It is an extremely popular method of contraception and one with which most women around the world are familiar and comfortable. The increased range of routes of administration has added to the advantages of combined hormonal contraception. Its non-contraceptive benefits (see below) add to its popularity.

Table 3.1 Contraindications to combined hormonal contraception – UK Medical Eligibility Criteria Categories 3 and 4

UK Medical Eligibility Criteria Category 3 conditions for combined hormonal contraception
Category 3 conditions (risks generally outweigh the benefits)

Fully, or nearly fully, breast-feeding and between 6 weeks and 6 months postpartum.

Before 21 days postpartum (regardless of infant feeding method)

Smoking <15 cigarettes/day and age 35 or over, or stopped smoking < one year ago

Obesity BMI 35–39 kg/m^2

Multiple risk factors for arterial cardiovascular disease

Adequately controlled hypertension

BP > 140–159 mmHg systolic and 90–94 mmHg diastolic

Family history of VTE in a first-degree relative aged <45

Immobility (unrelated to surgery)

Known hyperlipidaemias

Migraine without aura if aged 35 or over

Past history of migraine with aura at any age

Undiagnosed breast mass (initiation only)

Cancer of known gene mutation associated with breast cancer

Past breast cancer – 5 years without recurrence

Diabetes with retinopathy, nephropathy, neuropathy, other vascular disease or of more than 20 years duration (depending on disease severity may be category 4)

Current symptomatic or medically treated gallbladder disease

Past COC-related cholestasis

Mild compensated cirrhosis

Drugs which induce liver enzymes (e.g. rifampicin, rifabutin, St John's Wort, griseofulvin and certain anticonvulsants)

UK Medical Eligibility Criteria Category 4 conditions for combined hormonal contraception
Category 4 conditions (Unacceptable health risk and should not be used)

Breast-feeding <6 weeks postpartum

Smoking 15 or more cigarettes/day and aged 35 or over

Obesity BMI 40 kg/m^2 or over

Multiple risk factors for arterial cardiovascular disease

Blood pressure 160 mmHg systolic or over and 95 mmHg diastolic or over

Hypertension with vascular disease

History of/or current VTE

Major surgery with prolonged immobilization

Known thrombogenic mutations

History of or current ischaemic heart disease

History of or current stroke

Valvular and congenital heart disease complicated by pulmonary hypertension, atrial fibrillation, history of sub-acute bacterial endocarditis

Migraine with aura at any age

Gestational trophoblastic neoplasia (hCG elevated)

Table 3.1 (Continued)

UK Medical Eligibility Criteria Category 4 conditions for combined hormonal contraception
Category 4 conditions (Unacceptable health risk and should not be used)
Current breast cancer
Diabetes with retinopathy, nephropathy, neuropathy, other vascular disease or of more than
20 years duration (depending on disease severity may be category 3)
Viral hepatitis (active disease)
Severe decompenstaed cirrhosis
Liver tumour benign or malignant
Raynaud's disease – secondary with hyperanticoagulant

DISADVANTAGES

The disadvantages of combined hormonal contraceptives lie in their associated risks and side effects. The other major disadvantage is their short action compared to the intrauterine method, contraceptive implants and, to a lesser extent, progestogen-only injectable contraceptives. As discussed earlier, perfect use of contraceptive methods which require daily action by the user is uncommon. Likewise, continuation rates of combined hormonal contraceptives are disappointingly low. In a US study of over 1600 women starting or restarting the combined oral contraceptive pill, 28% of women had stopped using the pill within 6 months.[3] Discontinuation was most likely in the first 2 months and the commonest reason was irregular bleeding. Forty-two per cent of women who stopped using the combined pill did so without consulting a doctor. In that same study nausea (7%), weight gain (5%), breast tenderness (4%), and headaches (4%) were the other main reasons for discontinuation.

MINOR SIDE EFFECTS AND THEIR MANAGEMENT

Combined hormonal contraception has an effect on almost every system in the body. The list of potential side effects published in the Patient Information Leaflet by the manufacturers is long. It is generated from clinical trials in which women using a drug keep a detailed record of any ill-health during the period of follow-up. Researchers encourage participants to record any problems including those for which they take medication; so, for example, headache, abdominal pain and mood change are all commonly reported. A large cohort of women not using any method of contraception would be likely to report the same minor health problems with the same frequency over a similar period of time. There is, of course, a tendency for people who are taking any medication to blame illness on that drug. Women will often come to the clinic complaining of a variety of minor ailments which they attribute to the pill. In truth most of them are probably unrelated but it can be hard to persuade women that this is the case. Side effects which are probably genuinely related to estrogen and progestogen include breast tenderness, chloasma and nausea and, of course, breakthrough bleeding. Perhaps more disputable, but possibly related, is fluid retention; and unlikely to be related to the combined pill are most of the rest of the common side effects. Although referred to as 'minor' because they are not life threatening, these side effects are commonly associated with discontinuation and so should not be dismissed. While a 'cure' for the side effect is often not possible, women are much more likely to be reassured that the side effect is not dangerous if they feel that their concerns are being taken seriously and, when appropriate, investigated.

Many textbooks discuss in detail how a change of pill preparation can help specific conditions. The advice is often unhelpful and as stated earlier it is much more likely that changing to a different brand of pills coincides with the natural resolution of the condition or a change in the life circumstances of the woman, circumstances which in themselves were causing the ill-health. In an attempt to take a scientific approach to the management of side effects there are five questions to be asked.

1. Is it likely that the side effect would benefit from a change in the dose of estrogen?
2. Is it likely that the side effect could benefit from a change in type of progestogen?
3. Is it likely that the side effect would benefit from a change in both the dose of estrogen and the type of progestogen?
4. Would a change in the route of administration of combined hormonal contraception be of benefit?
5. Should the woman be advised to change to a different method of hormonal contraception or to a non-hormonal method?

• Breakthrough bleeding

Among UK women (regardless of contraceptive use), the self-reported cumulative incidence of inter-menstrual bleeding (IMB) over 1 year is 17%. When IMB occurs during oral contraceptive use it is traditionally called breakthrough bleed (BTB). The commonest cause of BTB is missing pills. Other causes include smoking, drug interactions and *Chlamydia* infection. BTB tends to improve with time and, unless there are obvious underlying causes, in the first 3 months of pill use women should be warned to expect it and be reassured that it will likely settle. If it does not, a careful history should be taken, including questions about missed pills, smoking and use of other drugs including over-the-counter preparations. Examination to exclude cervical conditions (ectropion, polyps, malignancy), and testing for *Chlamydia* infection should be undertaken before trying a pill with a different dose of estrogen or type or dose of progestogen, continuous administration of the pill or a different route of administration. See Figure 3.1 for management of breakthrough bleeding.

The risk of BTB occurring during use of the combined pill depends on the degree of suppression of endogenous ovarian activity. It is more likely to occur in women who have evidence of follicular development during pill taking. This in turn is certainly related to the amount of estrogen in the pill (and the duration of exposure to exogenous estrogen) and possibly related to the type and dose of progestogen. In a randomized controlled trial comparing two oral contraceptive formulations containing either 30 μg or 20 μg ethinyl estradiol, BTB was significantly more likely to occur with the lower-dose pill. Pill brands containing 23 days of active tablets or brands which include a few days of estrogen alone during the pill-free interval are associated with a greater degree of ovarian suppression and less likelihood of follicle growth. They should be associated with less BTB. In a comparison of two pills, both containing 20 μg ethinyl estradiol, with either 100 μg levonorgestrel or 500 μg norethisterone, BTB appeared to be significantly less in the LNG-containing pill. There has been no robust direct comparison between third- and second-generation progestogens and there appears to be no significant difference when one third-generation progestogen is compared directly with another. If it is available the combined contraceptive vaginal ring appears to have much better bleeding patterns than the pill.

• Chloasma

A brownish pigment to the skin of the face occurs in some women using hormonal contraception, particularly after excessive exposure to sunlight. It can occur with both estrogen and progestogen and it takes a long time to fade once hormonal contraception has been stopped. Mild chloasma can be hidden by the use of cosmetics but most women find it distressing. There is no point in changing to a different brand of combined pill and probably, once told that progestogen-only contraception *may* do the same thing, women will be reluctant to change to the POP. The only solution if chloasma is severe is to change to a non-hormonal method of contraception.

• Breast tenderness

Breast tenderness is common among women taking the pill and can occur cyclically. It may be due to either estrogen or progestogen. It tends to improve with time and if the woman can be reassured and persuaded to continue the method (and the brand of pill), the problem may resolve or at least become tolerable. Fear of breast cancer is a common cause of discontinuation of the pill. While breast examination is not a good way to exclude breast cancer it can be extremely reassuring. There is no evidence for superiority of any particular progestogen in managing mastalgia although the anti-mineralocorticoid effects of drospirenone and its effect

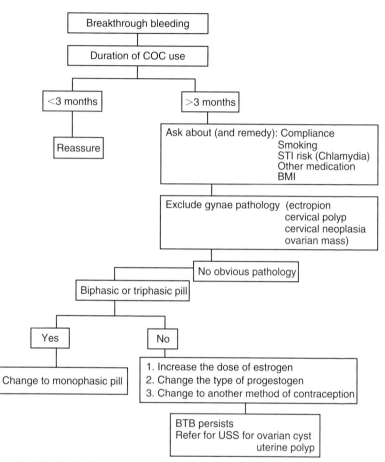

Figure 3.1 Algorithm for the management of breakthrough bleeding

on fluid retention may be of theoretical benefit. It may make sense to try a lower dose of estrogen. Once again, if mastalgia persists a change of method may be the only solution.

• Nausea

Nausea is surprisingly uncommon among women using combined hormonal contraception and when it does occur it tends to settle over the first 3 months of use. In the small minority of women in whom it is troublesome nausea on combined oral contraception is an indication to change the route of administration and in the UK the only alternative is the combined contraceptive patch.

• Fluid retention

Women commonly complain of fluid retention in the latter half of the spontaneous menstrual cycle and it is a common feature of the premenstrual syndrome. It is thought to be related to progesterone when it occurs as part of the PMS constellation. Some women complain of fluid retention on the combined pill. The combined pill containing drospirenone may be associated with less fluid retention since drospirenone has anti-mineralocorticoid activity.

• Weight gain

Weight gain – whether caused by the contraceptive method or not – is a common reason for discontinuation of all methods. Women – and men – gain weight during their reproductive lives. In an observational study of 1697 Brazilian women using a copper intrauterine device (IUD) the mean weight of the cohort was 58.5 kg when the IUD was inserted.[4] After 5 years of follow-up, mean weight was 61.2 kg and after 7 years it was 62.4 kg. It is possible that hormonal contraceptives, through a variety of mechanisms including (among others) stimulation of the renin-angiotensin system, altered carbohydrate metabolism or increased appetite, might cause weight gain.

In a recent Cochrane review, Gallo and colleagues[5] reviewed 570 published reports of weight change among users of combined hormonal contraception. No statistically significant differences in weight change were identified when contraceptive users were compared with non-users. Five of the 69 trials comparing two different formulations of combined pill did however demonstrate significant weight gain but the largest mean difference was 1.8 kg after 1 year. The authors of the review concluded that the evidence is insufficient to rule out any effect of combined hormonal contraception on weight change but that it is unlikely that there is any large effect.

MAJOR (SERIOUS) SIDE EFFECTS

The pill is among the most researched drugs in the world and it is extremely safe. In a 25-year follow-up of 46 000 women in the UK the overall risk of death from any condition was the same among women using the combined pill as it was among never-users.[6] Among women who are currently using the pill or who had used it within the last 10 years, use was associated with an increased risk of death from only two conditions, cervical cancer (relative risk 2.5) and cerebral vascular disease (relative risk 1.9). Despite the concerns about breast cancer this study did not show an increased risk of death among users or ex-users of the combined pill. Of course, some of the serious risks associated with the combined pill are not fatal and serious morbidity is also a major consideration.

• Cardiovascular disease

Cardiovascular disease is very uncommon among women of reproductive age but combined hormonal contraceptives increase the tendency to thrombosis in both the venous and arterial circulation. It is almost certainly the estrogen which causes this increased risk since it does not appear to be elevated among women using progestogen-only contraceptives, even high-dose methods. The risk of cardiovascular disease, particularly venous thromboembolism, is also increased during pregnancy and the risks of contraceptive methods must always be balanced against the relative risks associated with being pregnant. The associated increased risk of cardiovascular disease (CVD) among women using CHC is reflected in the medical eligibility criteria (Table 3.1) in which conditions which are also associated with an increased risk of CVD are almost all categorized as category 3 or 4. For an excellent review of hormonal contraception and cardiovascular disease see Curtis and Marchbanks.[7]

The most common serious consequence of use of combined hormonal contraception is venous thromboembolism (VTE). VTE is much more common than stroke or heart attack although much less likely to be fatal; in women who are not pregnant and not using CHC the risk is 5 per 100 000 woman-years. Women using the combined oral contraceptive pill who have no other known risk factors for cardiovascular disease are at increased risk of VTE. The data are almost non-existent for women using combined injectables, transdermal preparations and vaginal rings but for now it is sensible to assume that there is no difference between the four routes of administration. The risk of VTE is three to six times that of women not using combined hormonal contraception and is highest in the first year of use probably as a result of the unmasking of unrecognized thrombogenic mutations. Pill users who have factor V Leiden mutations have up to 20 times the risk of VTE compared with women who have the mutation but who do not take the pill. However, as the prevalence of mutations is relatively low and the number of women using the pill enormous, routine screening is not considered to be cost-effective. The risk of VTE among combined oral contraceptive pill users is probably increased by obesity and may be increased by immobilization and air travel but not by smoking and hypertension. The acrimonious debate over a differential risk of CVD with different types of progestogen still rumbles on. The risk of VTE among women using combined pills containing a third-generation progestogen appears to be almost doubled (25/100 000 woman-years) compared to women using second-generation progestogen pills (15/100 000 woman years). There is biological plausibility for the difference; oral contraceptive use appears to reduce the efficiency with which activated protein C down-regulates in-vitro thrombin formation. This effect is more pronounced in women using a combined pill containing desogestrel compared with one containing levonorgestrel. In absolute terms however the difference is very small (one to two extra cases per 10 000 woman-years), while the risk of VTE during pregnancy is 60/100 000 woman-years. The risk of VTE is also increased in conditions associated with underlying thrombogenic disorders such as Raynaud's disease.

• Myocardial infarction

A meta-analysis of 23 studies of COC use and myocardial infarction (MI) estimated an overall increased risk of 2.5 for current users compared with never users.[8] The risk was inversely related to the dose of estrogen but was nonetheless increased for women using low-dose pills. The absolute risk of myocardial infarction among young women is of course extremely small. Smoking and hypertension both substantially increase the risk of myocardial infarction among CHC users and there may be an increased risk among women with diabetes, elevated cholesterol and a history of pregnancy-induced hypertension or pre-eclampsia (and all these are reflected in the UKMEC, Table 3.1). The increased risk does not appear to be related to age and resolves rapidly once the pill has stopped. There is still debate over a differential risk of myocardial infarction in association with different types of progestogen as the results of studies are inconsistent and the confidence intervals are wide. If there is a difference it is unlikely to be clinically important.

• Stroke

The risk of ischaemic stroke is increased among current users of the combined pill (RR 2.7). There is some evidence for an increased risk among past users but no apparent relationship with duration of use. Smoking and hypertension increase the risk of ischaemic stroke among pill users and the risk may also be increased among women who suffer from migraine. Most studies have found no statistically significant increase in the risk of haemorrhagic stroke among combined oral contraceptive users although the risk may be increased among women once they reach 35 and over and if they smoke or have hypertension.

• Migraine

Migraine is associated with an increased risk of ischaemic stroke and the risk appears to be further increased among migraine sufferers who use combined hormonal contraception. Migraine with aura is generally thought to represent a greater risk of stroke and is a category 4 condition for CHC (i.e. it should not be used). In reality it can be hard to distinguish headache from migraine and migraine with aura from migraine without. Many women claim to suffer from migraine. Symptoms of aura include homonymous visual disturbances, unilateral paraesthesia and/or numbness, unilateral weakness and aphasia or speech disorder. The key to diagnosing aura is that these symptoms appear *before* the headache (and sometimes even instead of it). A past history of occasional episodes of migraine, particularly during puberty, is not uncommon and the UKMEC recommends that a careful trial of the combined pill may be considered.

CANCER

• Breast cancer

Combined oral contraceptive use has long been thought to be associated with an increased risk of breast cancer and a meta-analysis of data from over 50 000 women with breast cancer and 100 000 controls published in 1995 showed a relative risk of 1.24.[9] The increased risk takes 10 years to decline to that of non-users. A more recent case controlled study involving 8000 women in the USA suggested no increased risk of breast cancer, however, the upper limit of the confidence interval was in keeping with the much larger study published in 1995. The risk of breast cancer appears to be independent of the dose of estrogen and of the duration of use of the pill. It is not influenced by family history or age at first use.

• Cervical cancer

The combined pill is associated with an increased risk of squamous carcinoma of the cervix but it is often suggested that the association may simply be the result of inadequate adjustment of differences in sexual behaviour. In women with persistent infection with human papilloma virus (HPV) infection who use hormonal contraception for more than 5 years the relative risk of cervical cancer is increased up to fourfold. Hormonal contraceptive use for longer than 10 years, even among women who are HPV negative, may double the relative risk of cervical cancer. In the RCGP study ever-users of the combined pill were 2.5 times more likely to die from cervical cancer than never users.[6] Women who use hormonal contraception and have to attend a health professional for supplies are, however, a captive population for cervical screening. This continues to be one of the arguments raised against making combined oral contraception available over the counter.

• Liver cancer

Use of the combined pill is associated with an increased risk of liver cancer but only in populations with a high rate of hepatitis B infection. Among others, the absolute risk of liver cancer is extremely small.

CLINICAL MANAGEMENT

Most women who take the combined pill (and use the other combined hormonal contraceptive preparations) are young and fit. When starting a woman on the pill for the first time it is important to take a good medical history and to update this history at annual review. The key to history-taking is to identify existing conditions which might be exacerbated by use of combined hormonal contraception or which, because of the use of concomitant medication, may reduce the effectiveness of the contraceptive. It is important to ask specifically about risk factors for cardiovascular disease and cancer given the risks associated with combined hormonal contraception discussed earlier. Given that many women use hormonal contraception into middle age it is important too to take a good family history in order to identify any increased risk of conditions which may appear in later life, such as breast cancer.

It is not necessary to undertake routine physical examination of women before they start using hormonal contraception. The measurement of blood pressure is mandatory and an assessment of BMI (body mass index) is strongly recommended since a high BMI is a contraindication to combined hormonal contraception (see Table 3.1). Physical appearance, including severe acne, hirsutism, etc., may be of benefit in deciding which method of contraception is most likely to suit an individual woman. Routine breast and pelvic examination are not indicated unless something in the woman's history suggests that one or other of these should be undertaken. Not only are they poor tools for screening women for pathology, they also deter them from returning for further supplies of contraception if they think they have to undergo an examination regularly. A careful sexual history should be taken in order to assess the risk of sexually transmitted infection (see Chapter 18).

WHICH PILL?

The Faculty of Family Planning and Reproductive Health Care in the United Kingdom recommends that the pill of first choice should be a monophasic preparation containing 30 µg ethinyl estradiol with either norethisterone or levonorgestrel as the progestogen.[10] This recommendation is based on the following reasons. Breakthrough bleeding is more common with preparations which contain 20 µg of ethinyl estradiol; there is no evidence to support the use of bi- or triphasic pills; and, in general, pills containing the so-called second-generation progestogens are cheaper than those containing third-generation or other progestogens. This said, the key to effectiveness of any method of contraception is compliance and continuation and as discussed above these are determined by acceptability. If a young woman asks for a particular brand of pill, all things being equal, it may be expedient to provide the preparation for which she is asking since she is less likely to come back complaining of unwanted side effects or to stop using the method without consulting a health professional.

PRACTICAL PRESCRIBING

The manufacturers of hormonal contraceptives provide summaries of product characteristics (SPC) which give information on the licensed indications for the method. They make recommendations on how contraceptives should be administered, when to start them and what to do when pills (or patches) are missed. It is widely agreed that the SPC tends to err very much on the side of caution, making recommendations for contraceptive use which are unnecessarily restrictive. In response to this the World Health Organization produced a set of evidence-based recommendations to guide health professionals and women on how to use contraception safely and effectively. These Selected Practice Recommendations for contraceptive use were adapted by the Faculty of Family Planning and Reproductive Health Care and are available on the faculty website. The recommendations are often at odds with guidance given in the SPC and so strictly speaking many of these recommendations are outside the terms of the product license. Nevertheless the Faculty and WHO guidance do reflect common practice in contraceptive prescribing.

In general when a woman is starting combined hormonal contraception for the first time it is sensible to advise her to start on the first day of her next menstrual period. This will ensure maximum effectiveness and may also reduce the likelihood of breakthrough bleeding in the first cycle of use. The UK Selected Practice Recommendations however recommend that combined oral contraception *can* be started on any day up to the fifth day of the menstrual cycle without the need to use a backup method of contraception (such as condoms) or abstinence. When a woman starts the pill beyond day 5 of the menstrual cycle she should be advised to use backup contraception for the first 7 days.

Most oral contraceptive pills, the contraceptive patch and the vaginal ring are taken/used every day for 21 days followed by 7 days without medication (or with the placebo pill) when a withdrawal bleed is likely to occur. The next packet of pills (patch/ring) should then be started and continued for another 21 days. In the absence of a withdrawal bleed women should be advised to start their course of contraception as instructed and can be reassured that if they have not forgotten to take pills (or replace the patch at the appropriate time) they are highly unlikely to be pregnant. If a withdrawal bleed does not occur after the next 21-day course of treatment then they should seek advice. Women should be advised that breakthrough bleeding (see above) is common during the first 3 months of use of combined hormonal contraception and can be ignored. A follow-up visit 3 months after the first prescription of the combined oral contraceptive pill is generally regarded as good practice since it allows measurement of blood pressure, discussion of any problems and the reinforcement of messages about effective use. Once established on a particular brand of hormonal contraceptive pills (or on the patch or ring), and provided there are no relative contraindications to continued use and no plans for a pregnancy within the next year, women can be given 12 months supply of pills. They should be instructed to come back at any time should problems arise.

All women starting the pill should be advised what to do when pills are missed. Instructions for missed pills have undergone various changes over the last few years in internationally driven attempts to make them more evidence-based and less restrictive. The advice is based on evidence relating to how many pills can be missed before there is significant risk of the resumption of ovarian activity and ovulation. Despite the cautious view of many practitioners, possibly fuelled by fear of litigation, the evidence is extremely reassuring that a number of pills can be missed before contraceptive efficacy is jeopardized. The evidence for the current recommendations is largely derived from data taken from women using oral contraceptive pills containing 30–35 µg ethinyl estradiol. Pills containing 20 µg ethinyl estradiol may have less of a suppressive effect on ovarian activity and ovulation may, theoretically, be more likely after missed pills. For this reason WHO and Faculty guidance on missed pills provides the recommendation for pills containing 30 µg ethinyl estradiol or more and pills containing 20 µg ethinyl estradiol. The algorithm is shown in Figure 3.2 but can be summarized as follows:

- Whenever a woman realizes that she has missed pills, the essential advice is **just keep going**. She should take a pill as soon as possible and then resume her usual pill-taking schedule. If she is taking pills containing 30–35 µg EE she only needs to use additional contraceptive protection if she misses three pills or more. If using pills containing 20 µg or less EE, she needs to use additional contraceptive protection if she misses two or more. (A simple aide memoire is the phrase 'two for twenty, three for thirty.')
- If three or more 30 µg pills or two or more 20 µg pills are missed she should take a pill as soon as possible but she should also use condoms or abstain from sex until she has taken pills for 7 days in a row.
- Whichever dose of pill is being used, if pills were missed in week 3 of the packet then a pill-free interval should be omitted.
- Confusion arises over when to use emergency contraception. If pills are missed in the second or third week, EC is not indicated since ovulation will not occur until some time after the missed pills and the woman should be using additional precautions and/or missing the PFI. EC is only indicated if pills are missed in the first week since this risks extending the PFI to 9 or 10 days or longer and ovulation may occur despite restarting the next packet of pills.
- If more than three pills are missed the woman should be regarded as though she has been taking the pill so erratically that it will not be effective. Other precautions need to be taken *and* EC may be indicated.

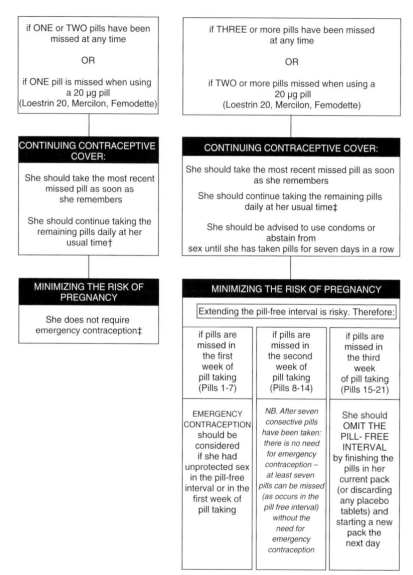

if ONE or TWO pills have been missed at any time	if THREE or more pills have been missed at any time
OR	OR
if ONE pill is missed when using a 20 µg pill (Loestrin 20, Mercilon, Femodette)	if TWO or more pills missed when using a 20 µg pill (Loestrin 20, Mercilon, Femodette)

CONTINUING CONTRACEPTIVE COVER:

She should take the most recent missed pill as soon as she remembers

She should continue taking the remaining pills daily at her usual time†

CONTINUING CONTRACEPTIVE COVER:

She should take the most recent missed pill as soon as she remembers

She should continue taking the remaining pills daily at her usual time‡

She should be advised to use condoms or abstain from sex until she has taken pills for seven days in a row

MINIMIZING THE RISK OF PREGNANCY

She does not require emergency contraception‡

MINIMIZING THE RISK OF PREGNANCY

Extending the pill-free interval is risky. Therefore:

if pills are missed in the first week of pill taking (Pills 1-7)	if pills are missed in the second week of pill taking (Pills 8-14)	if pills are missed in the third week of pill taking (Pills 15-21)
EMERGENCY CONTRACEPTION should be considered if she had unprotected sex in the pill-free interval or in the first week of pill taking	NB. After seven consecutive pills have been taken: there is no need for emergency contraception – at least seven pills can be missed (as occurs in the pill free interval) without the need for emergency contraception	She should OMIT THE PILL- FREE INTERVAL by finishing the pills in her current pack (or discarding any placebo tablets) and starting a new pack the next day

† Depending on when she remembers her missed pill she may take two pills on the same day (one at the moment of remembering and the other at the regular time) or even at the same time.

‡ Any pills missed in the last week of the previous packet should be taken into account when considering emergency contracepton.

Figure 3.2 Missed pill advice. From: First Prescription of Combined Oral Contraception (July 2006, updated January 2007), Copyright Faculty of Family Planning and Reproductive Health Care

TRICYCLING PILLS

The 21/7-day combined oral contraceptive pill regimen gives women a withdrawal bleed every month – and this regimen has been retained with the patch and ring. Increasingly, particularly in the Western world, women prefer amenorrhoea since avoiding regular menses avoids the common side effects associated with menses (dysmenorrhoea, PMS), avoids the social inconvenience of menstruation and saves money on sanitary protection. Taking the pill for three consecutive packets followed by a 7-day withdrawal bleed (tricycling) has been common in the UK for many years. In the US a 3-month preparation of the pill is now marketed. One pharmaceutical company now markets a continuous preparation which women can take for years on end without having withdrawal bleeds. There is no evidence that continuous use of combined hormonal contraception is any way harmful or associated with increased risks of cardiovascular disease or cancer. Some health professionals are reluctant to recommend tricycling or continuous pill use (mainly because they are ignorant of the basis of the standard regimen), and many women have reservations about continuing pill use because they feel that it is unnatural. In reality it is monthly menstruation that is unnatural and simply a consequence of modern contraception. When contraception was unavailable the vast majority of women were either pregnant (and amenorrhoeic) or lactating (and amenorrhoeic) or postmenopausal (and amenorrhoeic) or dead. When this is explained to them, many women feel relieved to know that they can use hormonal contraception continuously and skip menstrual periods either on an occasional basis, for example when they are going on holiday, or as a matter of routine.

CONTRACEPTION FOR SPECIAL GROUPS

• Women taking enzyme–inducing drugs

Drugs which induce the production of liver enzymes interfere with efficacy of combined hormonal contraception by increasing the rate of metabolism of both the estrogen and the progestogen. The Faculty of Family Planning and Reproductive Healthcare publishes excellent evidence-based guidance on drug interactions with all hormonal contraceptives.[11] Use of enzyme-inducing drugs is a category 3 condition for the combined oral contraceptive pill. The Faculty recommends that women taking liver enzyme-inducing drugs but wishing to use the combined pill should use a regimen containing at least 50 μg ethinyl estradiol (a combination of pills containing 20 and 30 μg if necessary) together with condoms until 4 weeks after the drug has been stopped. The combined contraceptive patch (at the usual dose) should also be used with a back-up method.

• Young people

In the UK the average age of first intercourse is 16, and sex before 16 is common. Young people need easy access to highly effective methods of contraception and the combined pill is relatively popular (see Chapter 14).

• Older women

In much of the Western world the age of first childbirth is approaching 30, second partnerships are common, and increasing numbers of women use hormonal contraception, and particularly combined hormonal contraception, until they reach the menopause. Because the risks of both cardiovascular disease and breast cancer increase with age, many health professionals become increasingly reluctant to prescribe combined hormonal contraception for women over the age of 35 and certainly over the age of 40. However, as women approach the peri-menopause menstrual dysfunction becomes increasingly common and the non-contraceptive benefits of combined hormonal contraception, particularly on the menstrual cycle, become increasingly acceptable and desirable. Many women who take the combined pill in their 40s use it not just for contraception but for the control of menstruation and they are extremely reluctant to stop using it if there are contraindications. Many health professionals tend to reduce the dose of estrogen when prescribing combined pills for older women and sometimes change to a third-generation progestogen-containing pill. In the meta-analysis by Khader and colleagues[8] the risk of myocardial infarction was lower with pills containing $20\mu g$ EE than with $30\mu g$ pills, however the differential risks of different progestogens remains controversial. Since we do not have the answer, it is probably best to discuss the increasing risks of combined hormonal contraception with women who wish to continue using it into their late 40s and even early 50s and to discuss which dose of estrogen and which progestogen could be used. Combined hormonal contraception suppresses ovarian activity and menstruation unless it is stopped for 7 days when a withdrawal bleed occurs. It also provides estrogen replacement therapy. Thus the common signs of the menopause, irregular menses and eventually amenorrhoea and vasomotor symptoms, are largely masked by combined hormonal contraception and if a woman continues to use it into her early 50s she will not know whether she still needs contraception or not. When a COC-user is around the age of 50 years, the POP or a barrier method should be substituted. This will then allow assessment of the menstrual cycle and any menopausal symptoms. In the absence of subsequent menstruation, an FSH concentration can be measured. If this is within the menopausal range, the barrier method or POP should be continued for 1 more year provided there is no further menstrual bleeding. If FSH concentration is within the pre-menopausal range, the woman should continue the barrier method or POP and follow the general rules for stopping contraception.

REVERSIBILITY

There is no evidence that past use of the pill has any effect on fertility. Once the pill is stopped normal fertility resumes rapidly. So-called post-pill amenorrhoea is almost always the consequence of a pre-existing condition (such as polycystic ovarian syndrome) which has been masked by use of the pill and its associated regular withdrawal bleeds. Combined hormonal contraception may however exacerbate hyperprolactinaemia since estrogen stimluates the lactotrophes to secrete prolactin.

OUTCOME OF PREGNANCY

There is no evidence for a teratogenic effect of combined hormonal contraception.

NON-CONTRACEPTIVE BENEFITS

Although contraceptives are primarily intended to prevent pregnancy, some, particularly hormonal methods, have other health benefits. For some women the additional benefits play a role in method choice, and there is some evidence that they increase compliance and continuation rates. Girls who complain of dysmenorrhoea before starting the combined pill are eight times more likely to use the pill consistently than girls without dysmenorrhoea. Although the evidence of benefit applies only to oral contraceptives it is unlikely to be any different with other routes of administration.

• Menstrual dysfunction

The artificially induced monthly withdrawal bleeds associated with CHC tend to be lighter and much more predictable than natural menstrual bleeds. If packets of pills (or combined patches) are taken without a break, amenorrhoea can also be induced by combined hormonal methods. Women with heavy or painful periods, anovulatory dysfunctional uterine bleeding, pre-menstrual symptoms, endometriosis or menstrual migraine all clearly benefit from amenorrhoea. Even when used as a 21/7 regimen there is evidence to suggest that use of the combined pill is associated with measurably lower blood loss, and fewer hospital consultations for menstrual problems.

• Malignant disease

Combined oral contraceptives protect against ovarian cancer and benign ovarian cysts. A meta-analysis of studies estimated a relative risk of 0.64 (95% CI 0.57–0.73) among ever-users compared with never users[12] and the risk of death from ovarian cancer was significantly reduced in the RCGP study. The reduction in risk is related to the duration of use (after 5 years the risk of ovarian cancer seems to be halved) and lasts for 10 years or more after pill use ceases. The protective effect may be reduced if low-dose pills are used but is still significant and may prevent more deaths than those due to the increase in breast cancer attributed to the pill. Use of the combined pill is also associated with a decreased risk of endometrial cancer. Protection continues for up to 15 years after discontinuation.

Women who have never used the combined oral contraceptive pill may also have a reduced risk of colorectal cancer.

While reduction in the risk of cancer almost certainly has no influence on an individual's choice of contraceptive method, the benefits in terms of public health may be important.

• Other conditions

Acne

A Cochrane review concluded that the combined pill can improve acne. There is no evidence to suggest that the type of progestogen in the pill makes a difference since most of the benefit is due to estrogen.[13] Pills containing an anti-androgen (drospirenone or cyproterone acetate) should theoretically be of particular benefit since acne is associated with hyperandrogenism.

Bone mineral density

Use of the combined hormonal contraceptive pill is associated with small increases in bone mineral density (BMD). This probably has little clinically significant effect on fracture risk or postmenopausal osteoporosis. However, for women with oligo-amenorrhoea who are of normal weight, the pill appears to be beneficial in preventing BMD loss and simultaneously provides contraception. It does not benefit BMD in women with anorexia nervosa and may even be detrimental.

Benign breast disease

A number of observational studies suggested that combined oral contraceptive pills used in the 1970s had a protective effect against benign breast disease. More recent studies have been less consistent. Modern pills contain lower doses of both estrogen and progestogen than those used in the 1970s and it is possible that the benefit for BBD is diminished, or lost, with lower doses of steroids.

REFERENCES

1. Potter L, Oakley D, de Leon-Wong E, Canamanr R (1996) Measuring compliance among oral contraceptive users. Fam Plann Perspect 28: 154–158.

2. Faculty of Family Planning & Reproductive Healthcare Clinical Effectiveness Unit (2005) The use of contraception outside the terms of the product licence. J Fam Plan & Reprod Healthcare 31: 225–242.

3. Rosenberg MJ, Waugh MS (1999) Oral contraceptive discontinuation: a prospective evaluation of frequency and reasons. Am J Obstet Gynecol 179: 577–582.

4. Hassan DF, Petta CA, Aldrighi JM, Bahamondes L, Perrotti M (2003) Weight variation in a cohort of women using copper IUD for contraception. Contraception 68: 27–30.

5. Gallo MF, Grimes DA, Schultz KF, Helmerhorst FM (2004) Combination estrogen-progestin contraceptives and body weight. Systematic review of randomized controlled trials. Obstet Gynecol 103: 359–373.

6. Beral V, Hermon C, Kay C, Hannaford P, Darby S, Reeves G (1999) Mortality associated with oral contraceptive use: 25 year follow up of a cohort of 46 000 women from Royal College of General Practitioners' oral contraception study. Brit Med J 318: 96–100.

7. Curtis KM, Marchbanks PA (2005) Hormonal contraception and cardiovascular safety. In Glasier A, Wellings K, Critchley H (eds) Contraception and contraceptive use. RCOG Press.

8. Khader YS, Rice J, John L, Abueita O (2003) Oral contraceptive use and risk of myocardial infarction: a meta-analysis. Contraception 68: 11–17.

9. The Collaborative Group on Hormonal Factors in Breast Cancer (1996) Breast cancer and hormonal contraceptives: a collaborative re-analysis of individual data on 53,297 women with breast cancer and 100,239 women without breast cancer from 54 epidemiological studies. Lancet 347: 1717–1727.

10. Faculty of Family Planning & Reproductive Health Care Clinical Guidance (2006) First Prescription of Combined Oral Contraception. www.ffprhc.org.uk

11. Faculty of Family Planning & Reproductive Healthcare Clinical Effectiveness Unit (2005) Drug interactions with hormonal contraception. J Fam Plan & Reprod Healthcare 31: 139–151.

12. Riman T, Nilsson S, Persson IR (2004) Review of epidemiological evidence for reproductive and hormonal factors in relation to the risk of epithelial ovarian malignancies. Acta Obstet Gynaecol Scand 83: 783–795.

13. Arowojolu AO, Gallo MF, Grimes DA, Garner SE (2004) Combined oral contraceptive pills for the treatment of acne. The Cochrane Database of Systematic Reviews.

FURTHER READING

Courtland Robinson J, Plichta S, Weisman CS, Nathanson CA, Ensminger M (1992) Dysmenorrhea and use of oral contraceptives in adolescent women attending a family planning clinic. Am J Obstet Gynecol 166: 578–583.

4 Progestogen–only pill

Marian P Everett

Chapter contents

The progestogen-only pill (POP) is a safe, effective and convenient method of contraception, yet is only used by approximately 5% of women in the UK.[1] Many women are unaware that there are different types of oral contraception, and the main group of women prescribed the POP are those who want an oral method but for whom estrogen is contraindicated, often because they are older or have medical contraindications. However the development of a new POP containing a higher dose of progestogen has now made the POP a more effective option for many younger women as well.

TYPES OF POP

There are currently five POPs available in the UK (Table 4.1). Four of these contain the older second-generation progestogens. The newest preparation contains a third-generation progestogen, desogestrel. All the preparations are marketed in blister packets; each pill is marked with the day of the week and the packs are marked with an arrow indicating the order of usage.

MODE OF ACTION

1. An effect on cervical mucus, rendering it impenetrable to sperm – the main mode of action of the older-type pills.

Table 4.1 Types of progestogen–only pill available in the UK 2006/07

Brand name	Progestogen	Dose (μg)	Pills per packet
Femulen	Etynodiol diacetate	500	28
Micronor	Norethisterone	350	28
Norgeston	Levonorgestrel	30	35
Noriday	Norethisterone	350	28
Cerazette	Desogestrel	75	28

2. An effect on the endometrium, making it unfavourable for implantation.
3. An effect on ovulation.

The dose of progestogen (desogestrel) in the newest POP is enough to prevent follicular development and maturation and ovulation in over 97% of cycles.[2]

Other POPs contain progestogens at much lower bioactive doses and their effect on ovulation varies among individual women and from cycle to cycle. Follicular development and ovulation are unaffected in up to 40% of cycles and regular menses continues. In 10–16% follicle development is completely suppressed so there is no prospect of ovulation, contraception is 100% and amenorrhoea results. In the remaining cycles follicle growth, either without ovulation or with inadequate luteal phase progesterone secretion, results in fluctuating amounts of estrogen secretion and bleeding is irregular.[3]

EFFICACY

Efficacy of the older-type POP appears to be related to the age of the user, probably reflecting compliance. It varies from 0.3 per 100 woman-years (wy) in women over 35 years old to 4.0 per 100 woman-years for younger users. POP use during breast feeding is highly effective (0.3/100 wy) because of the added effects of breast feeding on fertility.

The efficacy of the desogestrel-containing POP in clinical trials was 0.17 per 100 woman-years in non-lactating women, which is of comparable efficacy to combined oral contraception – which also inhibits ovulation in most or all cycles. If ovulation is inhibited, failure associated with less than perfect compliance is less likely. This makes the desogestrel-containing POP an effective option for younger women.

CONTRAINDICATIONS

There are relatively few scientific data to aid clinical decision-making in women with medical conditions in respect of the POP. The Faculty of

Family Planning and Reproductive Health Care (FFPRHC) have adapted the World Health Organization Medical Eligibility Criteria for all methods of contraception to reflect UK practice.[4] This forms the basis of appropriate prescribing of the POP in the UK (Table 4.2).

INDICATIONS FOR USE

The POP is indicated for women who choose to use oral contraception but for whom estrogen is contraindicated. It may be particularly useful in the following situations:

1. Women with a past history of VTE or with a known familial thrombophilia. The POP has no significant effects on clotting, fibrinolytic activity or platelet aggregation and may safely be used for women with a past history of thrombosis.
2. Breast feeding. The POP does not affect the volume of milk, and the amount of progestogen transferred in the milk to the baby is extremely small.
3. Women with risk factors for arterial disease:
   - Smokers over the age of 35 years
   - Women with controlled hypertension
   - Women with diabetes
   - Women with focal migraine
   - Women over 35 years with non-focal migraine
   - Women with high BMI (over 35)
   - Women with chronic systemic diseases, e.g. systemic lupus erythematosus.

TAKING THE POP

• History

Prior to starting the POP, a full history should be taken with details of past medical history, current drug therapy, gynaecological and obstetric history, menstrual history, previous contraceptive usage and current requirements.

• Examination

Pelvic or breast examination is not necessary prior to prescribing the POP, unless the history indicates it is required. Cervical screening should be carried out in accordance with the national programme. Blood pressure (BP), weight, height and body mass index (BMI) should be recorded as a baseline. Following the initial assessment BP should be monitored annually.

Table 4.2 UK medical eligibility criteria for prescribing of the POP (Category 3 & 4 conditions)

Category 4 conditions

There are very few absolute contraindications to POP, the following are considered to represent an unacceptable health risk if POP is used

1. Pregnancy
2. Current breast cancer

Category 3 conditions

These are conditions in which the theoretical or proven risks usually outweigh the advantages but the method may be used with added caution if other methods are inappropriate or unacceptable

1. Severe decompensated liver disease or active viral hepatitis
2. Liver tumours; both benign adenoma and malignant hepatoma
3. Recent trophoblastic disease; until the levels of human chorionic gonadotrophin return to normal
4. Women on long term liver enzyme inducing drugs such as antiepileptics; enzyme inducing drugs do decrease circulating levels of progestogens and women using POP would require additional precautions
5. Women who develop ischaemic heart disease or stroke whilst taking POP should be advised that the risks outweigh the benefits and they should discontinue
6. Breast cancer; after discussion with the woman's oncologist, the POP may be used with caution once the woman has been in remission for 5 years

Common category 2 conditions worth highlighting

Conditions in which the advantages of using the method generally outweigh the theoretical or proven risks.

1. Serious side effects on the combined pill which are not clearly due to estrogen, e.g. cholestatic jaundice
2. Women with diabetes, both insulin-dependent and non-insulin-dependent

Common category 1 conditions worth highlighting

1. Structural heart disease. Young women with serious congenital heart disease now survive and will require contraception. The POP may be prescribed even where there is an increased risk of arrhythmias
2. Past history of ectopic pregnancy. The POP reduces the risk of pregnancy both intra- and extrauterine. A method that prevents ovulation is desirable; the desogestrel-containing POP would be the optimal choice if estrogen was contraindicated
3. A past history of venous thromboembolism, (VTE) current VTE on anticoagulants or a family history of VTE or known thrombophilia

• Starting regimens

The FFPRHC has adapted the WHO Selected Practice Recommendations for Contraceptive Use[5] for the UK into clinical guidance which is evidence-based and represents best practice.[6] This clinical guidance differs from the POP manufacturers' patient information and Summaries of Product Characteristics (SPC) leaflets and therefore is outside the terms of the product licence. It is unlikely that the SPC will be amended to reflect this UK evidence-based guidance.

1. The POP can be started on day 1 to day 5 of the cycle without additional precautions.
2. The POP can be started at any time in the cycle if it is reasonably certain that the woman is not pregnant:
   a. there has been no sexual intercourse since the start of the last menstrual period
   b. she is within 7 days of the start of her last menstrual period
   c. she is already using a reliable method of contraception
   d. she is fully or partially breast feeding, amenorrhoeic and less than 6 months postpartum
   e. she starts within 4 weeks postpartum
   f. she starts within 7 days of an abortion or miscarriage.
   In any of the above situations, extra precautions or abstinence should be recommended for 48 hours after commencing the POP.
3. Following abortion or miscarriage, the POP can be started on the day of a surgical termination or second stage of a medical abortion (induced or spontaneous if less than 24 weeks). No additional contraception is required. If started after more than 7 days advise additional contraception or abstinence for 48 hours.
4. Postpartum, contraception is not needed prior to day 21. If the POP is started on day 21 no additional contraception is needed. If commenced on days 21–28 advise additional contraception or abstinence for 48 hours. If started after day 28 then pregnancy must first be excluded.
5. Breast feeding, again contraception is not needed before day 21, start as above.
6. Changing from the combined pill, start any time during active pill taking or on the day following the last active pill, no extra protection is required.
7. Changing from a progestogen-only injectable or implant, the POP may be started at any time up to 14 weeks from the previous injection or on or before the day of removal of the implant; no additional precautions are required.

• Daily pill taking

The POP should be taken every day at the same time of day continuously without a break. There are no pill-free intervals as with the combined pill, and bleeding, if it occurs, will be on pill days and not correlated with any particular stage of the packet.

The older POPs are not as effective in preventing pregnancy in young women as the combined pill. It is clearly essential to explain the higher failure rate to these women. Efficacy depends on meticulous attention to pill taking, particularly for the older type POP, following the 3-hour or 12-hour rule depending on which POP is prescribed (see below).

• Missed or late pills

The POP must be taken regularly every 24 hours. The woman may be up to 3 hours late with any pill, i.e. 27 hours since the last pill. In this situation she should take her late pill as soon as possible, take the next pill at the usual time, continue with the rest of the pack and she does not need additional protection.

If however she is more than 3 hours late this is a 'missed' pill, she should take the missed POP as soon as possible, take the next POP at the usual time and use additional contraception or abstain for 48 hours. The cervical mucus changes are fully effective within 48 hours of taking the POP.[6] If unprotected intercourse has occurred at any time in the 48 hours since the previous pill was taken, then emergency contraception should be advised.

The desogestrel-containing POP, however, has a '12-hour' rule and may be taken up to 12 hours late, i.e. 36 hours since the last pill was taken. If it is taken within this 12-hour margin then the woman should be advised to continue with the rest of the pack as normal. If the desogestrel-containing POP is taken more than 12 hours late, then advise the use of additional precautions or abstinence for 48 hours and again if unprotected intercourse has occurred within this 48-hour window emergency contraception should be offered.

• Other factors affecting efficacy

1. Vomiting within 2 hours of pill taking, the woman should be advised to take another POP immediately. If vomiting persists then this should be managed as in missed pills and additional protection or abstinence advised until 48 hours after normal pill taking is resumed.
2. Severe diarrhoea for more than 24 hours should also be managed as for missed pills.
3. Weight: it is common practice in the UK to advise women weighing more than 70 kg to take two of the older-type POPs together every day. There is no direct evidence to support this practice, but there

Table 4.3 Drugs which may interact with the POP

Antibiotics	Antidepressants	Antiepileptics	Antifungals	Antiretrovirals	Other
Rifampicin	St John's Wort	Topiramate	Griseofulvin	Amprenavir	Bosentan
Rifabutin		Carbamazepine	Imidazoles	Efavirenz	Modafinil
		Oxcarbazepine	Triazoles	Nelfinavir	Tacrolimus
		Phenytoin		Nevirapine	
		Primidone		Ritinavir	
		Phenobarbitone			

is evidence that levonorgestrel implants (which are independent of compliance for their effectiveness) are less effective in obese women.[7] There is no evidence that this practice is in any way harmful and the FFPRHC in the UK suggests as a good practice point that women taking the POP containing levonorgestrel, etynodiol diacetate or norethisterone who weigh more than 70 kg should take two pills together on a daily basis. Women taking the desogestrel-containing POP only need take one pill daily irrespective of their weight.

4. Liver enzyme-inducing drugs. This includes antibiotics, antiretrovirals and anti-epileptic drugs as well as some 'over-the-counter' medications (Table 4.3). These drugs may all reduce the level of active progestogen circulating and thereby affect efficacy of the POP.

ADVANTAGES

A safe and effective method of contraception with a failure rate of 0.3–4 per 100 woman-years.

1. The desogestrel-containing POP is very effective even in young women due to its effects on inhibition of ovulation
2. It can be used during lactation as it has no effect on the quality or quantity of breast milk and has no effects on the baby.
3. It has minimal effects on metabolic parameters including glucose tolerance and lipid profile, and may safely be used in women with diabetes and risk factors for arterial disease.
4. It has no measurable effects on blood clotting and it may safely be used in women with a past history of VTE.
5. It may be used in women with contraindications to estrogen such as focal migraine with aura or high blood pressure.
6. There is no evidence of increased risks of any malignancy.

7. It can be used by women who experience estrogenic side effects with the combined pill.
8. It may protect against ascending pelvic infection due to the cervical mucus changes but this is not proven.

It may be used safely by older women until the age of 55 years at which time they may be assumed to be postmenopausal (96% of women will be at least 1 year post menopausal at age 55). Any changes in bleeding patterns at this age would need to be viewed with a higher index of suspicion for pathology and investigated appropriately.[7]

DISADVANTAGES

1. Women using the older types of POP must be meticulously careful with pill taking. This is less important with the desogestrel-containing POP.
2. The main disadvantage with all progestogen-only contraception is the effect on bleeding patterns; with the POP this ranges from complete amenorrhoea to chaotic and unpredictable bleeding. This is the main reason women discontinue the POP. It is impossible to predict what the bleeding pattern will be for any individual woman, however irregular bleeding often settles with increasing age.
3. Side effects such as weight gain, mood swings, acne, headaches and loss of libido are occasionally reported by women taking the POP.
4. The development of functional ovarian cysts may cause pain and require investigation. These occur in a small minority of women and are due to the persistent unruptured follicles which then gradually enlarge and become symptomatic.
5. The POP does not protect against the acquisition of sexually transmitted infection and HIV (though it may partially protect against ascending pelvic infection). The additional use of condoms should be recommended if appropriate.

SPECIAL CONSIDERATIONS

1. Adolescents
   The combined pill is the standard choice of oral contraception for adolescents but if estrogen is contraindicated then the POP and in particular the desogestrel-containing POP may be prescribed instead.

   Gross obesity (a BMI of over 35) may preclude some young women from using the combined pill and if oral contraception is desired then the desogestrel-containing POP may be prescribed.

2. Older women

   The POP is an ideal contraceptive choice for older women. It is safe, highly effective, has few side effects, and may be continued until age 55 years if necessary. It does not mask menopausal symptoms and if required FSH levels can be checked whilst a woman is taking the POP. An FSH concentration of over 30 IU/L on two occasions at least 2 months apart is indicative of menopause. Women should continue with contraception thereafter for 1 more year if over 50 years and for 2 more years if under 50.

3. Breast feeding

   The combined pill is contraindicated in lactating women but the POP is highly effective and safe for the baby. Studies on neonatal blood have not shown any detectable circulating levels of progestogen. All POPs are highly effective during lactation, whatever the age and weight of the mother.

4. Women with multiple risk factors for arterial disease

   This includes women who smoke and are over 35 years old, women with controlled hypertension or rising blood pressure on combined oral contraception, women with a history of angina or complicated diabetes, women with managed hypercholesterolaemia, both focal migraine and non-focal migraine in women over 35 years.

5. Past history of VTE or women with increased risk factors such as a known thrombophilia, immobilization, or before and after major surgery.

6. Chronic systemic diseases such as sickle-cell disease, which may be improved with less crises (although Depo-Provera® would be an even better choice), systemic lupus which is not exacerbated by progestogen as it may be with estrogen.

7. Women who wish to take oral medication yet want the lowest possible dose of hormones.

REFERENCES

1. Office for National Statistics (2005/6) Omnibus Survey Report No. 30 Contraception and Sexual Health, 2005/06. Available at www.statistics.gov.uk

2. Rice CF, Killick SR, Dieben T, Coelingh Bennink H (1999) A comparison of the inhibition of ovulation achieved by desogestrel 75 µg and levonorgestrel 30 µg daily. Human Reproduction 14: 982–985.

3. McCann MF, Potter LS (1994) Progestin-only oral contraception: a comprehensive review. Contraception 50: S159–S188.

4. UK Medical Eligibility Criteria for Contraceptive Use (UKMEC 2005/2006) Faculty of Family Planning and Reproductive Health Care 2006.

5. WHO Selected Practice Recommendations for Contraceptive Use (2nd Edition) (2004) Geneva, Switzerland: WHO.

6. FFPRHC (2002) UK Selected Practice Recommendations for Contraceptive Use. London UK: FFPRHC. http://www.ffprhc.org.uk

7. FFPRHC (2005) Guidance (Jan05) Contraception for women aged over 40 years. J FFPRHC 31(1): 51–64

FURTHER READING

FFPRHC (2003) Clinical Effectiveness Unit. New product review (April 2003). Desogestrel-only pill (Cerazette). J FPRHC 29(3): 162–164.

Progestogen–only injectables

Diana Mansour

Chapter contents

The first long-acting, reversible hormonal contraceptive preparation to be developed was a depot intramuscular injection of progestogen. Its safety record now covers 40 years of prescribing and it is the contraceptive choice of 3% of women in the UK and more than 27 million women worldwide in over 130 countries.

There are two progestogen-only injectable (POI) contraceptive methods available: depot medroxyprogesterone acetate (DMPA, Depo-Provera®) and norethisterone enanthate (NET-EN, Noristerat®/Norigest®). There is no limitation to the duration of use of DMPA in the UK, however NET-EN is licensed only for short-term use in women who need contraception following rubella immunization or whose partners have recently undergone a vasectomy.

MODE OF ACTION

POI inhibit ovulation through suppression of the hypothalamic/pituitary/ovarian axis causing a reduction in luteinizing hormone and to a certain extent, follicle-stimulating hormone concentrations. Their additional mechanisms of action include endometrial suppression (preventing implantation), increasing cervical mucus viscosity (inhibiting sperm penetration) and adversely affecting sperm motility/function.

EFFICACY

POI are highly effective in preventing pregnancy as they do not rely on daily action. The National Institute for Health and Clinical Effectiveness (NICE) Guidance in Long-Acting Methods of Contraception quotes a failure rate of less than four women per 1000 becoming pregnant over a 2-year period if the injectables are given at the recommended intervals.[1] If they fail there is no evidence that there is an increased risk of congenital abnormalities.

CONTRACEPTIVE BENEFITS

1. Convenient, effective, reversible methods with little dependence on the user.
2. Unrelated to intercourse.
3. Safe – no reported attributable deaths.
4. Safe for breast-feeding mothers (first injection of DMPA should be postponed until 6 weeks after delivery to reduce the likelihood of heavy, prolonged bleeding). Lactation is not inhibited.
5. Fully reversible although some delay in return to fertility.
6. Freedom from side effects associated with estrogen, e.g. venous thromboembolism.
7. Discrete, non-visible contraception.

NON-CONTRACEPTIVE BENEFITS

1. Amenorrhoea helpful for women with premenstrual symptoms, ovulation pain and heavy or painful periods.
2. Can be used in women with sickle cell disease (evidence suggests a reduction in sickle cell crises).
3. May protect against pelvic inflammatory disease although will not prevent sexually transmitted infection (STIs).
4. Reduce the risk of extrauterine pregnancies as POI inhibit ovulation.
5. Fewer functional ovarian cysts as there is ovarian quiescence.
6. May relieve endometriosis-related pain.
7. May reduce fibroid formation and growth.
8. Can reduce the risk of endometrial cancer by five-fold with the protective effect lasting at least 8 years after cessation.[2]

Table 5.1 Disadvantages of progestogen–only injectables

1. Given intramuscularly, therefore cannot be removed if adverse effects occur
2. Irregular, prolonged or infrequent vaginal bleeding and amenorrhoea
3. Weight gain is commonly reported (up to 2 kg in the first year)
4. Progestogenic adverse effects – mood change, lassitude, loss of libido, bloating and breast tenderness
5. Delay in return of fertility
6. May adversely affect bone mineral density but in adults this is usually recovered when the injectable is discontinued

---

DISADVANTAGES

There are some potential disadvantages to using progestogen-only injectables that lead to early discontinuation (Table 5.1). Approximately one in two women will have stopped the method within the first year of use with between 30–40% citing bleeding problems as the main reason. This highlights the importance of informed counselling.

SPECIFIC SIDE EFFECTS AND COMPLICATIONS

• Disturbances in menstrual pattern

The association between progestogen-only contraception and altered/irregular vaginal bleeding is well established. Amenorrhoea is common with DMPA and NET-EN (around 55% of users at 1 year and 70% at 2 years with DMPA) as these methods inhibit ovarian follicle formation and ovulation. Many women find amenorrhoea highly acceptable. Careful pre-treatment counselling and reassurance that a period is not necessary for good health is required.

In up to 10% of women bleeding may be frequent and irregular but rarely is it heavy. Within the first 3 months of use around 30% of women may complain of prolonged bleeding episodes (>10 days) with this decreasing to around 10% at 12 months. The cause for this is poorly understood. Pathology (STIs, cervical or endometrial abnormalities) should be ruled out if abnormal bleeding persists.

Treatment to control excessive bleeding is required in around three occasions per 100 woman-years of use. Supplementary estrogen (if not contraindicated) stops individual bleeding episodes in almost all cases. Two or more packets of a 30-μg combined oral contraceptive pill (COC) can be given cyclically. If estrogen is contraindicated then mefenamic acid (500 mg twice daily) may be useful; however the effect may short lived. Practitioners sometimes give the next injection early to induce ovarian quiescence but there is no evidence that this helps.

DMPA-users may find that it takes 6–12 months before a regular cycle is re-established. Continuing menstrual disturbances should be investigated. NET-EN produces a similar bleeding pattern to DMPA but with a lower rate of amenorrhoea.[3]

• Weight gain

Most women's weight fluctuates over time but some women may gain weight rapidly after the first injection of DMPA or NET-EN and continue to gain moderate amounts of weight during use. Patient information leaflets report weight gain of 5–8 lb within the first year of using DMPA increasing to 14–16 lb after 4–6 years. There is evidence that users of POI (DMPA) gain more weight than women using the levonorgestrel intrauterine system or copper intrauterine device. Users of NET-EN and DMPA gain similar amounts of weight.

Weight gain associated with DMPA has been studied in obese and non-obese adolescents.[4] From the start of this study obese adolescent girls gained significantly more weight than did obese girls starting the COC or controls (mean weight gain at 18 months was 9.4 kg, 0.2 kg and 3.1 kg respectively). Weight gain in the obese subjects was related to duration of use. Weight gain in non-obese girls was also greater with DMPA (4.0 kg in DMPA users, 2.8 kg in those taking the COC and 3.5 kg in controls).

Possible weight gain should be discussed pre-treatment. The main mechanism appears to be an increase in appetite not a slowing of the metabolic rate. Dieting and exercise will help but many women find this difficult to maintain. This weight increase is not associated with fluid retention and diuretics are ineffective.

It is safe to use progestogen-only injectables in obese women with no reported increase in serious adverse events or loss of efficacy.

• Bone mineral density

The administration of DMPA creates a relative hypo-estrogenic state with serum estradiol levels within the early follicular phase range. Bone mineral density (BMD) generally decreases over time particularly within the first few years of use of DMPA, after which it appears to plateau. There are very little data investigating fracture risk; one small study found no significant association.[5]

Most studies use BMD as a surrogate for bone health and suffer from serious methodological problems including the recruitment of heterogeneous populations to each study arm, BMD measured at different sites using a variety of methods and few prospective longitudinal studies. Those longitudinal studies that have been published report high drop-out rates and only a few involve young women.

In summary the current studies suggest that DMPA users have a lower mean BMD compared to non-users and their BMD continues to decline over

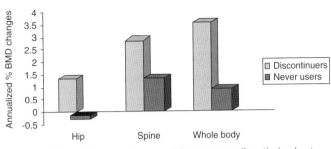

Figure 5.1 Change in bone mineral density among adolescent women discontinuing depot medroxyprogesterone acetate (data from Ref. 7)

time. The deficits are usually within one standard deviation of the mean BMD of non-users and the clinical relevance of this is uncertain. BMD loss in DMPA users is around 2–3% in the first few years slowing to less than 1% in subsequent years.

There is evidence that BMD starts to recover especially in the spine when DMPA is discontinued with rates generally higher than for non-users (**Figure 5.1**). One study in adults compared former DMPA users and never-users. Thirty months after discontinuation both groups had similar BMD levels at the spine and hip.[6] Another study investigating adolescents reported similar mean BMD levels of discontinuers and never-users after 12 months.[7] If women discontinue using DMPA before their menopause limited evidence suggests they have a similar BMD as postmenopausal never-users.

Caution needs to be exercised therefore in those women who have lifestyle and/or medical risk factors that put them at increased risk of low BMD (amenorrhoeic athletes, heavy smokers, women with anorexia nervosa, perimenopausal women and those on long-term corticosteroid treatment).

In light of available evidence, the Committee on Safety of Medicines in the UK advised the following:[8]

1. In adolescents, DMPA may be used as first-line contraception but only after other methods have been discussed with the patient and considered to be unsuitable or unacceptable.
2. In women of all ages, careful re-evaluation of risks and benefits of treatment should be carried out in those who wish to continue use for more than 2 years.
3. In women with significant lifestyle and/or medical risk factors for osteoporosis, other methods of contraception should be considered.

This advice is compatible with current UK Medical Eligibility Criteria (UKMEC) advice.[9]

The potential adverse effects of pregnancy/lactation on bone and the social and economic consequences for the adolescent caused by unintended pregnancy must be considered. Further research is needed to clarify the relationship between DMPA and fracture risk and on the extent of recovery of BMD after discontinuation especially in adolescents and long-term users.

• Progestogenic side effects

Bloating, mastalgia, headaches, mood swings, acne and low libido are recognized progestogenic side effects and are mentioned in patient information leaflets for hormonal contraceptives. There is little evidence, however, to indicate that POI are associated specifically with mood change, loss of libido, acne or headaches.

• Delay in return of fertility

POI do not cause permanent infertility. However DMPA and NET-EN users usually experience a delay in return to fertility with the delay being longer in women receiving DMPA. This delay is due to persistence of progestogen in the circulation. Mean time to conception has been reported to be 9 months after the last DMPA injection (the true delay therefore being 5.5 months) with 78% of couples having conceived at 1 year and 92% at 2 years after discontinuation.[10]

Pregnancies have been reported as early as 14 weeks after the last injection with the mean time to ovulation being 5.3 months. Therefore on discontinuation, even if amenorrhoea persists, another method of contraception should be used immediately to avoid an unplanned pregnancy.

• Cardiovascular risks

Some studies have suggested that DMPA and NET-EN administration cause a lowering of high-density lipoprotein and a rise in low-density lipoprotein with no significant change in blood pressure. Endothelial function may also be adversely affected. A World Health Organization Task Force concluded that long-term DMPA use induces moderate changes in lipid metabolism which are unfavourable in terms of risk for atherosclerosis.[11] However, these are all surrogate markers for cardiovascular disease and long-term use of DMPA is not associated with an increased risk of stroke, myocardial infarction or venous thromboembolism.

The UK Medical Eligibility Criteria conclude that the theoretical or proven risks outweigh the advantages if POI are used in women with current vascular disease or multiple cardiovascular risk factors (UKMEC 3).[9]

• Cancer risks

Data from several studies suggest no increased risk of breast cancer in previous users of DMPA or with increasing duration of DMPA use. However in current or recent users (within the previous 5 years) the risk appears to double. These findings may have occurred as a result of surveillance bias or acceleration in growth of pre-existing tumours.[12] However, studies of postmenopausal women taking combined HRT have implicated progestogens in the increased risk of breast cancer.

There is little evidence to suggest that POI increase the risk of cervical intraepithelial neoplasia or cancer or any other reproductive cancers.

SELECTION OF USERS

The following women are suitable for POI:

1. Women who wish to use an injectable contraceptive method.
2. Women for whom estrogen is contraindicated.
3. Forgetful pill takers.
4. Women with sickle cell disease.
5. Women with fibroids, endometriosis-related symptoms or menstrual cycle problems.
6. Women with epilepsy (frequency of seizures may be reduced).
7. Breast-feeding women.
8. Women requesting contraception immediately after medical or surgical abortion in the first and second trimester.
9. Women with learning difficulties – this is a vulnerable group which may require a contraceptive method that does not rely on tablet taking, may reduce premenstrual disturbance of their mental state and reduces/stops menstrual loss.

CONTRAINDICATIONS

The UK Medical Eligibility Criteria give comprehensive guidance to prescribers on the contraindications to use of POI (**Box 5.1**).[9]

DRUG INTERACTIONS

Liver enzyme-inducing drugs do not appear to interfere with hepatic clearance of DMPA as elimination of medroxyprogesterone acetate is reliant on hepatic blood flow. However, the summary of product characteristics for NET-EN suggests that these drugs may affect its efficacy.

DMPA may interfere with warfarin metabolism, therefore the international normalized ratio (INR) should be carefully monitored. The risk of haematoma formation at the injection site, however, is a reason to advise alternative methods of contraception.

PRE-TREATMENT COUNSELLING

Structured and detailed pre-treatment counselling ensures that potential users are fully informed and can make an appropriate decision to use a particular

---

Box 5.1 UKMEC category 3 & 4 conditions for POI

Category 4 conditions –there is an unacceptable risk if this method is used
1. Current breast cancer
2. Acute porphyria (may provoke attacks)
3. Pregnancy

Category 3 conditions – the potential or proven risks outweigh the advantages
1. Past history of breast cancer and no evidence of current disease for 5 years
2. Recent trophoblastic disease (as with all contraceptive steroids, DMPA and NET-EN should be avoided until human chorionic gonadotropin is undetectable). Subsequently injectables may be an excellent way of preventing pregnancy in the 2-year follow-up period
3. Benign liver adenoma or malignant hepatoma, severe past progestogen-associated cholestatic jaundice
4. Severe cirrhosis (de-compensating)
5. Active viral hepatitis
6. Unexplained/undiagnosed vaginal bleeding (suspicious of a serious condition)
7. Multiple risk factors for cardiovascular disease
8. Current history of ischaemic heart disease
9. History of cerebrovascular accident
10. Diabetes for more than 20 years, or diabetes with micro-vascular/renal disease
11. Current venous thromboembolism (on anticoagulants)
12. Hypertension with vascular disease
13. Continuation of POI if new onset of migraine with aura

Caution should also be applied in the following circumstances:
1. When potential users are planning a pregnancy in the next year
2. If irregular vaginal bleeding/amenorrhoea is culturally unacceptable
3. In those with significant risk factors for osteoporosis

---

contraceptive method with studies showing improved acceptance and contraception continuation rates.

After discussing contraceptive options, taking a medical, sexual and family history, recording the weight and height and checking the blood pressure the following points should be discussed before giving the first injection:

1. Discuss weight gain and bleeding patterns.
2. Explore why contraceptive methods have been discontinued in the past.
3. Discuss the efficacy and safety of using injectables.
4. Detail the non-contraceptive benefits.

5. Explain in an unbiased way the nuisance side-effects and how they may be resolved.
6. Discuss the delay in return to normal fertility and regular menstruation following administration of the injection.
7. Make contingency plans if side-effects are experienced, e.g. telephone help lines to improve access to a health professional.
8. Arrange a follow-up appointment in 11–12 weeks time.
9. Address any worries or concerns before a final decision is made.
10. Provide written information, e.g. Family Planning Association leaflet.

ADMINISTRATION

Depo-Provera® is a microcrystalline suspension of 150 mg MPA given in a deep intramuscular injection into the gluteal region (the deltoid is an alternative site in overweight women). It is administered 12-weekly.

Noristerat is an oily preparation of 200 mg NET-EN, administered 8-weekly. It too is given as an intramuscular injection and should be warmed close to body temperature prior to administration.

Both methods should be given within the first 5 days of the menstrual cycle otherwise an additional contraceptive method/abstinence is required for 7 days. With both compounds the injection site should not be massaged as this sometimes dissipates the depot, resulting in higher initial blood levels and a potential risk of shortened duration of action.

It is advisable to take the woman's blood pressure as an opportunistic screen prior to giving DMPA or NET-EN.

FOLLOW-UP

1. Blood pressure and weight can be checked at intervals recommended for women in their reproductive years.
2. Continued use should be reviewed every 2 years in line with the CSM guidelines.
3. Caution is advised in continuing to use POI in women over 40. Alternative methods should be discussed in women over 45 years.
4. Any abnormal vaginal bleeding should be investigated prior to giving the first injection and endometrial pathology excluded if it occurs in women over 40 after prolonged amenorrhoea.

OVERDUE INJECTIONS

DMPA is normally given every 12 weeks, however some clinics routinely call women back at 11 weeks. This allows a 2–3-week safety window if there is a delay in attending the appointment.

The patient information leaflet for DMPA advises that health professionals should check women are not pregnant if 89 days or more (12 weeks and 5 days) have elapsed since the last injection. The next injection can then be given but a barrier method of contraception or abstinence is advised for the next 7 days. FFPRHC guidance however recommends that injections may be given up to 2 weeks late without extra contraceptive protection.[13] If 14 weeks or more have elapsed since the last injection, provided the woman is not pregnant DMPA is given and an additional method or abstinence is advised for 7 days. This advice is outside the UK Marketing Authorization for DMPA, therefore informed consent should be sought and the discussion fully documented.

REFERENCES

1. Long-acting reversible contraception, National Institute for Health and Clinical Excellence, Clinical Guideline 30 developed by the National Collaborating Centre for Women's and Children's Health, London, 2005.

2. World Health Organization (1991) Collaborative Study of Neoplasia and Steroid Contraceptives. Depot medroxyprogesterone acetate (DMPA) and risk of endometrial cancer. Int J Cancer 49: 186–190.

3. Draper BH, Morroni C, Hoffman M, et al. (2006) Depot medroxyprogesterone versus norethisterone oenanthate for long-acting progestogenic contraception. Cochrane Database Syst Rev 3: CD005214.

4. Bonny AE, Ziegler J, Harvey R, et al. (2006) Weight gain in obese and nonobese adolescent girls initiating depot medroxyprogesterone, oral contraceptive pills or no hormonal contraceptive method. Arch Pediatr Adolesc Med 160: 40–45.

5. Lappe JM, Stegman MR, Recker RR (2001) The impact of lifestyle factors on stress fractures in female Army recruits. Osteoporosis Int 12: 35–42.

6. Scholes D, La Croix AZ, Ichikawa LE, et al. (2002) Injectable hormone contraception and bone density: results from a prospective study. Epidemiology 13: 581–587.

7. Scholes D, LaCroix AZ, Ichikawa LE, et al. (2005) Change in bone mineral density among adolescent women using and discontinuing depot medroxyprogesterone acetate contraception. Arch Pediatr Adolesc Med 159: 139–144.

8. Committee on Safety of Medicines (2006) Updated prescribing advice on the effect of Depo-Provera Contraception on bone. Published by the MHRA, November 2004 http://medicines.mhra.gov.uk 24 November 2006.

9. The UK Medical Eligibility Criteria for Contraceptive Use (UKMEC 2005/2006). Faculty of Family Planning and Reproductive Health Care, London, July 2006. www.ffprhc.org.uk.

10. Pardthaisong T (1984) Return of fertility after use of the injectable contraceptive Depo Provera: updated data analysis. J Biosoc Sci 16: 23–34.

11. Kongsayreepong R, Chutivongse S, George P, et al. (1993) A multicentre comparative study of serum lipids and apolipoproteins in long-term users of DMPA and a control group of IUD users. World Health Organization. Task Force on Long-Acting Systemic Agents for Fertility Regulation Special Programme

of Research, Development and Research Training in Human Reproduction. Contraception 47: 177–191.

12. Skegg DC, Noonan EA, Paul C, Spears GF, Meirik O, Thomas DB (1995) Depot medroxyprogesterone acetate and breast cancer. A pooled analysis of the World Health Organization and New Zealand studies. JAMA 273: 799–804.

13. Faculty of Family Planning and Reproductive Health Care (2006) UK Selected Practice Recommendations for Contraceptive Use. http://www.ffprhc.org.uk/ 26 November 2006.

ACKNOWLEDGEMENT

The author would like to acknowledge the assistance of Dr Zara Haider in the preparation of this chapter.

6 Progestogen–only implants

Martha Hickey

Chapter contents

Contraceptive implants are registered in over 60 countries and used by millions of women. They provide fertility control that is safe, long-acting and rapidly reversible. The efficacy is comparable to that of sterilization.

Subdermal contraceptive implants deliver progestogens from non-biodegradable polymer capsules or rods placed under the skin avoiding first-pass liver metabolism. Rods contain a matrix, which is a mixture of steroid crystals and polymer, while capsules contain free steroid crystals. Both deliver a controlled release of low-dose steroids with high bioavailability.

The six rod system Norplant®, first licensed in 1983, was withdrawn from the market in the UK in 1999 and the US in 2002 by the manufacturers, primarily due to difficulties associated with removal. Modern implants with fewer rods and a preloaded applicator are much easier to insert and remove. Jadelle® and Implanon® are approved in many countries. They have been expensive to develop and market, have high up-front costs and require training in techniques of insertion and removal.

Subdermal implants should be provided as a choice amongst other long-term methods. They are an attractive option for young women, women who cannot use estrogens and women who wish contraception for an extended period of time and who are also willing to accept unpredictable vaginal bleeding. Service provision should include a good geographical distribution of adequate numbers of trained counsellors, health providers who are trained in insertion and removal as well as management of side effects. There should not be any restrictions to removal. There is a possibility that biodegradable devices or those that can be self-removed will be available in the future.

TYPES OF CONTRACEPTIVE IMPLANT

• Levonorgestrel implants

Norplant® (Fig. 6.1) comprised six Silastic® capsules (2.4 mm by 3.4 cm) each containing 36 mg of levonorgestrel inserted subdermally in a fan pattern in the upper arm. They released levonorgestrel at a rate of 80 µg/24 h during the first 6–10 months declining to 30 µg/24 h maintained for 5 years when 69% of the original steroid load still remains. Norplant® was highly effective, with a 5-year cumulative pregnancy rate of 3.9%. Levonorgestrel is cleared from the circulation within 120 hours of implant removal. Norplant is no longer manufactured.

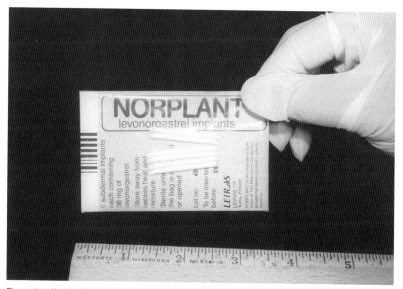

Figure 6.1 Norplant® – six capsules. Courtesy of Office of Public Information Population Council

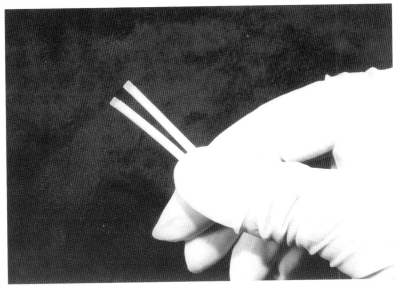

Figure 6.2 Jadelle® – two rods. Courtesy of Office of Public Information Population Council

Jadelle® (Fig. 6.2) is identical to Norplant® but has two rods and was initially approved as a 3-year method. Extension of use to 5 years is approved in over 30 countries. Contraceptive effectiveness and clinical data of Norplant® and Jadelle® are almost identical.

• Etonorgestrel implants

Implanon® is approved for use in over 40 countries, including many European Union countries, Australia, Indonesia, Canada and the USA. It is licensed for 3 years use.

Implanon® (Fig. 6.3) is a non-biodegradable single semi-rigid rod (40 × 2 mm) with an ethylene-vinyl acetate co-polymer (EVA), core, containing 68 mg of etonorgestrel, surrounded by a rate-limiting EVA membrane. The initial release rate of around 60–70 μg/day slowly decreases to around 30–40 μg/day at the end of the second year and to 25–30 μg/day at the end of the third year.

Maximum serum levels of etonorgestrel are attained on day four after insertion. Low body weight is associated with higher serum etonorgestrel levels. After removal, etonorgestrel serum levels become undetectable within 1 week.

• Other types of implant

Several other types of implants are available or are in development (Table 6.1). A single, silastic 35-mm contraceptive capsule, Uniplant® containing 38 mg

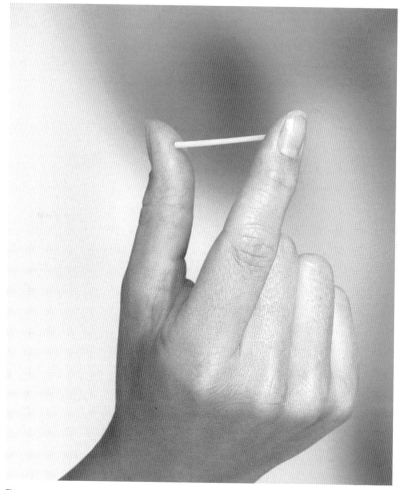

Figure 6.3 Implanon® implant. Courtesy of Organon

nomegestrol acetate and effective for 1 year has been developed in France. Nomegestrol acetate is a 19-norprogesterone derivative which suppresses ovulation and alters the characteristics of cervical mucus.

An implant developed by the Population Council uses a single rod releasing Nestorone®, a potent 19-norprogesterone derivative which suppresses ovulation. It is inactive when ingested orally since it is rapidly inactivated by hepatic first-pass metabolism and may be particularly suited for use by breast-feeding mothers since there is no transmission via breast milk.

Table 6.1 Comparison of contraceptive implants

Trade name (developer)	Progestogen	Number of rods/capsules	Dimensions of rods/capsules	Duration of effectiveness
Norplant® (Population Council) no longer available	Levonorgestrel	Six silicone capsules	34 mm × 2.4 mm	5–7 years
Jadelle® (Population Council)	Levonorgestrel	Two silicone rods	43 mm × 2.4 mm	3–5 years
Implanon® (Organon)	Etonorgestrel	One polymer (resin) rod	40 mm × 2 mm	3 years
Nestorone® (Population Council)	Nestorone	One silicone rod	40 mm	2 years
Elcometrine® (South to South Cooperation in Reproductive Health)	Nestorone	One silicone capsule	45 mm	6 months
Uniplant ®	Nomegestrol	One silicone capsule	35 mm	1 year

Sino-implant Domestic No. 1 and Sino-implant Domestic No. 2 are variations on Norplant and Jadelle respectively and are marketed in China and Indonesia.

There is a 6-month system registered in Brazil under the brand-name Elcometrine® approved for 6 months use to treat endometriosis.

All currently available implants require surgical removal. Biodegradable systems such as Capronor® (levonorgestrel in E-caprolactone polymer) and Annuelle® (cholesterol pellets containing norethindrone) have been developed to eliminate the need for removal. The possibility of not being able to remove degrading capsules is a major concern.

MECHANISMS OF ACTION

• Levonorgestrel implants

Levonorgestrel implants alter the quality of cervical mucus, inhibiting normal sperm penetration. They also disrupt follicular growth and ovulation causing a variety of changes that range from anovulation to insufficient luteal function. These effects vary between women and in the same user over time. Ovulation is uncommon during the first year but it becomes more frequent in subsequent years. The endometrium of Norplant® or Jadelle® users does not exhibit the orderly changes that characterize the normal endometrial cycle regardless of the occurrence of ovulation.

• Etonorgestrel implants

Etonorgestrel implants act primarily via suppression of ovulation. Although follicular development and estradiol production are initially suppressed, ovarian activity slowly increases after 6 months and mean estradiol levels are normal. Increased viscosity of cervical mucus and inhibition of sperm penetration may contribute to the high contraceptive efficacy of this implant.

Data on endometrial effects are limited. In at least some women, endometrial development is suppressed.

EFFECTIVENESS

A systematic review of contraceptive effectiveness of implants by the UK Health Technology Assessment Unit of the NHS found no difference in effectiveness between Norplant® and Jadelle® up to 5 years, or between Norplant and Implanon up to 3 years (Table 6.2).[1]

There were no pregnancies in the clinical trials of Implanon but method failures have now been reported and the failure rate is estimated to be 1 per 1000 users.

• Drug interactions

The effectiveness of progestogen-only implants may be reduced in women taking medications that affect the metabolism of progestogens (e.g. liver enzyme inducers) including rifampicin and certain anticonvulsants.

There have been a number of documented pregnancies in women taking liver enzyme-inducing drugs while using etonorgestrel implants. For short-term users, condoms should be used until 4 weeks after use of the liver enzyme inducers has ceased. Use of other contraceptives should be encouraged for women who are long-term users of any of these drugs.

Antiretroviral drugs (non-nucleoside reverse transcriptase inhibitors and protease inhibitors) may either decrease or increase the bioavailability of steroid hormones. Limited data suggest that potential drug interactions may alter safety and effectiveness of both the hormonal contraceptives and the antiretroviral drugs. The consistent use of condoms is recommended for preventing HIV transmission and may also compensate for any possible reduction in the effectiveness of the hormonal contraceptive.[2]

Table 6.2 Efficacy of implants

	Cumulative pregnancy rate (number of pregnancies per 100 women)	
Norplant®	First 3 years < 0.6	At 5 years 0.6–1.1
Jadelle®	First 3 years 0.3	At 5 years 1.1
Implanon®	0.1 per 100	
Uniplant®	0.9 per 100	

- ## Obesity

Obese women do not experience decreased effectiveness when using modern Norplant® 'soft' capsules or Jadelle®.

The effectiveness of Implanon® in overweight women has not been determined because women who weighed more than 130% of their ideal body weight were excluded from the trials. Both the manufacturers and regulatory bodies warn that Implanon may not provide effective contraception during the third year of use in overweight or obese women, with a comment that earlier replacement should be considered. In studies that included a small number of women weighing over 70kg, no pregnancies occurred in these women during Implanon use.[3]

CONTRAINDICATIONS

The UK Medical Eligibility Criteria give clear guidelines on contraindications to use of implants (Table 6.3).[4]

ADHERENCE AND CONTINUATION

Contraceptive implants are associated with high continuation rates and are generally well liked by users for their long duration of contraceptive protection, ease of use, high effectiveness, and reversibility. Implants may be a more acceptable long-term method than sterilization in cultures where sterilization is perceived to be related to loss of vitality, or of fertility in afterlife, or is otherwise in violation of religious beliefs. They are also useful to young women who want to delay childbearing and to women who have contraindications to the use of estrogens. The advantages and disadvantages of implants are summarized in Table 6.4.[4]

The most common reason for early removal of progestogen-only implants is altered bleeding patterns. Other reasons include exacerbation of acne, weight gain, breast tenderness, and headache but most adverse effects are not bothersome enough to lead to removal. In clinical studies, the great majority (around 80%) of implant users would use this method again and would recommend it to friends.[4]

A recent study of Implanon® users attending a community family planning clinic demonstrated 89% continuation rates at 6 months, 75% at 1 year, 59% at 2 years and 47% at 2 years and 9 months. 39% chose to use a second implant when the first one expired.[5]

ASSESSMENT AND COUNSELLING

Pregnancy must be excluded before implant insertion. Screening for sexually transmitted infections (STI) should be offered if appropriate (Chapter 18). Good-quality counselling before insertion as well as continuing support from healthcare staff during use are important prerequisites of both continuation of use and satisfaction of users (Table 6.5).

Table 6.3 UK Medical Eligibility Criteria for use of contraceptive implants

UK Category 4 (conditions which represent unacceptable health risks)
Known or suspected pregnancy
Breast cancer diagnosed within the last 5 years
Hypersensitivity to any of the components of the implant

NB. If any of these develop during use, the implant should be removed

UK Category 3 (condition where the risks usually outweigh the advantages)
Current venous thromboembolism
Continued use after myocardial infarction or stroke
Continued use after new onset of migraine with aura
Gestational trophoblastic neoplasia if hCG abnormal
Past history of breast cancer with no active disease for 5 years
Unexplained vaginal bleeding (if underlying pathological condition such as pelvic malignancy is suspected, it must be evaluated)
Active viral hepatitis (not including carriers)
Hepatic tumours (benign or malignant), primary sclerosing cholangitis, decompensated cirrhosis
Concurrent use with hepatic enzyme-inducing drugs

Category 3 for continuation of method if migraine with aura, stroke, ischaemic heart disease

UK Category 2 (condition where the advantages usually outweigh the risks)
Multiple risk factors for arterial cardiovascular disease
Current or past history of myocardial infarction or stroke (initiation)
Hypertension with vascular disease
Blood pressure (>160 mmHg systolic or >100 mmHg diastolic) unless other conditions which may predispose to arterial cardiovascular disease
Diabetes mellitus
Hyperlipidaemia
Past history of venous thromboembolism or pulmonary embolism
Known thrombogenic mutation
Surgery with immobilization
Undiagnosed breast mass (should be evaluated as soon as possible)
Migraine without aura (any new headaches or changes should be fully evaluated)
Cervical intraepithelial neoplasia
Gallbladder disease
Compensated cirrhosis, COC related cholestasis
Irregular, heavy or prolonged vaginal bleeding
Carriers of known gene mutation associated with breast cancer
Secondary Raynauds disease with lupus anticoagulant
Antiretroviral therapy for HIV

Table 6.4 Advantages and disadvantages of implants

Advantages	Disadvantages
Highly effective, long-acting, reversible	Provides no protection from STI including HIV
Rapidly reversible – no effect on future fertility	Insertion and removal require trained personnel (may be costly and/or difficult to access in a timely fashion)
No day-to-day action required	
Dissociation of use from intercourse	Risks of procedure include bruising, scarring (note if history of keloid scarring), infection, bleeding and rarely vasovagal reactions
Efficacy unaffected by gastrointestinal upset	
Possible reduced dysmenorrhoea in Implanon users	Risks of difficult removal if inserted incorrectly or major weight gain after insertion
Reduced total menstrual loss	Possible side effects also include weight change, headaches, acne, breast tenderness, alteration in vaginal bleeding pattern
No evidence of effect on bone density	
No apparent adverse effect on breast milk volume or consistency, infant growth or development	Discontinuation not entirely under user control

Table 6.5 Assessment/counselling points

- Exclude pregnancy before insertion, consider timing with regards to current method of contraception or time of menstrual cycle
- Explain mechanism of action
  Implanon – primarily by inhibition of ovulation
  Jadelle – inhibition of ovulation and prevention of normal sperm transport
- Duration of use: 1–5 years depending on implant and advise the woman to return when it is time for it to be removed and/or be replaced
- Details of procedure of insertion and removal
- Advantages and disadvantages of method (see above)
  including side effects and possible complications
- Inform that many women will experience a change in bleeding pattern which may persist
  Jadelle® approximately 65% will experience altered bleeding patterns
  Implanon® approximately 20% will experience amenorrhoea
  approximately 45% will have infrequent, frequent or prolonged bleeding
- Adequate and balanced information on alternative methods
- High efficacy, which may be reduced if certain concomitant medication is used (e.g., phenytoin, phenobarbital, primidone, carbamazepine, rifampicin, and possibly also oxcarbazepine, topiramate, felbamate, ritonavir, nelfinavir, griseofulvin and the herbal remedy St John's Wort)
- Advise her to return at any time to discuss side-effects, problems or if she changes her mind/wishes to conceive
- Prevention of sexually transmitted infections (i.e. dual protection)

• Future fertility

Rapid resumption of fertility is particularly advantageous for women who are spacing their pregnancies. Most women resume normal ovulatory cycles during the first month after implant removal. There are no long-term effects on future fertility, rates of miscarriage, stillbirth or ectopic pregnancy, sex ratios or congenital malformations.[6]

• Ectopic pregnancy

The absolute risk of ectopic pregnancy during use of contraceptive implants is very low, because of the high effectiveness of the method. Norplant users had no increase in the rate of ectopic pregnancies compared with women using IUDs, oral contraceptives, condoms, or no method.[6]

• Use in lactation

The safety and efficacy of all currently available implants have been evaluated during lactation. They do not significantly appear to influence breastfeeding duration, milk output and composition, or infant growth. The potential effect of steroids on later development of the infant remains controversial. Small amounts of contraceptive steroids are excreted in breast milk and concerns about the exposure of infants during the first 6 weeks of life persist. Since Nestorone® does not appear to pass via breast milk this may become the preferred progestogen for use during lactation.[7]

COMPLICATIONS AND ADVERSE EVENTS

• Complications of insertion and removal

The reported rates of complications from implant removal range between 0.2% and 7.0% and include impalpability of the implant, broken or damaged implant, and difficult localization. Breakage or deep placement of implants and the formation of a fibrous capsule can lead to difficult removals. Complications are reduced and removal times shorter with Jadelle and Implanon compared to Norplant.

Implant migration is rare. Traumatic peripheral neuropathy and other neurovascular injuries have been reported. Nerve injury can result in impaired sensation, severe localized pain or neuroma formation.[3]

• Disruption of menstrual bleeding patterns

Disturbances of vaginal bleeding patterns are almost inevitable in users of subdermal progestogen-containing implants. For an individual user, it is impossible to predict how a contraceptive implant will alter bleeding patterns. Amenorrhoea occurs more commonly in Implanon® users compared with levonorgestrel implant users. A range of patterns may occur and there are no devices that can guarantee regular bleeding or amenorrhoea.

Prolonged and irregular bleeding are major reasons for rejection and discontinuation of these methods. Effective pre-treatment counselling appears to improve continuation rates. Even with prolonged or frequent bleeding, the average total blood loss is similar or less than in normally menstruating women.

Irregular bleeding is a simple nuisance, but also causes concerns about possible health effects and leads to socio-cultural problems. Amenorrhoea may be tolerated (even enjoyed) by educated women who have received adequate information and counselling but for others, it deprives them of the regular reassurance that they are not pregnant and may have other negative connotations. Some of the socio-cultural inconveniences may be resolved by supportive counselling and explanation that the irregular bleeding is not monthly 'menstrual flow'.[4]

Because irregular bleeding may also be a feature of infection and (rarely) of malignancy, this symptom may also prompt additional unnecessary investigations, such as high vaginal and endocervical bacteriology, cervical cytology, colposcopy, or even endometrial biopsy.

It has been suggested that the transmission of STI (including HIV) may be increased in men exposed to menstrual blood and in women who are currently menstruating. However a large observational study in Uganda demonstrated that hormonal contraception use was not associated with an increased risk of HIV acquisition in women.[8]

Mechanism of disrupted bleeding patterns

The exact mechanism of progestogen-induced bleeding disturbances is not completely understood, but does not appear to undermine contraceptive efficacy. There is a great deal of individual variation in bleeding patterns between users and within the same user over time. These can only be partly explained by variations in ovarian activity, and changes in the endometrial vasculature that may explain breakthrough bleeding have been demonstrated.

Effective and acceptable treatments are unlikely to be developed without a fuller understanding of the factors underlying this bleeding.[9]

• Management of abnormal bleeding patterns

The development of an effective treatment regimen which would improve both short- and long-term bleeding patterns, without compromising contraceptive efficacy or producing side effects, would be of great clinical benefit and may improve both acceptability and continuation rates.

Currently, there is no effective long-term management for bleeding disturbances (Table 6.6). Treatments that have been tested include vitamin E, oral or transdermal estradiol, oral levonorgestrel, combined oral contraception, aspirin, non-steroidal anti-inflammatory drugs (NSAIDs), doxycycline and the anti-progesterone, mifepristone. Some have proved ineffective. While some were able to reduce the duration of a bleeding episode, none resulted in long-term improvement in bleeding patterns once treatment was discontinued.[9]

Table 6.6 Management of altered bleeding patterns

Amenorrhoea

Consider the rare possibility of pregnancy

Counsel women that amenorrhoea does not require any treatment

If this is unacceptable, implant removal and guidance in choosing an alternative method

Irregular/frequent/prolonged bleeding

Counsel women that this is common with use of implants and not harmful

If bleeding is heavy, persistent or occurs after a period of amenorrhoea, consider other causes including sexually transmitted infections and gynaecological conditions

If the woman desires treatment options available include:

Non-steroidal anti-inflammatory drugs, e.g. mefenamic acid 500 mg bd for 5 days

ibuprofen 800 mg tds for 5 days

If medically appropriate, ethinylestradiol 50 μg for 21 days or combined oral contraceptive pill (>30 μg ethinylestradiol) for 20 days

If this is unacceptable and/or treatment is not effective – implant removal and guidance in choosing an alternative method

---

• Non–menstrual side effects

A review of 55 observational studies found no increase in the rates of adverse outcomes, including pelvic inflammatory disease, loss of bone mineral density, anaemia, thrombocytopaenia, and death in implant-users compared with non-users. Few studies have had adequate numbers of participants or length of follow-up to examine adequately the risk of serious conditions (cardiovascular events, HIV and neoplastic conditions) with contraceptive implant use. In addition, these studies primarily included women of good health and therefore provide no information about contraceptive implant use in women with pre-existing medical conditions.

The most frequent non-menstrual adverse events during use of implants, in the range of 15–25% in clinical trials, are headache, lower abdominal pain, weight gain and acne. Most of these adverse events have each led to discontinuation of the method in less than 3% of the users.[10]

Weight gain

A gradual increase in body weight of 1.5–2% per year has been observed in users of levonorgestrel implants. At two years, about 60% had gained 1 kg and 37% gained 3 kg. This was greater than the mean of 0.3 kg per year typical of US women of similar age. For continuing implant users, there was an overall average 5-year weight gain of 2.5 kg which was significantly higher than the gain of 1.5 kg in the comparison group. In contrast a retrospective non-comparative study in France reported no change in weight.[11]

Ovarian follicles/cysts

Persisting follicular growth and delayed follicular atresia predisposes to the development of ovarian cysts. Persistent ovarian follicles or cysts that will spontaneously regress are common during use of low dose progestogen-only contraceptives and become more frequent with duration of use. They are not pathological and providers should be aware of the transient nature of these cysts and avoid unnecessary interventions.[10]

Metabolic effects

The effects of hormonal contraceptives on metabolic variables are related to the type and dose of the contraceptive steroid. Studies have not reported any statistically significant effects on thyroid function tests, carbohydrate or lipid metabolism and do not appear to increase the risk of complications from diabetes mellitus.

Bone density

No negative effect of Norplant® or Implanon® on bone density has been identified. There is no information available on the effect of progestogen-only implant use on fracture risk.

Breast cancer

The Women's CARE study, a large study of breast cancer risk associated with use of hormonal contraceptives, found that the use of neither depo-medroxyprogesterone acetate nor progestogen-only implants is linked with an increased breast cancer risk.[12]

IMPLANT INSERTION AND REMOVAL[2,8]

• Timing of insertion

Ideally, implants should be inserted from Day 1 to Day 7 (inclusive) of the menstrual cycle without the need for additional contraception.

Implants can be inserted at any other time of the cycle if it is reasonably certain that the client is not pregnant, but additional contraception is required for 7 days.

• Implant insertion

Implants are inserted subdermally, usually under local anaesthesia with the use of a trochar, usually in the inner aspect of the non-dominant arm (see Figure 6.4).

Implanon®

- The implant is inserted subdermally in the medial aspect of a subject's upper non-dominant arm, 6–8 cm above the elbow in the

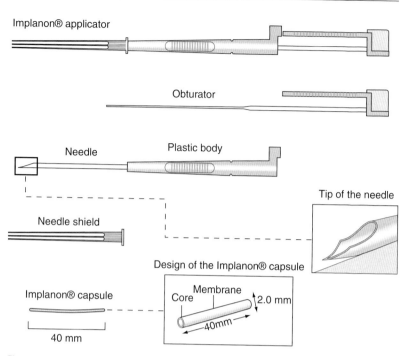

Figure 6.4 Implanon – a single capsule with a disposable inserter

groove between the biceps and triceps (sulcus bicipitalis medialis), using a specially designed preloaded disposable applicator (Figure 6.5). The use of the applicator differs from that of a classic syringe. When inserting the Implanon, the obturator of the applicator remains fixed whilst the cannula is retracted from the arm.

- It is strongly recommended that healthcare providers be trained.
- Information and detailed instructions of insertion and removal of Implanon are available from the manufacturers (Organon).

Jadelle®

- The rods are inserted under the skin of the inner side of the upper arm.
- In some countries, a pre-loaded disposable inserter is available. Elsewhere, the rods are loaded in a reusable trocar.
- In either technique, a local anaesthetic is injected and the clinician makes a small incision – about 3 mm long – using either the disposable inserter or the trocar.
- The rods are placed subdermally in the shape of a V opening toward the shoulder.

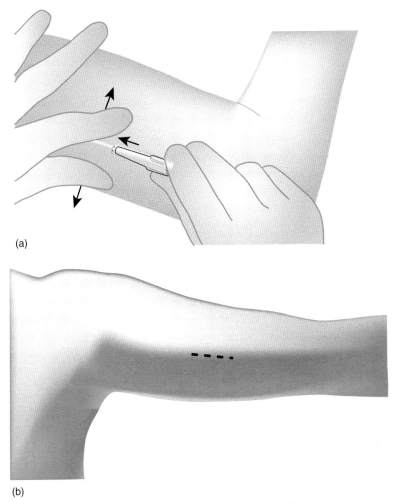

(a)

(b)

Figure 6.5 (a) Insertion of Implanon®; (b) appropriate location of Implanon®

Apply sterile gauze to the wound which usually does not required sutures. Palpate the implant to make sure that the procedure has been completed successfully. Both the provider and the woman should be certain that they can palpate the implant after insertion.

If the implant(s) cannot be palpated, the woman should be advised to use another method of contraception until the presence of the implant(s) can be verified (see localization of implants section).

To minimize bruising, a pressure dressing/gauze bandage should be applied and left in place for 24 hours. Ask the woman to allow the wound to heal and not to manipulate the implant to prevent migration.

If the applicator is for single use only, it must be adequately disposed of, in accordance with local regulations for the handling of biohazardous waste.

Observe the woman for a few minutes for signs of syncope or bleeding from the insertion site. Explain that there might be some bruising and tenderness for the first few days after the anaesthetic wears off.

Advise the woman to keep the insertion area dry for 24 hours. The pressure bandage may be removed after 24 hours. Advise her to seek medical advice if she develops pain, discharge or swelling at the insertion site or fever.

Record in the woman's medical record the batch number of the inserted implant, the date of insertion and the arm in which the implant has been inserted. The woman should be given the date of when the implant has to be removed.

Follow-up depends on the practice of the particular clinic. She may be asked to return for periodic health checks or to report if problems arise.

• Implant removal

If the implant is easily palpable

- Removal, using a 'pop-out' technique, is facilitated by the rigidity of the device and takes a few minutes.
- Place a small amount of local anaesthetic under the distal tip of the implant(s).
- Make a 2–3 mm incision over the distal tip of the implant(s).
- Gently push the implant(s) toward the incision until the tip is visible.
- Incise the sheath surrounding the implant(s).
- It has been found that a fibrous capsule generally forms around contraceptive implants. This thin sheath can be either sharply or bluntly dissected in order to free the rods/capsules and allow removal.
- If the implant(s) cannot be pushed into the incision, insert closed forceps and gently dissect the tissues around the implant and free it for removal.
- Grasp the bare implant(s) with fingers or forceps and remove.

If the implant is deep

- Do not attempt to remove the implant unless experienced in deep removals. Scarring and swelling from unsuccessful attempts will delay and increase the difficulty of future removal.

If the implant is impalpable

- Exclude pregnancy.
- Start additional contraception.
- Do not attempt to remove the implant.
- Localize with appropriate imaging techniques.

• Localization of implants

Jadelle® rods can be located through X-ray, ultrasound or compression mammography, all of which are painless procedures.

Radiography (X-ray or CT scanning) cannot be used to localize Implanon® rods as they are not radio-opaque. Studies of radio-opaque implants are being conducted.

All implants can be visualized by ultrasound and by MRI. Optimal visualization is achieved with the use of a higher-frequency linear array transducer. However, when the implant has been inserted intramuscularly or subfascially, ultrasound examination is more useful.

If an Implanon® implant cannot be localized by palpation, ultrasound or MRI, it should be verified whether the rod is actually present in the body. This can be achieved by determining serum etonogestrel levels. The manufacturer should be contacted and correct procedures for sampling and processing sought. Currently, results can be obtained within 4 weeks.

REFERENCES

1. French RS, Cowan FM, Mansour DJA, et al. Implantable contraceptives (subdermal implants and hormonally impregnated intrauterine systems) versus other forms of reversible contraceptives: two systematic reviews to assess relative effectiveness, acceptability, tolerability and cost-effectiveness. Health Technology Assessment 2000; Vol. 4:No.7 Online. Available: http://www.hta.nhsweb.nhs.uk/fullmono/mon407.pdf 1st December 2006.

2. Faculty of Family Planning & Reproductive Health Care. UK Medical Eligibility Criteria For Contraceptive Use (UKMEC 2005/2006). Online. Available: http://www.ffprhc.org.uk/admin/uploads/UKMEC200506.pdf 1st Dec 2006.

3. Organon EU (2006) Summary of Product Characteristics. Implanon: Implant for subdermal use. Online. Available: http://smpc.organon.com/images/smpcimplanon.pdf 1st Dec 2006.

4. Ortayli N (2002) Users' perspectives on implantable contraceptives for women. Contraception 65: 107–111.

5. Lakha F, Glasier AF (2006) Continuation rates of Implanon in the UK: data from an observational study in a clinical setting. Contraception 74: 287–289.

6. Glasier A (2002) Implantable contraceptives for women: effectiveness, discontinuation rates, return of fertility, and outcome of pregnancies. Contraception 65: 29–37.

7. Diaz S (2002) Contraceptive implants and lactation. Contraception 65: 39–46.

8. Curtis KM (2002) Safety of implantable contraceptives for women: data from observational studies. Contraception 65: 85–96.

9. Weisberg E, Hickey M, Palmer D, et al. (2006) A pilot study to assess the effect of three short-term treatments on frequent and/or prolonged bleeding compared to placebo in women using Implanon. Hum Reprod 21: 295–302.

10. Brache V, Faundes A, Alvarez F, et al. (2002) Nonmenstrual adverse events during use of implantable contraceptives for women: data from clinical trials. Contraception 65: 63–74.

11. Gupta S (2006) Obesity and female hormones. The Obstetrician and Gynaecologist 8: 26–31.

12. Strom BL, Berlin JA, Weber AL, et al. (2004) Absence of an effect of injectable and implantable progestin-only contraceptives on subsequent risk of breast cancer. Contraception 69: 353–360.

ACKNOWLEDGEMENT

The author would like to acknowledge the assistance of Dr Maria Garefalakis in the preparation of this chapter.

7 Intrauterine devices

Meera Kishen

Chapter contents

Intrauterine contraceptive devices (IUDs) are an effective, safe and convenient contraceptive option for many women. There are currently about 100 million users worldwide, most of them in China. In the UK, it is estimated that around 5% of women aged 16–49 years use a copper IUD.[1] The IUD has been the subject of adverse publicity in the past and, in particular, there has been concern about an association between IUD use and increased risk of pelvic inflammatory disease (PID). Recent research on IUD use has been reassuring and has clarified many of the old concerns.

TYPES OF INTRAUTERINE DEVICE

There are two types of IUD: inert and copper-bearing. The World Health Organization (WHO) does not recommend insertion of inert IUDs, because

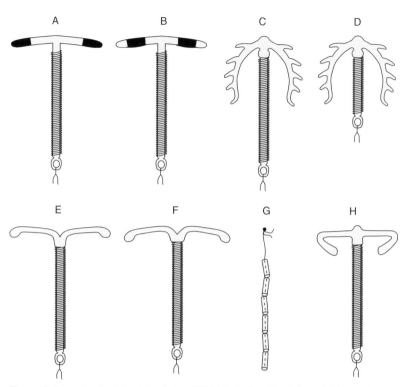

Figure 7.1 Copper-bearing intrauterine devices. (A) TT 380 slimline; (B) T Safe 380A; (C) Nova-T 380; (D) GyneFix; (E) Multiload Cu 375; (F) Multiload Cu 250; (G) Multiload 250 Short; (H) Flexi-T 300

copper-bearing devices are much more effective. Inert IUDs are no longer manufactured although some older women may still have them in situ.

IUDs come in many shapes and sizes (**Fig. 7.1**). All have one or two nylon filaments attached to the lower end to facilitate removal.

• Framed copper devices

Copper-bearing framed IUDs are generally licensed for use over 5–10 years. Currently in the UK, banded T devices such as the T Safe 380A and TT Slimline 380 are licensed for 8–10 years of use. U-shaped devices such as Multiload 250 and Multiload 375 are licensed for 5 and 8 years respectively. The Nova-T 380 and Flexi T 380 are licensed for 5 years. The surface area of the copper determines the effectiveness and active life of the device.

• Frameless copper devices

A frameless copper intrauterine implant, GyneFix (**Fig. 7.2**) has been developed in an attempt to reduce common side effects associated with

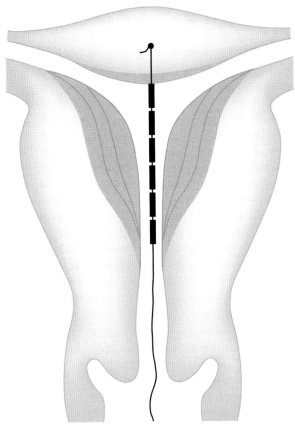

Figure 7.2 GyneFix at insertion. The line drawings represent different cavity shapes

framed copper IUDs. GyneFix consists of a non-biodegradable, monofilament, polypropylene thread and six copper beads providing a total surface area of $330\,mm^2$. The upper and lower beads are crimped onto the thread to keep the others in place. A knot at the upper end of the filament serves as an anchor which is implanted into the fundal myometrium. The device is licensed in Europe for 5 years.

MODE OF ACTION

All IUDs cause a foreign body reaction in the endometrium, with increased prostaglandin production and leucocyte infiltration. This reaction is enhanced by copper, which affects endometrial enzymes, glycogen metabolism and estrogen uptake. Copper also inhibits sperm transport, reducing the number of spermatozoa reaching the upper genital tract. Alteration of uterine and tubal fluid impairs the viability of the gametes. Both sperm and ova retrieved from copper-bearing IUD-users show marked degeneration.[2] Hormonal surveillance shows no evidence of early pregnancy in users of modern copper-bearing IUDs. Prevention of fertilization rather than implantation is the main mode of action for devices with more than $300 \, mm^2$ of copper, except when they are used for emergency contraception.

EFFECTIVENESS

IUDs are extremely effective at preventing pregnancy with pregnancy rates at 1 year of 2–3% with early inert and copper-bearing devices to less than 0.5% with newer devices which contain over $300 \, mm^2$ of copper. Overall failure rates at 5 years are around 2%. Failure rates are even lower in older women whose natural fertility is declining. Ectopic pregnancy rates with modern copper IUDs are lower than in women using no contraception. For all devices, the rates of pregnancy, spontaneous expulsion and removal for bleeding tend to fall with continuing use.

ADVANTAGES

• Compliance and continuation

IUDs require very little compliance for successful use. It is a method of contraception that is unrelated to coitus, which makes it attractive to many users. Any copper-bearing IUD inserted in a woman over 40 years of age can be left in situ until the menopause without concern regarding its continued effectiveness.

• Cost

Copper-bearing devices are extremely inexpensive. They provide contraception for up to 10 years and are therefore highly cost-effective. Framed copper-bearing devices cost around £10 each and the frameless GyneFix around £20. Copper IUDs are more cost effective than oral contraceptives even at one year of use and are the most cost effective of all long-acting contraceptive methods.[3]

• Reversibility

Return of fertility is rapid following IUD removal. Studies show a mean time to pregnancy following IUD removal of 3 months.

DISADVANTAGES

• Bleeding patterns and pain

Menstrual bleeding and pain are the most common reasons for removal of a copper IUD, with a cumulative discontinuation rate of around 24% at

5 years. Intermenstrual spotting/light bleeding and heavier and prolonged periods are common in the initial 3–6 months of IUD use. Rates of discontinuation due to bleeding and pain are similar for different types of framed IUDs and the frameless GyneFix.

• Infection

The overall PID rate in IUD-users is around 1.4–1.6 cases per 1000 woman-years of use which is double the risk compared to women using no method of contraception. Although a six-fold increase in the risk of PID has been noted in the 20 days following insertion (9.7 per 1000), the overall risk is low. Beyond the first 3 weeks, the risk remains very low. This initial increased risk is considered to be related to the introduction of organisms into the uterine cavity at the time of insertion, especially if the woman has an undetected infection or if the operator fails to use proper aseptic technique.

• Expulsion

Spontaneous expulsion of framed copper IUDs is not uncommon and occurs in around 1 in 20 insertions in the first year of use, particularly in the first 3 months. Expulsion rates in subsequent years remain low. There appears to be little difference in expulsion rates between different framed IUDs. The timing of insertion as well as the expertise of the person inserting the device may have some influence on expulsion rates. Postplacental IUD insertion is associated with higher expulsion rates.

• Perforation

Perforation of the uterus is rare (around 1 per 1000 insertions). There appears to be no difference in perforation rates with different framed IUDs or the GyneFix. The risk of perforation is increased if an IUD is inserted between 48 hours and up to 4 weeks postpartum. There is little evidence to support the view that the risk of perforation is greater in women who have a caesarean delivery or breast feed. The skill of the clinican inserting the device may influence perforation rates.

WHO CAN USE AN IUD?

The copper IUD is a first choice method of contraception for a woman in a mutually monogamous relationship even if she is nulliparous. It is particularly appropriate for women who have difficulties complying with regular contraceptive use. Immediately reversible, the IUD is well suited to women who are spacing pregnancies. It also offers long-term effective contraception to those who may have completed their families but wish to avoid or defer sterilization. Copper-bearing devices are highly effective as emergency contraception (Chapter 11).

Table 7.1 Medical Eligibility Criteria for IUD use (adapted from UKMEC[4,5])

Summary of the main features	
Unrestricted use (UKMEC1)	Benefits generally outweigh the risks (UKMEC 2)
Age – 20 years and over	Menarche to under 20 years
Parous women	Nulliparous women
Postpartum – 4 or more weeks (1)	Less than 48 hours postpartum
First trimester TOP	Second trimester TOP
Past ectopic pregnancy	Uterine anatomical abnormalities (2)
History of pelvic surgery	Heavy or prolonged bleeding/dysmenorrhoea
Past PID with subsequent pregnancy	Past PID without subsequent pregnancy
Cervical ectropion	Vaginitis without purulent cervicitis
Cervical intraepithelial neoplasia	Continuation in women with current PID (3)
Diabetes mellitus	Treated PID or STI within the last 3 months (4)
Uterine fibroids (with normal cavity)	HIV positive women and women with increased risk of STI (5)
	Complicated valvular heart disease
Risks outweigh the benefits (UKMEC 3)*	Unacceptable health risk (UKMEC 4)
Postpartum insertion between 48 hours and 4 weeks	Pregnancy
Current VTE on anticoagulants	Current gestational trophoblasic disease
Ovarian cancer (initiation)	Known pelvic tuberculosis (initiation)
Known pelvic tuberculosis (continuation)	Immediate post-septic abortion
	Puerperal sepsis
	Undiagnosed vaginal bleeding
	Distorted uterine cavity
	Current PID or purulent cervicitis (initiation)
	Endometrial/cervical cancer (initiation)

(1) Including women who are breast-feeding, not breast-feeding or post-caesarean section.
(2) Where there is no distortion of uterine cavity.
(3) For IUD users with PID, appropriate antibiotics should be started. There is no need to remove the IUD unless symptoms fail to resolve.
(4) Women who are HIV positive may be offered an IUD after testing for bacterial STIs.
(5) After consideration of other methods, a woman may use an IUD within 3 months of treated PID provided she has no signs or symptoms.
* Provision of a method to a woman under UKMEC 3 requires expert clinical judgement and/or referral to a specialist contraceptive provider.

There are four UKMEC categories (see Chapter 2) for IUD use outlined below (Table 7.1). For almost all women the benefits of using an IUD outweigh the risks.

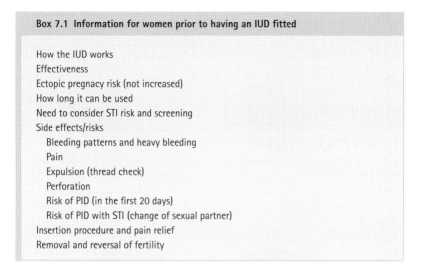

Box 7.1 Information for women prior to having an IUD fitted

How the IUD works
Effectiveness
Ectopic pregnacy risk (not increased)
How long it can be used
Need to consider STI risk and screening
Side effects/risks
   Bleeding patterns and heavy bleeding
   Pain
   Expulsion (thread check)
   Perforation
   Risk of PID (in the first 20 days)
   Risk of PID with STI (change of sexual partner)
Insertion procedure and pain relief
Removal and reversal of fertility

WHAT INFORMATION SHOULD WOMEN RECEIVE?

It is essential that women are given accurate, evidence-based information relating to the IUD along with information on all contraceptive methods available to ensure informed choice. The information should be presented clearly, the woman's understanding of the information checked and any questions clarified (Box 7.1). Leaflets should be used to assist information sharing during the consultation.

WHICH DEVICE?

A banded T device such as the Copper T 380A (or TT Slimline 380) is the gold standard among copper IUDs in terms of efficacy and duration of action and should be the first consideration for any woman requesting long-acting intrauterine contraception, However factors such as a woman's previous experience with IUD use, e.g. menorrhagia, or technical reasons at fitting, e.g. a tight internal os, uterine length shorter than 6.5 cm may lead to choice of other devices.

CLINICAL ASSESSMENT

Providers must ensure a woman's suitability for an IUD based on good clinical assessment and informative counselling. The assessment of a woman prior to IUD-fitting should include a detailed clinical history including sexual history, pelvic examination and investigations to exclude reproductive tract infection as appropriate.

• History

History should include details of age, past contraceptive use, menstrual history, past obstetric and gynaecological history, past history of STI/pelvic infection, and nature and duration of current relationship. Age and sexual activity are important factors in STI risk assessment.

• Examination

1. Examine the vagina and cervix with a speculum to exclude abnormality and infection.
2. If indicated, take endocervical or vaginal swabs to exclude sexually transmitted infections (eg. Chlamydia, gonorrhoea).
3. Undertake pelvic examination to determine the size, shape and position of the uterus.

INSERTION

A calm, unhurried environment will assist the woman to relax during the procedure thus facilitating insertion and minimizing discomfort. The correct insertion technique substantially reduces the risk of expulsion and perforation. Analgesia should have been discussed with the woman prior to the procedure. Equipment required for the procedure is listed in Box 7.2.

• Timing of insertion

An IUD may be inserted at any time during the menstrual cycle if pregnancy can be excluded by careful history taking and assessment including a

---

Box 7.2 Equipment required for IUD insertion

Essential
  Good light source
  Bivalve speculum
  Bacteriological swabs (as appropriate)
  Cotton wool/gauze swabs
  Clean (non-sterile) gloves
  Disposal bags for used instruments and clinical waste
  Sterile 10-inch sponge-holding forceps
  Sterile malleable uterine sound graduated in centimetres
  Sterile 12-inch tissue forceps or single-toothed tenaculum with blunted tips
  Pair of scissors (long enough to allow the threads to be cut)

Desirable
  Syringe/needles and local anaesthetic (for cervical block)
  Cervical dilators

---

pregnancy test where appropriate (Table 7.2). Insertion during menses has conventionally been recommended because pregnancy is unlikely, the internal os is slightly open (possibly making insertion easier) and post-insertion bleeding is disguised by menses. However, there are disadvantages; expulsion rates are slightly higher as uterine contractility is increased, some women prefer not to be examined during menstruation and this timing can pose logistic difficulties for a clinic service. In all circumstances a copper IUD is efffective immediately following insertion.

For IUD insertion as an emergency method of contraception, see Chapter 11.

• Insertion technique

As the method of insertion is different for each device, the manufacturer's instructions should be followed carefully.

1. Employ a 'no-touch' technique throughout the procedure. The part of the sound and the loaded introducer which enter the uterus must not be touched, even by a gloved hand, at any time. Hence, use of clean gloves (non-sterile) is sufficient.
2. Expose the cervix with a speculum following bimanual examination of the pelvis while the woman lies preferably in a modified lithotomy position.
3. Wipe the cervix clean of any mucus or discharge and grasp the cervix with a tenaculum/12-inch atraumatic Allis' forceps. Apply gentle traction to straighten the uterocervical canal.
4. Pass a uterine sound gently to determine the depth and direction of the uterine cavity and the direction and patency of the cervical canal. If cervical spasm/resistance is encountered, local anaesthetic administration and dilatation of the cervical os may need to be considered.

Table 7.2 Timing of insertion

Category	Recommendations
Women with regular periods	Anytime in the menstrual cycle, if reasonably certain she is not pregnant
Women who are amenorrhoeic	Anytime at her convenience, if reasonably certain she is not pregnant
Postpartum (including post caesarean section)	From 4 weeks postpartum
Post TOP (first and second trimester)	At the time of surgical termination or as soon as possible
Switching from another method of contraception	Anytime, if reasonably certain she is not pregnant

5. Load the device into the introducer in such a way that it will lie flat in the transverse plane of the uterine cavity when released. The device should not remain in the introducer tube for more than a few minutes as it will lose its 'memory' and become distorted in shape.

6. Carefully insert the introducer tube through the cervical canal; release the IUD according to the specific instructions for each device, and withdraw the introducer.

7. Some operators sound the cervical canal to exclude low placement of the device.

8. Trim the IUD threads with long scissors to about 3 cm from the external os.

IUDs must be inserted and removed by appropriately trained personnel who should keep their skills updated.

The technique of GyneFix insertion is simple but different from that of framed IUDs. Special training in the insertion technique is recommended to ensure proper implantation into the fundus.

• Problems at insertion

Syncope and bradycardia

Severe pain associated with vasovagal syncope – 'cervical shock' – is rare, but may be caused by dilatation of the internal cervical os with the sound or introducer. Appropriate use of analgesia (surface analgesia by gel/spray or intra- or para-cervical block) can reduce the incidence of cervical shock.

The vasovagal episode is usually transient and self-limiting and the insertion procedure can be completed safely. If severe, insertion may have to be abandoned and the woman resuscitated. If the woman fails to recover quickly with basic resuscitation manoeuvres, the IUD may have to be removed to facilitate recovery.

If a woman develops a bradycardia during the insertion procedure:

1. The procedure must be stopped and the foot end of the bed elevated and oxygen administered.

2. A clear airway must be maintained – by supporting the chin or use of a face mask. Any tight clothing, especially around the neck, should be loosened.

3. Pulse, blood pressure and breathing should be monitored.

If the bradycardia is persistent (<40 beats per minute as a general guide):

4. The IUD should be removed.

5. Atropine 0.6 mg should be administered intravenously.

If the woman becomes unconscious:

6. Call for help/ambulance to transfer the woman to hospital.
7. Check and maintain airway, breathing and circulation.

Epileptic attacks

These are sometimes precipitated by IUD insertion, especially in women with a past history of epilepsy. Rectal diazepam should be available and administered to control seizures.

Perforation

This is rare and occurs in no more than around 1 per 1000 insertions. Careful insertion technique can prevent most perforations. Perforation may be partial, with part of the IUD piercing the uterine or cervical wall, or complete, with the IUD passing through the uterine wall into the peritoneal cavity. Most perforations occur at the time of insertion and go unnoticed. Perforations occur most often at the uterine fundus and heal quickly without any treatment. Copper-bearing devices cause an intense inflammatory reaction within the peritoneal cavity leading to adhesions.

Failure to insert

This may be due to client anxiety, poor operator technique or anatomical abnormality of the cervix or uterus. If unusual difficulty is encountered, the procedure should be abandoned and the woman asked to return at a later date to see a more experienced clinician. Care should be taken to provide interim contraception for the woman.

• Resuscitation

1. A trained assistant should always be present at IUD insertion to monitor vital signs during the procedure.
2. The necessary equipment and drugs to deal with cervical shock/convulsions/cardiac arrest should always be available in IUD clinics (**Box 7.3**).
3. All clinicians fitting IUDs must be trained and updated in basic resuscitation skills.

• Instructions following insertion

Most women do not experience any problems following IUD insertion. Some report mild-to-moderate lower abdominal pain. Women are generally advised to rest for a few minutes following IUD insertion. Simple analgesics often relieve pain. She should be instructed to check the IUD threads often in the first few weeks of use and thereafter monthly at the end of her period.

Box 7.3 Contents of a resuscitation box

Essential
  Pocket mask with one-way valve
  Atropine (0.6 mg/mL ampoules)
  Adrenaline (epinephrine) (1 in 1000 solution −1 mg in 1 mL ampoules)
  Selection of needles and syringes

Desirable
  Rectal diazepam (10 mg in 2.5 mL suppositories)
  Oxygen with mask and reservoir bag

If she is unable to feel threads or feels the tip of the device in the cervical canal, she should be advised to use condoms until she has returned for review and assessment.

Before the woman leaves the clinic, she should be given:

• A written record of the date and type of IUD inserted.

• Clear information regarding symptoms which should make her return for review.

• Follow-up

A follow-up visit after the first menses or 3–6 weeks after IUD insertion is recommended to exclude perforation, expulsion and infection. A vaginal examination is advisable. There is no need for further routine reviews. The woman should be advised to return if she experiences problems or when she wishes to have the IUD removed or changed.

REMOVAL

An IUD can be removed at any time in the menstrual cycle. If the woman does not wish to become pregnant in that cycle, she should avoid intercourse in the 7 days prior to removal or the IUD should be removed during menstruation and alternative contraception started immediately. If, for any reason, the IUD has to be removed without application of the '7-day rule', emergency contraception must be considered. Removal of GyneFix is simple and is by the same technique as for framed devices.

If threads break during removal, the cervical canal can be explored gently with straight artery forceps to check if the lower end of the device has descended into the canal. If the device remains totally within the uterine cavity, exploration of the cavity with a long, thin, curved forceps or a 'hook' may be carried out to locate and remove the device. This should be done only by clinicians experienced in intrauterine instrumentation.

IUD CHANGE

IUDs should not be replaced before the recommended intervals as removal and re-insertion increase the risk of failure, expulsion and infection. In a woman aged 40 or over, copper-bearing IUDs may be left unchanged until 12–24 months after the final menstrual period.

COMPLICATIONS AND THEIR MANAGEMENT

• Bleeding and pain

Increased menstrual bleeding, often with pain, is the commonest problem associated with IUD use.

For the first few months, intermenstrual bleeding or spotting may occur, but decreases with time. Pre- and post-menstrual spotting is also common.

Copper-bearing devices increase the amount of bleeding by around 25% but there is great individual variation. Non-steroidal anti-inflammatory drugs (NSAIDs) are used with varying success. If intolerable menorrhagia persists, the IUD should be removed and other methods including a hormone-releasing intrauterine system considered (see Chapter 11).

Pain may persist for a few days following insertion. IUD use may cause or exacerbate dysmenorrhoea which may be alleviated by NSAIDs. Pelvic pain other than dysmenorrhoea must be investigated to exclude possibilities such as incorrect placement of the device, ectopic pregnancy or infection.

• Vaginal discharge

Increased watery or mucoid discharge is common in IUD users and women may be concerned as discharge is usually perceived to be associated with infection.

If profuse, persistent or offensive discharge is reported, vaginal and endocervical swabs should be taken to exclude infection. Bacterial vaginosis is commoner among IUD-users than among women not using an IUD. It usually responds to a short course of oral metronidazole but often recurs.

• Pelvic infection

The diagnosis of PID associated with IUD use is notoriously inaccurate as it is usually based on clinical criteria. Patients with vaginal discharge and/ or uterine pain are commonly labelled as suffering from PID – particularly if they have an IUD in place – although symptoms do not by themselves signify infection.

A woman is most likely to develop PID just after IUD insertion. Analysis of 13 WHO clinical trials found that women were 6.3 times more likely to develop PID in the 20 days following IUD insertion than at any later time.[6] This risk can be minimized by appropriate screening and by meticulous attention to preventing infection during the insertion procedure. There is no rationale for routine antibiotic cover for all women undergoing IUD insertion; it will have no effect on the future risk of IUD-users acquiring STIs which remains the main cause of PID related to IUD use. Health professionals should encourage women to seek medical help promptly if symptoms appear, especially in the first month post-insertion.

Actinomycosis

The presence of actinomyces-like organisms (ALOs) in the cervical smears of IUD-users sometimes creates concern as clinicians have associated this with a potential risk of pelvic actinomycosis. *Actinomysis israelii* is a normal commensal of the female genital tract and is not predictive or diagnostic of any disease. In the absence of symptoms, there is no indication to routinely remove the IUD or treat with antibiotics. In a symptomatic woman, the IUD should be removed with appropriate antibiotic treatment and referred to a specialist in reproductive health care for further assessment.

• Pregnancy

Intrauterine pregnancy

In the rare event of a woman becoming pregnant with an IUD in situ, she has a higher risk of spontaneous early or mid-trimester pregnancy loss (which may be associated with sepsis), premature labour and increased perinatal mortality if the device is left in situ. If pregnancy is confirmed in a woman with an IUD up to 12 weeks gestation, the device should be removed if the threads are accessible. If the threads are not seen or felt at the cervical os, the presence or absence of the IUD within the uterus should be confirmed by ultrasound scan. If the woman wishes to continue with the pregnancy, she can be reassured that there is no evidence for an increased risk of congenital malformation.

After 12 weeks gestation, the threads have usually been drawn up into the enlarged uterine cavity. Even if they are visible, there is a greater likelihood of the device being firmly wedged alongside the pregnancy. The device should be left in place.

At delivery, the IUD is usually expelled with the placenta and membranes. If not, an ultrasound examination and/or abdominal X-ray should be carried out early in the puerperium to locate it.

Ectopic pregnancy

If a woman using an IUD is suspected of being pregnant, the possibility of ectopic pregnancy should always be considered. Modern IUDs are highly effective and reduce the risk of all types of pregnancy including ectopic pregnancy, particularly when compared with women not using contraception. However, when pregnancy occurs with an IUD in situ, the risk of it being an ectopic pregnancy is increased as IUDs provide more protection against intrauterine than extrauterine pregnancy.

The symptoms of ectopic pregnancy – pain and menstrual irregularity – may be mistakenly attributed to PID or even to the IUD itself. Classical symptoms of pregnancy such as amenorrhoea may be absent. The diagnosis should be suspected if there is any unexplained pelvic pain, lower abdominal cramps, any irregular bleeding and especially if a period is scanty, late or missed (see Chapter 20). Sensitive β-hCG tests that are currently available for clinic-based urinary testing are likely to confirm a pregnancy even at low levels of hCG. If the clinical picture is suspicious of an ectopic pregnancy, even if the pregnancy test is negative, the woman must be referred for urgent gynaecological assessment.

• Lost threads

Threads not visible

If threads are not visible at the time of examination, the following possibilities should be considered:

1. Threads drawn into the uterine cavity – alongside the device in a normal or an enlarged uterus (exclude pregnancy).
2. Expulsion of the device.
3. Delayed perforation/transmigration of the device.

To locate missing threads

1. Carefully expose the cervix, in good light, as this will allow short threads in the cervical canal to be seen in many cases.
2. Some clinicians opt to instrument and explore the endocervical canal or uterine cavity. This will retrieve the threads in up to 50% of cases. The cervical canal should be sounded at the end of the procedure to confirm that the device has not been brought down.
3. Alternatively, ultrasonography should be performed to locate the position of the missing IUD. The woman should be advised that she should use another form of reliable contraceptive until the intrauterine position of the device has been confirmed. If the IUD is present in the uterine cavity on ultrasound, the woman can be reassured that she has contraceptive protection and no further action is required.
4. If IUD removal is desired, one or more of a variety of IUD retrievers, such as an IUD hook or Patterson alligator forceps, may be used to retrieve the device itself after confirming the presence of the device.

• Lost devices

Expulsion

Most spontaneous expulsions occur in the first year of use, especially in the first 3 months after insertion, and often during a menstrual period. Hence women should be instructed to check threads at the end of periods, especially in the first year. They should be advised to return for review if they are unable to feel the threads, can feel the tip of the device, experience unexplained pelvic pain or intermenstrual bleeding as these may signify expulsion.

Complete expulsion of the device may be diagnosed if the threads are not seen on examination and if ultrasound examination of the pelvis and/or X-ray of the abdomen fail to reveal the presence of the IUD in the uterus or the abdominal cavity. If the woman wishes, another IUD may be inserted. Second insertions, even of the same type of IUD, are not associated with higher expulsion rates.

Partial expulsion is much more common than complete expulsion. The end of the vertical stem is found protruding from the cervical canal. If the device is found partially expelled, it should be removed, and if the woman wishes, another inserted immediately. If for any reason it is not possible to re-insert the device at that visit, the need for emergency contraception should be considered.

Perforation

Perforation of the uterus is rare and almost always occurs during insertion. In large clinical trials, perforation rates of 1.3 per 1000 insertions have been reported. The management involves:

1. If perforation is recognized prior to insertion, usually no treatment is required as fundal perforations heal quickly without further complications.
2. If perforation is recognized during or just after insertion of the device, the procedure should be stopped and the device removed immediately.
3. If the perforation is recognized within a few days or weeks after insertion, the device should be removed by laparoscopy or laparotomy.
4. If the perforation is not recognized at insertion and is diagnosed only when the woman presents some time after insertion with missing threads, the device is usually always surgically removed. Lost inert devices have remained in the peritoneal cavity for years without producing problems. However, they do tend to migrate and may be found anywhere in the abdomen. Open or linear devices theoretically cause few problems but closed devices could cause intestinal obstruction. Copper-bearing devices cause a sterile inflammatory reaction and rapidly become adherent to the omentum or bowel.

Displacement of intrauterine device within the uterine cavity

Occasionally, rotation of the IUD within the uterine cavity can occur. This will cause pain and bleeding and will necessitate removal of the device.

There is no evidence to suggest that asymptomatic downward displacement of the IUD within the uterine cavity increases the failure rate of the device. Hence there is no need to remove or replace devices which are considered to be subfundal clinically by noting the lengthening of the IUD threads or by ultrasound scan, provided the lower end of the device is clearly above the cervical internal os. Routine scans to check IUD position are unnecessary.

REFERENCES

1. Office for National Statistics 2005/06.

2. World Health Organization (1997) Intrauterine devices. Technical and managerial guidelines for services. WHO: Geneva.

3. National Institute for Health and Clinical Excellence (NICE) (2005) Long-acting reversible contraception: the effective and appropriate use of long-acting reversible contraception. http://www.nice.org.uk/pdf/CG030fullguideline.pdf.2005

4. Faculty of Family Planning and Reproductive Health Care Clinical Effectiveness Unit (2007) FFPRHC Guidance on intrauterine contraception. (in preparation)

5. Faculty of Family Planning and Reproductive Health Care Clinical Effectiveness Unit (2006) UK Medical Eligibility for Contraceptive Use. http://www.ffprhc.org.uk/admin/uploads/UKMEC 200506.pdf.2006

6. World Health Organization (2004) Medical Eligibility Criteria for Contraceptive Use. Third edition. WHO: Geneva.

8 Intrauterine systems

Ailsa E Gebbie

The original rationale behind the development of an intrauterine system (IUS) was that direct administration of a progestogen into the uterine cavity might reduce myometrial contractility and thereby lower the risk of expulsion of an intrauterine device (IUD). In fact, the IUS has far surpassed these early expectations and provides highly effective contraception in combination with very significant non-contraceptive benefits. It offers women the advantages of both hormonal and intrauterine contraception, avoiding many of their disadvantages. The major non-contraceptive benefit of the direct release of progestogen into the uterine cavity by an IUS is to reduce menstrual bleeding significantly.

TYPES OF INTRAUTERINE SYSTEM

• Progestasert®

The first hormone-releasing IUS to be available commercially was a T-shaped device which released 65 μg progesterone daily and lasted for only 1 year

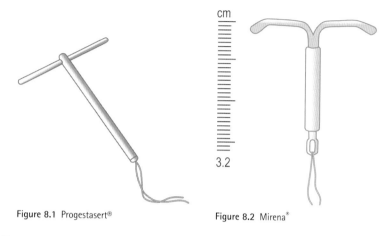

Figure 8.1 Progestasert®

Figure 8.2 Mirena®

(Progestasert®). It was associated with a higher than normal rate of ectopic pregnancy and has not been widely used (Figure 8.1).

• Mirena®

The most popular IUS releases levonorgestrel (Mirena®) and is widely available throughout the world (Figure 8.2). It was first developed in Finland in the late 1970s and was licensed for use in the UK in 1995. It is modelled on a standard T-shaped frame with a central silastic sleeve which is impregnated with 52 mg of levonorgestrel. Release of hormone is via a rate-limiting silastic membrane at a dose of approximately 20 µg per day for at least 5 years.

New low-dose versions of a Mirena® which release 5 or 10 µg per day on devices with shorter stems and smaller arms are being studied. These IUS are designed for post-menopausal use in conjunction with estrogen.

• FibroPlant®

The most recent modification in IUS is based on the frameless copper device, GyneFix® (Chapter 7), which is implanted directly into the uterine fundus with a knot (FibroPlant®). It releases 14 µg levonorgestrel per day (Figure 8.3).

• Other types of IUS

Other modifications of IUS are in various stages of development and trials, using different progestogens and varying sizes and shapes of plastic frame. Novel intrauterine systems which release antiprogestogens are also currently being tested and could potentially be 'bleed-free' contraceptive strategies of the future.

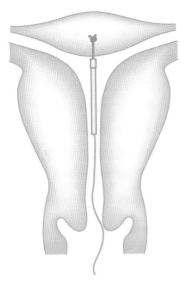

Figure 8.3 Fibroplant®

MODE OF ACTION

• Local effects

The main mode of action of an IUS is primarily to exert a potent hormonal effect on the endometrium and cervical mucus, which inhibits sperm migration. In addition, an IUS may also have a 'foreign body effect' in the uterine cavity which inhibits implantation but this is of much less contraceptive importance than the hormonal effect. In studies, fertilized eggs have not been recovered from the reproductive tract of women using IUS which supports a mechanism of action prior to fertilization.

The endometrial histology of an IUS user is characterized by severely atrophic glands and decidualized stroma. In addition, there is a typical appearance of large thin-walled blood vessels present within the superficial endometrium, which is also found of users of other low-dose progestogen methods of contraception. This abnormal vascular response may explain the problems of unscheduled bleeding associated with these methods.

With Mirena®, the local levonorgestrel concentrations in the endometrium are 1000-fold higher than with either an implant or oral combined pill. This exerts a very potent effect with some limited local diffusion into myometrium and perhaps other pelvic tissues.

• Systemic effects

There is evidence that a Mirena® is associated with varying degrees of anovulation in the first year of use. Thereafter over 85% of women will have normal hormonal cyclical activity which is comparable to users of copper intrauterine devices. Bleeding patterns with a Mirena® do not reflect ovarian function but represent the local effects of levonorgestrel on the endometrium.

An IUS will not affect the onset of menopause or the occurrence of menopausal symptoms. It simply masks the changes in bleeding pattern which chacteristically occur at that time.

INDICATIONS FOR USE AND EFFECTIVENESS

In the UK and many other European countries, a Mirena® is licensed for:

- Contraceptive use
- Treatment of menorrhagia
- Use as part of an HRT regimen.

• Contraception

An IUS is ideal for women who wish a very high level of protection against pregnancy with a method that is completely reversible. In common with all intrauterine contraception, it is a method independent of intercourse which requires no regular action on the part of the user.

Quoted failure rates for a Mirena® are around 1–2 per thousand users per year which is more effective than copper IUDs. The risk of ectopic pregnancy with a Mirena® is also extremely low at around 0.02 per 100 woman-years over 5 years.

• Menorrhagia

The potent hormonal effect of an IUS on the endometrium dramatically reduces menstrual bleeding. In randomized trials, women with menorrhagia experience around 90% reduction in menstrual blood loss (Figure 8.4).

Mirena® is a highly effective medical management of menorrhagia and allows women to avoid surgical procedures. It has been shown to be more effective than oral progestogens or mefanamic acid in reducing menstrual blood loss but slightly less effective than endometrial ablation.[1] There is some indirect evidence that since it was introduced into the UK, hysterectomy rates have fallen.[2]

• Hormone replacement therapy

An IUS can be used to provide the progestogen component of a hormone replacement therapy (HRT) regimen. The selected estrogen with the route of delivery of choice can be added for symptom relief and the potent local effect of the intrauterine progestogen provides a high degree of endometrial protection.

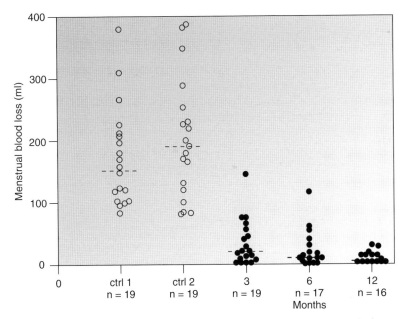

Figure 8.4 Bleeding patterns with Mirena® for menorrhagia. Menstrual blood loss in menorrhagic women at two control periods (ctrl) and after 3, 6 and 12 months of use
(Reproduced with permission from Andersson K, Rubo G (1990) Levonorgestrel-releasing intrauterine device in the treatment of menorrhagia. BJOG 690–694.)

A woman who already uses an IUS for contraception can simply add in estrogen when she becomes menopausal. Alternatively an IUS can be inserted de novo in menopausal women who wish this particular HRT combination.

Users of Mirena® combined with estrogen for an HRT regimen will experience more days of bleeding and spotting initially than users of conventional sequential HRT but thereafter often achieve complete amenorrhoea (Figure 8.5). This combination is very acceptable to women who otherwise would experience regular withdrawal bleeds with a standard sequential HRT.

ADVANTAGES

• Contraceptive benefits

1. High contraceptive efficacy with guaranteed compliance; no motivation required from the user.
2. Rapid return of fertility on removal.

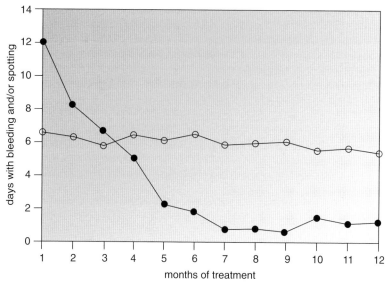

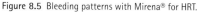

months of treatment

Figure 8.5 Bleeding patterns with Mirena® for HRT.
Mean number of days with bleeding/spotting each month in perimenopausal women during estrogen-progestogen treatment. One group (open circles) treated cyclically in 3-week periods with 2 mg estradiol valerate a day and 250 µg levonorgestrel for the last 10 days. Another group (solid circles) was treated with 2 mg estradiol valerate without interruption and had a Mirena®.
(Reproduced with permission from Andersson K, Mattsson L, Rybo G, Stadberg E (1992) Intrauterine release of levonorgestrel – a new way of adding progestogen in hormone replacement therapy. Obstet Gynecol 79: 963–967)

3. Very low serum hormone levels which minimizes side effects. The serum levonorgestrel levels associated with a Mirena® are a quarter of those of the equivalent progestogen-only pill.

- **Gynaecological benefits**

1. Substantial reduction in menstrual blood loss. Thereby causes a rise in haemoglobin and prevents anaemia.
2. Reduction in dysmenorrhoea.
3. Reduction in size of small fibroids although an IUS is often not effective in the presence of large fibroids, particularly if they are situated near the endometrial cavity.
4. May reduce the pain and bleeding associated with endometriosis.
5. Has been shown to reverse endometrial hyperplasia.

6. Can be used as an adjuvant to the drug tamoxifen to prevent endometrial hyperplasia.[3] Tamoxifen is widely used in women with breast cancer and has a known association with endometrial abnormalities.

7. Very likely to reduce risk of endometrial cancer but no direct evidence for this at the present time.

8. Can be useful as part of a strategy to help premenstrual syndrome (PMS). Women with PMS often have co-existing menstrual problems and an IUS can also be combined with high-dose estrogen specifically to help pre-menstrual mood symptoms (see Chapter 21).

9. Can be used in women with bleeding disorders who have heavy periods.

• Other benefits

1. A potentially lower risk of pelvic inflammatory disease than in users of copper IUDs. This was found in most but not all studies.

2. Women using an IUS are less likely to have actinomyces-like organisms (ALOs) reported on their cervical smear than copper IUD users.

3. No significant effect on weight or blood pressure.

4. No apparent effect on risk of breast cancer.[4]

DISADVANTAGES

• Bleeding problems

1. Unpredictability of the bleeding pattern following insertion of an IUS. Most women will experience several months of persistent and erratic bleeding initially which gradually settles with time.

2. The oligo-amenorrhoea that women subsequently develop will not be viewed positively by women who dislike the lack of menstrual bleeding and worry about the possibility of pregnancy or menopause.

• Progestogenic side effects

Despite very low circulating concentrations of hormone with an IUS, some women will still notice progestogen-related side effects.

1. Breast pain. May be a problem initially but tends to settle.

2. Acne. Women with moderate or severe pre-existing acne must be warned that this could worsen and be unacceptable to them.

3. Mood swings. Usually not severe and tend to settle with time.

4. Persistent follicular ovarian cysts. These are usually asymptomatic or can occasionally cause pain. They almost always will settle with time.

• Emergency contraception

An IUS should **not** be used for emergency contraception as failures have occurred in this situation. It is thought that the serum progestogen levels with an IUS are too low to exert immediate effects on ovarian function. If it is appropriate, a copper IUD should be offered and the woman can switch over to an IUS at a later stage if she wishes.

COST

1. A Mirena® currently costs around £90 in the UK and is significantly more expensive than a copper IUD (the cheapest are around £10). However, if a Mirena® remains in situ for the full duration of its lifespan, it is a very cost-effective method of contraception and is cheaper than many hormonal methods.[5]

2. In randomized trials, a Mirena® has found to be cost effective as an alternative to hysterectomy for the medical management of menorrhagia.[6]

WHO CAN USE AN IUS

Table 8.1 gives the Medical Eligibility Criteria for IUS use which the Faculty of Family Planning and Reproductive Health Care (FFPRHC) has adapted from the WHO Medical Eligibility Criteria for Contraceptive Use (WHOMEC) for UK practice.[7]

For almost all women the benefits of using an IUS outweigh the risks.

• Special considerations

Use in nulliparous women

Although the IUS has over the years mainly been used by parous women, nulliparous women are increasingly choosing it for its high efficacy and menstrual benefits. Young age and nulliparity are not contraindications per se. As with a copper IUD, a careful sexual history is required prior to insertion of an IUS to identify women at potentially higher risk of sexually transmitted infection that might best be advised to avoid an intrauterine method (see Chapter 7).

The continuation rates of Mirena® in nulliparous women are equal to those of parous women and are better than in nulliparous combined pill users. [8]

Postpartum use

An IUS has no effect on lactation and no 'daily remembering' for the woman during the postpartum period.

Table 8.1 Medical Eligibility Criteria for IUS use (adapted from UKMEC)

Unrestricted use (UKMEC1)	Benefits generally outweigh the risks (UKMEC2)
Age – 20 years and over	Menarche to under 20 years
Nulliparous and parous women	Second trimester TOP
Postpartum – 4 or more weeks (1)	Uterine anatomical abnormalities (2)
First trimester TOP	Cervical intraepithelial neoplasia
Past ectopic pregnancy	Past PID without subsequent pregnancy
History of pelvic surgery	Vaginitis without purulent cervicitis
Past PID with subsequent pregnancy	Continuation in women with current PID (3)
Cervical ectropion	Diabetes
Endometriosis	HIV positive women and women with increased
Smokers and obese women	risk of STI (4)
	CV disease (stroke, lipid disorders)
	History of VTE
	Known thrombogenic mutations
	Complicated valvular heart disease

Risks outweigh the benefits (UKMEC3)	Unacceptable health risk (UKMEC4)
Postpartum insertion between 48 hours and 4 weeks	Pregnancy
	Current gestational trophoblastic disease
Current VTE (on anticoagulants)	Known pelvic tuberculosis (initiation)
Ovarian cancer (initiation)	Immediate post-septic abortion
Known pelvic tuberculosis (continuation)	Puerperal sepsis
	Undiagnosed vaginal bleeding
Current ischaemic heart disease (continuation)	Distorted uterine cavity
	Current PID or purulent cervicitis (initiation)
Migraine with aura	Endometrial/cervical/breast cancer (initiation)
Liver tumours	
Active liver disease	
Past breast cancer with no active disease	

(1) Including women who are breast-feeding, not breast-feeding or post-caesarean section.

(2) Including fibrids with no distortion of uterine cavity.

(3) For IUS users with PID, appropriate antibiotics should be started. There is no need to remove the IUS unless symptoms fail to resolve.

(4) After consideration of other methods, a woman may use an IUS within 3 months of treated PID provided she has no signs or symptoms.

With Mirena®, approximately 0.1% of the maternal dose of levonorgestrel reaches the infant in breast milk and no adverse effects on infant growth or development have ever been detected.[9]

CLINICAL MANAGEMENT

• Insertion procedure

Insertion of an IUS follows exactly the same principles as insertion of a copper IUD (see Chapter 7).

The Mirena® is marketed with a special disposable introducer which has been developed for ease of use (**Figure 8.6**). It has a wider diameter in its insertion tube (4.7 mm) than some of the older copper IUDs but this diameter is similar to the 'gold standard' copper-banded devices.

Difficulty may be experienced with fitting of a Mirena® in a nulliparous woman due to a tight cervical os and small uterine cavity. Use of local anaesthesia prior to insertion may be helpful. Either the stem or the arms of the system may be too large to fit comfortably within a small nulliparous uterus causing more pain and bleeding than would be normally expected.

• Management of bleeding problems

Erratic bleeding is extremely common following insertion of an IUS and almost always will settle within a few months. Women must be very carefully counselled in advance about this or they will want to have the IUS removed because they perceive it has 'not worked'.

There is no particularly effective strategy to deal with persistent bleeding other than waiting for it to settle spontaneously. A combined pill can be given for a few months if the woman is suitable for this.

If an older woman is having an IUS inserted for gynaecological reasons, it may be appropriate to investigate her prior to insertion with pelvic ultrasound and an endometrial biopsy. A woman who has an IUS inserted for menorrhagia may find that the bleeding often takes even longer to settle than when an IUS is inserted in a woman with a normal bleeding pattern.

If a woman with an IUS suddenly develops significant bleeding problems after several years she should be investigated. Infection and malignancy must be excluded. Endometrial polyps can occasionally arise in the presence of an IUS and cause persistent bleeding.

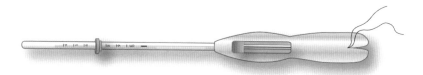

Figure 8.6 Mirena inserter

- ## Duration of use

  1. Contraception. A Mirena® is licensed for 5 years for contraception. If inserted at the age of 45 years or above, many clinicians advise that the Mirena® can remain unchanged for longer than 5 years if contraception is still required.
  2. Gynaecological indications. A Mirena® can remain in situ for as long as it remains effective, e.g. continues to relieve the symptoms of heavy menstrual bleeding, which may be several years more than the manufacturers' normal recommendation of 5 years.
  3. HRT regimen. If a Mirena® has been inserted for use as part of an HRT combination with estrogen, it must be changed 5-yearly to guarantee endometrial protection.

- ## Long-term use

There are now data from studies on women who have had three or four consecutive IUS for long-term contraception.[10] Bleeding patterns remain excellent and women do not have a return to persistent bleeding and spotting following exchange to a second or subsequent IUS.

Around 25% of Mirena® users will be amenorrhoeic by the end of the first 5 years of use and this rises to 60% after the second period of 5 years of use.[10]

REFERENCES

1. Cochrane Collaboration Database (2005) Progesterone or progestogen-releasing intrauterine systems for heavy menstrual bleeding 2005 19;(4): CD002126.

2. Reid P, Mukri F (2005) Trends in number of hysterectomies performed in England for menorrhagia: examination of health episode statistics, 1989 to 2002–3. BMJ 330: 938–939.

3. Gardner F, Konje J, Abrams K, et al. (2000) Endometrial protection from tamoxifen-stimulated changes by a levonorgestrel-releasing intrauterine system: a randomised controlled trial. Lancet 356(9243): 1711–1717.

4. Backman T, Rauramo I, Jaakkola K, et al. (2005) Use of the levonorgestrel-releasing intrauterine system and breast cancer. Obstet Gynecol 106(4): 813–817.

5. National Institute for Health and Clinical excellence (NICE) (2005) Long-acting reversible contraception: the effective and appropriate use of long-acting reversible contraception.

6. Hurskainen R, Teperi J, Rissanen P, et al. (2004) Clinical outcomes and costs with the levonorgestrel-releasing intrauterine system or hysterectomy for treatment of menorrhagia. Randomized trial 5-year follow-up. JAMA 291: 1456–1463. http://www.nice.org.uk/pdf/CG030fullguideline.pdf.2005

7. Faculty of Family Planning and Reproductive Health Care Clinical Effectiveness Unit (2006) UK Medical Eligibility for Contraceptive Use. http://www.ffprhc.org.uk/admin/uploads/UKMEC 200506.pdf.2006

8. Suhonen S, Haukkamaa M, Jakobssen T, Rauramo I (2004) Clinical performance of a levonorgestrel-releasing intrauterine system and oral contraceptives in young nulliparous women: a comparative study. Contraception 69(5): 407–412.

9. Heikkila M, Haukkamaa M, Lukkainen T (1982) Levonorgestrel in milk and plasma of breast-feeding women with a levonorgestrel-releasing IUD. Contraception 25(1): 41–49.

10. Ronnerdag M, Odlind V (1999) Health effects of long-term use of the intrauterine levonorgestrel-releasing system. A follow-up study over 12 years of continuous use. Acta Obstet Gynaecol Scand 78(8): 716–721.

9 Barrier methods

Madelaine Ward

Chapter contents

A barrier method of contraception is one that prevents spermatozoa gaining access to the female upper genital tract preventing fertilization. From earliest times, an extensive array of barrier methods has been used by couples attempting to control their fertility. Nowadays, both physical and chemical barrier methods still offer advantages in terms of safety and reversibility. The condom is known to prevent the spread of human immunodeficiency virus (HIV) and other sexually transmitted infections. The efficacy of these methods depends critically on quality of use and failure rates are reduced significantly when they are used consistently and correctly by well-motivated individuals.

A marked decline in the use of barrier methods occurred following the widespread availability of oral contraception in the 1960s and 1970s. Since the 1980s and the global pandemic spread of HIV infection into the heterosexual population, attention has returned to barrier methods. Promoting use of condoms to combat spread of the virus has contributed to the breakdown of many traditional taboos concerning the openness with which sexuality and contraception is discussed.

Selection of a barrier method of contraception is frequently a matter of compromise between the advantages and disadvantages. Any method of contraception is better than none, and the most effective method is the one the couple chooses to use. Barrier methods can be obtained from health professionals, without a prescription over the counter or via the internet. Health professionals can assist individuals to use barrier methods effectively. Failures with these methods do occur and a woman may be at risk of pregnancy or STIs and HIV following a burst condom or dislodgement of a diaphragm. Individuals using barrier methods must be informed when to use emergency contraception and where to obtain it (see Chapter 11).

FEMALE BARRIER METHODS

For hundreds of years women have prevented the access of sperm to the cervix by using various materials such as sponges and pads of cotton. Tops of lemons and limes were inserted into the vagina in a similar way to the modern diaphragm.[1] Today's caps did not appear until the 19th century. The German gynaecologist Hasse (using the pseudonym Mensinga) is credited with introducing the diaphragm in 1882 although Wilde described a rubber pessary made to a wax model of the patient's cervix almost 50 years earlier. In the 1920s Marie Stopes encouraged the use of cervical caps. In the 1950s, the diaphragm or 'Dutch cap' was the most commonly used device in the UK. However, by 2005, in Great Britain female barrier methods were used by only 1% of sexually active women aged 16–49 years and using contraception.[2]

• Diaphragms

A diaphragm consists of a thin, latex rubber or silicone hemisphere, the rim of which is reinforced by a flexible flat or coiled metal spring. The external diameter ranges from 55 to 95 mm, in 5 mm increments. In practice, most women use the 70–80 mm sizes (**Fig. 9.1**). Silicone diaphragms range from 60 to 90 mm in diameter.

Variations

1. The flat-spring diaphragm has a firm watch-spring (**Fig. 9.2A**), remains in the horizontal plane on compression and is easily fitted. It is suitable for the normal vagina and is usually tried first.

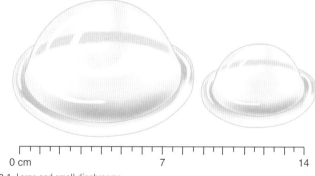

0 cm   7   14

Figure 9.1 Large and small diaphragms

2. The coil-spring diaphragm has a spiral coiled spring (**Fig. 9.2B**), is considerably softer than the flat-spring, and is particularly suitable for a woman with tight vaginal musculature who is sensitive to the pressure of the flat-spring type. With the largest sizes, handling and insertion may be slightly less easy because of a tendency to twist on compression.

3. The arcing diaphragm (**Fig. 9.3**) combines features of both the above and exerts strong pressure on the vaginal walls. It is particularly useful when the vaginal walls appear lax or the length and position of the cervix make reliable fitting of the commoner types of diaphragm difficult.

Mode of action

The diaphragm acts as a physical barrier during sexual intercourse to prevent sperm reaching the cervical mucus and the upper genital tract. It should lie diagonally across the cervix (see **Fig. 9.7**), reaching from the posterior vaginal fornix to behind the pubic symphysis. The largest comfortable size should be used as the vagina expands during sexual arousal.

Effectiveness

When a diaphragm is used perfectly, it is estimated to be between 94% effective however with typical use, the failure rate is 16 per HWY (100

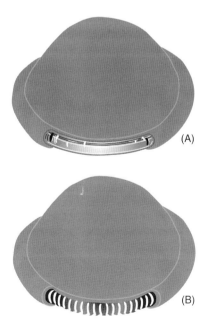

Figure 9.2 (A) Flat-spring diaphragm to show rim in cross-section; (B) Coil-spring diaphragm to show rim in cross-section

(A)

(B)

Figure 9.3 Arcing diaphragm

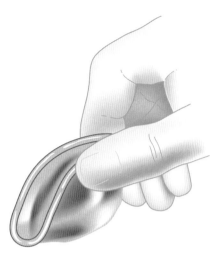

woman-years) (see Chapter 1). Higher efficacy is found when diaphragms are used by experienced users who have completed their families rather than by women who are spacing their pregnancies.

Because a sperm-tight seal between the rim of the diaphragm and the vaginal walls is impossible to achieve, the additional use of a spermicide is recommended in order to increase effectiveness.[3] However, as spermicides add greatly to the 'messiness' of the method, some women may choose to rely on the barrier function of the diaphragm alone.

Causes of failure, apart from poor motivation, are incorrect insertion or fitting, displacement during intercourse, and unnoticed defects in the diaphragm.

Indications

1. When a couple wish the woman to use a barrier method of contraception and find other contraceptive methods unacceptable.
2. When there are medical reasons that contraindicate hormonal contraception.
3. When a couple need intermittent, or infrequent, yet reliable contraception.

Contraindications

1. Poor vaginal muscular support or prolapse, although this may be overcome by careful assessment of the size and type of diaphragm fitted. Postpartum, fitting should be delayed until at least 6 weeks to allow muscle tone to return.

2. Psychological aversion or inability to touch the genital area.
3. Inability to learn insertion technique.
4. Lack of hygiene or privacy for insertion, removal and care of the diaphragm.

Advantages

1. No systemic side effects.
2. Effective when fitted and used correctly.
3. Does not interfere with lactation.
4. Spermicide provides extra lubrication if vaginal dryness is a problem.
5. Significant reduction in the risk of pelvic inflammatory disease relative to that of women using no method of contraception. Estimation of the degree of protection from the diaphragm alone is difficult as additional spermicide is almost always used and this may be the protective factor.
6. Reduction in the risk of pre-malignant disease and carcinoma of the cervix. Again, the use of spermicidal agents may be the actual protective factor.
7. Reusable and, depending on usage, durable.
8. Can be inserted up to 3 hours before intercourse.

Disadvantages

1. Requires premeditation, and thereby loss of spontaneity with intercourse.
2. Spermicide makes the method rather 'messy'.
3. May cause:
   a. Discomfort to the wearer or her partner during intercourse
   b. Loss of cervical and some vaginal sensation.
4. Has to be fitted and followed-up by trained personnel.
5. Does not provide protection against the transmission of HIV and other infections.
6. Sensitization to latex or spermicide may develop.
7. More frequent candidal infections, although the incidence of bacterial vaginosis is not increased.
8. Increased incidence of symptomatic urinary infection resulting from altered bladder neck angle and increased vaginal colonization with coliforms in diaphragm users. Women with recurrent urinary infections should be advised to use another method of contraception.
9. Toxic shock syndrome following prolonged retention of a diaphragm has been reported rarely.
10. Efficacy depends on correct use and sustained motivation.

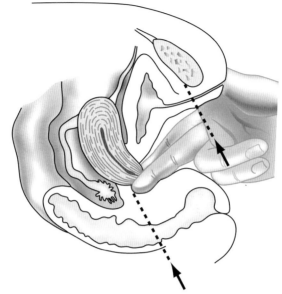

Figure 9.4 Estimating the size of diaphragm to be fitted

Fitting a diaphragm requires time and patience on the part of trained personnel. Models and diagrams of the female anatomy will often improve understanding. A vaginal examination should assess the following:

1. Position and condition of the uterus and cervix.
2. Length of vagina and muscle tone.
3. Measurement of the distance between the posterior fornix and the posterior aspect of the pubic symphysis.

Selection and fitting

1. A diaphragm, corresponding roughly in size to the distance between the posterior fornix and the symphysis pubis, is chosen (**Figs 9.4 and 9.5**).
2. With the woman supine, the labia are separated, the diaphragm is compressed and inserted into the vagina, downwards and backwards into the posterior fornix, before being released (**Fig. 9.6**).
3. The anterior rim is tucked behind the pubic symphysis and the position of the cervix checked to assure it is covered (**Fig. 9.7**).
4. Secure fitting is checked. When the woman strains down, the anterior rim of the diaphragm should not project or slip.

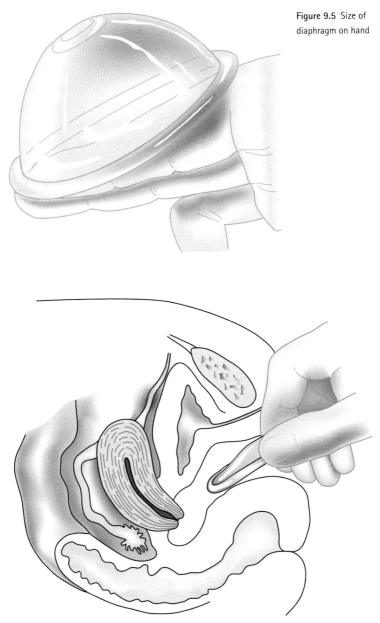

Figure 9.5 Size of
diaphragm on hand

Figure 9.6 Diaphragm being inserted

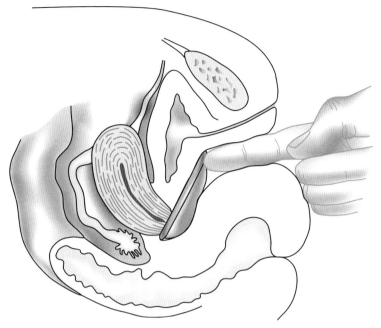

Figure 9.7 Checking the position of the diaphragm

5. Too large a diaphragm may project anteriorly, be immediately uncomfortable, or become uncomfortable or distorted after being worn (**Fig. 9.8A**).

6. If the diaphragm is too small, a gap will be felt between the anterior rim and the posterior surface of the symphysis pubis, or it may even be inserted in front of the cervix (**Fig. 9.8B**).

7. Persistent anterior protrusion of the diaphragm may be due to a mild cystocele, and may be discovered only after the woman strains or stands up. In this case, a cap other than a diaphragm is required.

8. The flat-spring diaphragm is usually used dome-upwards and, if reversed (to increase retention behind the pubic symphysis), is slightly more difficult to remove. The coil-spring type is normally recommended for use dome-downwards. However, there is no evidence that efficacy is affected by the direction in which the dome is inserted.

9. The diaphragm is removed by hooking the index finger under the anterior rim and pulling gently downwards.

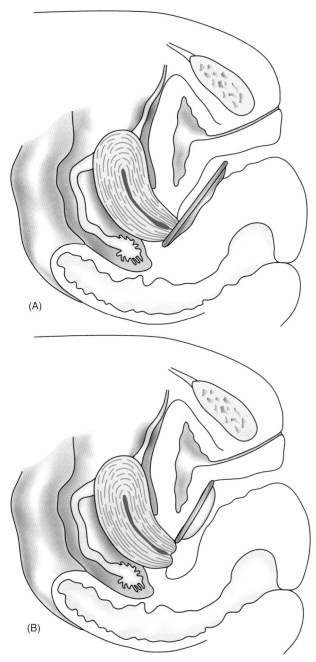

Figure 9.8 (A) Diaphragm too large; (B) Diaphragm too small

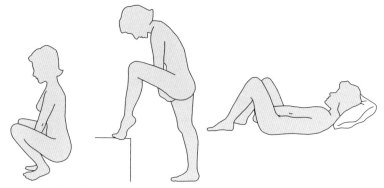

Figure 9.9 Positions for inserting a diaphragm

Teaching the woman

1. The woman has to wash her hands and empty her bladder before finding a suitable position, squatting, or with one foot on a chair, or occasionally lying on her back, according to her preference. She is first taught to locate the cervix which should be described as feeling similar to the tip of the nose (**Fig. 9.9**).

2. The instructor then inserts the diaphragm for the woman, allowing her to feel the cervix covered with the thin rubber or silcone. This is extremely important since correct placement of the diaphragm over the cervix is vital to its success.

3. The woman removes the diaphragm by hooking her finger under the anterior rim and pulling downwards (**Fig. 9.10**).

4. She is then taught to insert the diaphragm herself, the instructions being precisely those given for fitting by the instructor. Emphasis is placed on the downward and backward direction in which the compressed diaphragm is inserted into the vagina. After releasing the diaphragm, the correct covering of the cervix must always be rechecked (**Fig. 9.11**), as should the snug fit of the anterior rim behind the pubic symphysis.

5. Variation in the order of teaching these techniques may be required for some women, depending on their aptitude.

6. The partner may be willing and able to learn the technique of insertion on the woman's behalf.

Instructions for use

1. The diaphragm may be inserted at any convenient time prior to intercourse to minimize the loss of spontaneity.

2. Insertion of the diaphragm can be incorporated as part of the woman's regular nightly routine, whether or not intercourse is planned.

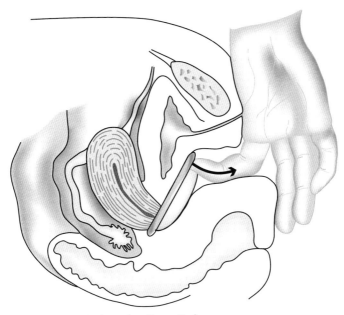

Figure 9.10 Removing the diaphragm (standing position)

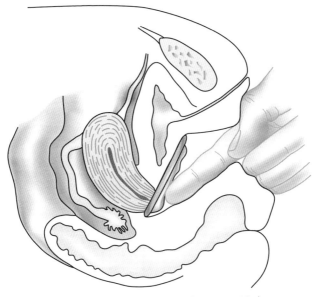

Figure 9.11 Checking the diaphragm covering the cervix (standing position)

3. To ensure maximum effectiveness, the diaphragm should always be used with spermicide.

4. A strip of cream approximately 2 cm long is placed on either side of the diaphragm prior to insertion and a little cream on the rim allows for an easier insertion.

5. If the diaphragm has been in place for more than 3 hours prior to intercourse, additional spermicide should be inserted into the vagina either by using an applicator or a pessary. The diaphragm should not be removed to re-apply the cream.

6. The diaphragm should be left in position for at least 6 hours after the last act of intercourse.

7. Care of the diaphragm is essential, after removal it should be washed in warm, soapy water and dried carefully. It should be restored to its normal rounded shape and stored in its container in a cool place. It should never be boiled. Perfumed soap, disinfectants or detergents should never be used to clean it, nor talcum powder to dry it.

8. Oil-based products can damage the latex diaphragms.

Follow-up

It is customary, but not mandatory, to provide a woman with a practice diaphragm for 1 week. This allows her to gain confidence in insertion, removal and care of the diaphragm and to assess whether it is comfortable. The diaphragm should not be used for contraception during this practice week. At the second visit, the woman should be asked to have the diaphragm in situ and then on vaginal examination the fit and covering of the cervix is assessed. The woman is advised to check regularly for holes or cracks. There is no evidence that colour change or the shape of the outer rim reduces the efficacy. It is recommended that the diaphragm should not be used during the menstrual period for women who have a history of toxic shock syndrome.

A diaphragm should be replaced annually or as soon as any defect develops. The size and fitting should be reviewed if a woman loses or gains 3 kg in weight, and after pregnancy, miscarriage, abortion or vaginal surgery.

Diaphragms under development

A 'Buffer-Gel' one-size disposable diaphragm made of polyurethane is being tested.

Similarly, a silicone diaphragm 'Silcs' with an arching ring and a finger cup on one side for easy removal is being developed.

• Cervical caps

Prentif cavity rim cervical cap

This cap is shaped like a thimble and is designed to fit closely over the cervix. It fits precisely on the cervix and is held in place by suction, not by

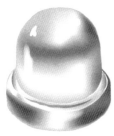

Figure 9.12 Cervical cap

spring tension, as in the diaphragm. It is made of firm latex with an integral thickened rim incorporating a small groove. This groove is intended to increase suction to the sides of the cervix. There are four sizes, based on the internal diameter of the rim, from 22 to 31 mm (**Fig. 9.12**).

Mode of action

By covering the cervix, the cap acts as a physical barrier to the entrance of sperm into the cervical canal.

Effectiveness

Perfect use failure rates vary from 9 (for nulliparous women) to 26/HWY (for parous women) while typical use failure rates are reported to be between 16 and 32/HWY (see Chapter 1).

Indications

In a woman unsuitable for the diaphragm, provided the cervix is normal and healthy, pointing down the axis of the vagina and not acutely backwards.

Contraindications

1. Short or damaged cervix.
2. Purulent cervical discharge suggesting infection.
3. Inability to reach the cervix with the fingers.

Advantages

1. Suitable for women with poor muscle tone and some cases of uterovaginal prolapse.
2. Not felt by the male partner.
3. No reduction in vaginal sensation.
4. Fitting unaffected by changes in the size of the vagina, either during intercourse or from changes in body weight.
5. Unlike a diaphragm, a cervical cap may remain in place for a maximum of 30 hours after intercourse.
6. Unlikely to produce urinary symptoms.

Disadvantages

1. Requires accurate selection of cap size and fitting to avoid displacement during intercourse.
2. Self-insertion and removal of a cervical cap are more difficult than with a diaphragm.
3. An unpleasant odour may develop if the cap is in situ for more than the recommended time.

Selection and fitting

1. The correct size is that which allows the rim to touch the vaginal fornices easily without a gap, comfortably accommodates the cervix, and is not displaced when the woman bears down.
2. With the woman in the supine position, the labia are separated, the rim of the cap is compressed and then guided along the posterior vaginal wall until the posterior rim is just behind the cervix. The thumb and first two fingers are used as illustrated in Figure 9.13.
3. The cap is allowed to open by removing the thumb and then it is pushed upwards onto the cervix with the fingertips (Fig. 9.14). A final check is made to ensure that the cervix is palpable through the bowl and that no gap is left above the rim.
4. The cervical cap is removed by inserting a fingertip between the rim of the cap and the cervix, easing the cap downwards and withdrawing it with the index and middle fingers.

Teaching the woman

The woman is taught to feel her cervix, and to insert and remove the cap, according to the instructions given above for fitting of the diaphragm. The spermicide should only be placed in the dome and the cap inserted around 20 minutes before intercourse.

Instructions for use and follow-up

1. Spermicidal cream should only fill one-third of the bowl of the cap.
2. In case the cap is displaced further, spermicide should be inserted into the vagina immediately prior to intercourse in the form of a pessary.
3. The position of the cervical cap should always be rechecked prior to each act of intercourse to ensure that accidental dislodgement has not occurred. If this has happened, emergency contraception is recommended.
4. The schedule of follow-up visits is the same as for the diaphragm.

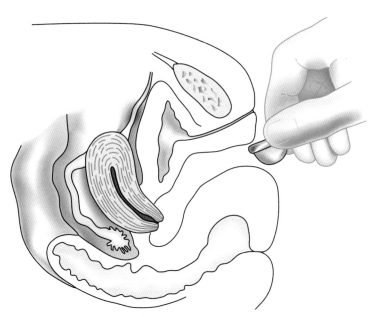

Figure 9.13 Cervical cap being inserted

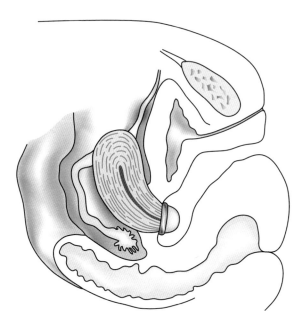

Figure 9.14 Cervical cap in situ

Figure 9.15 Vault cap (Dumas)

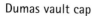

Dumas vault cap

This cap has an almost hemispherical bowl with a thinner dome through which the cervix can be palpated (Fig. 9.15). It is designed to fit into the vaginal vault, stays in place by suction, and covers, but does not fit closely to, the cervix. Five sizes range from 50 to 75 mm.

Indications

1. Woman wishes to have the convenience of a cap.
2. Unsuitability for, or inability to use, a diaphragm.
3. Unsuitability of the cervix because of its shape or position for a well-fitting cervical cap.

Selection, fitting and teaching

Instructions are precisely the same as for the cervical cap, with modifications only in the siting of the upper rim. The correct size should cover the cervix without exerting pressure on it, and fit snugly into the vaginal vault (Fig. 9.16).

Instructions for use and follow-up

These are identical to those of the cervical cap, with a spermicide being used to fill one-third of the bowl of the vault cap prior to insertion.

Vimule

This is a variation of the vault cap with a thimble-shaped prolongation of the dome (Fig. 9.17). There are three sizes – small (45 mm), medium (48 mm) and large (51 mm). The vimule has fallen into some disrepute because of its association with the development of vaginal abrasions, possibly because of the relatively sharp-edged rim.

Indications

It is used specifically for the woman requiring a vault cap to accommodate a cervix which is so long that it prevents suction being exerted by a cervical cap on the vaginal vault.

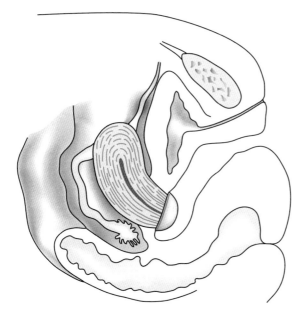

Figure 9.16 Vault cap
in situ

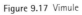

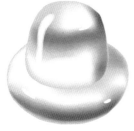

Figure 9.17 Vimule

Selection, fitting and teaching

Again, this is identical to that of the cervical cap apart from the exact siting
of the upper rim (Fig. 9.18). A vimule may often provide the solution for a
woman who proves difficult to fit with alternative 'caps'. A string attached
to the vimule facilitates removal during learning, but should be removed
once the user is confident.

Instructions for use and follow-up

These are identical to those for the cervical cap, with a spermicide being
used in the same manner.

Figure 9.18 Vimule in situ

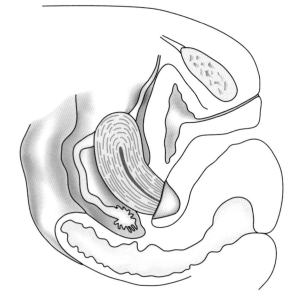

• Newer cervical devices

Lea's shield

This is a silicone, re-usable, one-size barrier with a removal loop (Fig 9.19). The Lea's shield is held in place by the vaginal muscles. Once inserted, it completely covers the cervix. When used in conjunction with spermicide, it can be left in situ for 48 hours and has a valvular device which allows the escape of cervical secretions or menstrual fluid and trapped air.

During fitting, the valve should be facing down and the thickest end of the shield inserted first ensuring that the loop is within the vagina. It must stay in position for 8 hours after the last act of intercourse.

Lea's shield is a new vaginal contraceptive that does not require clinician fitting.[4] It appears very acceptable to a small select group of women. It is available over the counter in North America and several European countries.

FemCap

This is a thin flexible silicone dome-shaped rubber cap similar to a US sailor's hat. It was designed to reduce dislodgements and give less pressure on the urethra than the cervical cap and diaphragm, respectively, and to require less clinician time for fitting.[5]

This cap is held in position by the vaginal walls to cover the cervix with the circular brim. The posterior brim adheres to the vaginal walls and is

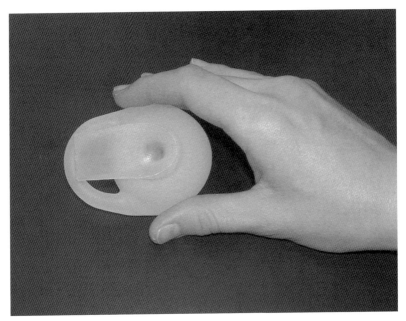

Figure 9.19 The Lea's Shield. Courtesy of the Cervical Barrier Advancement Society

designed to funnel ejaculatory fluids into a groove between the dome and the brim which acts as a reservoir for spermicide.[6]

The correct size should be determined by a health professional. The smallest size is 22 mm for nulliparous women, medium 26 mm for parous women who have not delivered vaginally, and largest 30 mm for women who have had a vaginal delivery.

Effectiveness

The 6-month Kaplan–Meier cumulative unadjusted typical use pregnancy probabilities were 13.5% among FemCap users and 7.9% among diaphragm users.[5] The FemCap can remain in situ for up to 48 hours and the manufacturers suggest it is usable for up to 2 years.

Oves cervical cap

This is a thin, flexible disposable silicone cap designed to remain in situ for up to 3 days. A small amount of spermicide is placed in the cap prior to insertion and spermicide need not be reapplied thereafter. A small loop on the rim facilitates removal. The Oves cap is available in Europe, and comes in three sizes: 26, 28, and 30 mm. There are little data on its efficacy.

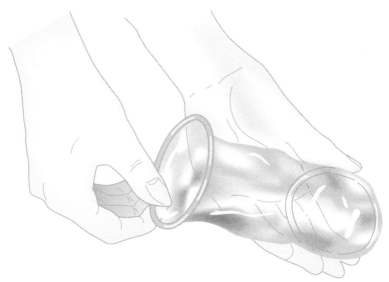

Figure 9.20 Female condom

• Female condom

This is a polyurethane sheath with its open end attached to a flexible polyurethane ring (**Fig. 9.20**). A removable polyurethane ring inside the condom serves as an introducer and holds the device in the vagina. The condom comes in a single size (15 cm long by 7.5 cm in diameter), with a silicone-based, non-spermicidal lubricant and is for single use only. It is available over the counter or by mail order under the trade name Femidom (UK), FC Female Condom (United States) and in over 100 countries world wide. Some clinics and general practitioners provide them free of charge. Initial adverse responses to female condoms decrease as couples become familiar with their use. A cheaper second-generation version made of nitrile instead of polyurethrane should be available in the near future.[7]

Mode of action

As with all barrier methods, female condoms prevent spermatozoa gaining access to the female upper genital tract.

Effectiveness

Data suggest that the female condom is as effective as the diaphragm. With consistent and correct use the failure rate is 5% while the typical use failure is 21% (see Chapter 1).

Indications

1. When a woman wishes to use a reversible, barrier method of contraception.
2. For maximum protection against sexually transmitted infections (STIs) including HIV when the male condom is unacceptable.

Contraindications

Some couples find female condoms psychologically unacceptable.

Advantages

1. An effective method of contraception that is controlled by the woman.
2. Available over the counter or the internet.
3. Affords very high protection against STIs by protecting the vulva and urethra.
4. Stronger than latex male condoms with less risk of splitting and not weakened by oil-based vaginal preparations.
5. Less diminution of sensation for the man than with latex condoms.
6. Can be inserted a long time (i.e. hours) in advance of intercourse and also left in some time after ejaculation thereby allowing less disruption of the sexual act.

Disadvantages

1. Unattractive appearance.
2. Altered sensation and a 'rustling' noise during intercourse.
3. Some initial difficulty with insertion may be experienced but this improves quickly with repeated use.
4. Can occasionally be pushed completely into the vagina or penetration can take place outside it.
5. Unsuitable for women who dislike touching their genitalia.

Instructions for use

1. To insert the condom the woman squats with one foot on a chair or lies down.
2. The sheath-covered inner ring is squeezed between thumb and other fingers to slide the condom into the vagina as if inserting a tampon.
3. Once the condom is in the vagina, the inner ring is pushed as high as possible so that it will remain there during intercourse.
4. The outer ring should lie closely against the vulva.

5. The penis should be guided into the condom to ensure that it does not enter the vagina outside the condom.
6. Immediately after intercourse, the outer ring is twisted and the condom gently pulled out keeping the semen inside.
7. The condom is wrapped in tissue and discarded in a bin and not down the toilet.

CONDOMS

The first condoms described historically were used for decoration and, thereafter, for protection against disease. In 1564, Fallopio, the Italian anatomist described the use of a linen sheath to protect the wearer from syphilis. With the development of vulcanized rubber in 1844 and then liquid latex in 1922, condoms could be inexpensively mass-produced resulting in worldwide availability and an effective, reversible male method of contraception.

The condom is recognized by such familiar names as Johnny, sheath, and protective. They may be purchased from supermarkets, vending machines, by mail order and the internet and are free of charge in contraceptive and sexual health clinics and some general practitioner surgeries. Embarrassment over asking for condoms should not prevent young persons from obtaining them. Condoms have been extensively promoted in the 'Safe Sex' campaign as an effective barrier against the spread of HIV. Prominent advertising has attempted to increase the public's awareness of the risks of unprotected intercourse and to encourage condom use. New trends in marketing and packaging condoms aim to increase consumer appeal and to escape from the association with clandestine sex.

Types

A large range of condoms is now available:

1. Made from fine latex rubber, polyurethane (strong thin plastic) or lamb intestine.
2. Larger sizes consisting of a circular cylinder (from 65–52 mm width, 180–206 mm long, 60–140 microns thick) with one closed, plain or teated end and an integral rim at the open end. Flared shape condoms are available for easier use.
3. Smaller sizes (49 mm width, 160–186 mm long, 50–75 microns thick).
4. Lubricated with a spermicide, coloured, flavoured, scented and textured variations to improve acceptability.
5. If allergies to latex exist, polyurethane condoms are available but are more expensive. They are very thin and adhere to the skin for improved sensation and are unaffected by oil-based lubricants.

6. Condoms which are thicker and exceed the British Standards are marketed primarily for anal intercourse in homosexual men to offer extra protection against infection with HIV.

7. 'Heightened Stimulation Condom' (sold under the trade name of Tingle in the UK) is 63 mm wide, 205 mm long and contains a lubricant which creates a mild tingling sensation for each person.

8. 'Enhanced Delayers' condoms have 5% benzocaine inside the condom or teat which temporarily desensitizes the nerve ending of the penis. In men who suffer premature ejaculation this can be of some assistance.

9. Condoms made from lamb intestine have improved sensitivity compared with latex condoms because they are thinnner but their efficacy against STIs is unknown.

Mode of action

Like all barrier methods, condoms prevent spermatozoa from reaching the female upper genital tract.

Effectiveness

The perfect-use failure rate for condoms is 2% in the first year of use with typical-use rates of 15%. Failure rates are consistently low when condoms are used perfectly by well-motivated individuals. In order to ensure high quality, the major manufacturers worldwide have established standards for size, resistance to breaking, freedom from defects, packaging and labelling. Users become technically more competent with experience and have fewer breakages. Tightness of condoms may be a factor in their failure and larger condoms may be needed by some individuals. If the condom is not used at the beginning of intercourse or is applied only just before ejaculation, pre-ejaculatory secretions may contain sufficient sperm to cause pregnancy. Poor practices such as snagging the condom with fingernails or rings, tearing the condoms while opening the pack, unrolling the condom prior to putting it on and re-using condoms obviously cause higher failure rates. There is no evidence that nonoxinol '9' lubricated condoms provide additional protection against pregnancy or STIs compared with other products.[8]

Indications

1. When a couple wish the man to use a reversible method of contraception.
2. During the period of instruction in the use of a cap.
3. Following pregnancy, before another method is adopted.
4. Condom promotion for 'safer sex' when used for personal protection against STIs, when a hormonal method is used to prevent pregnancy.

5. When other methods are unacceptable or additional contraception is required (e.g. when oral contraceptive pills have been forgotten).

Contraindications

1. When they are psychologically unacceptable.
2. Any malformation of the penis.
3. When either partner is allergic to latex rubber.

Advantages

1. Effective when used correctly and consistently.
2. Widely available, inexpensive and often provided free. No requirement to consult healthcare professionals.
3. Simple to use with no local or systemic side effects.
4. A very high level of protection against STIs, including HIV infection. Studies indicate that consistent use of condoms results in 80% reduction in HIV incidence.[9]
5. Protection against carcinoma and pre-malignant disease of the cervix.
6. Improvement of performance in some patients with premature ejaculation.

Disadvantages

1. Unattractive appearance.
2. Diminution of pleasurable sensation during intercourse, particularly transmission of body heat.
3. Requires application prior to coitus and prompt removal thereafter, which couples may find an unacceptable interruption to sexual activity.
4. Erectile difficulty may be increased, though some men in later years find the use of a condom helps to maintain an erection.
5. Availability and access especially for the young.

Instructions for use

1. The packet is checked for safety markings and the 'use by' date.
2. The condom is removed from the packet and unrolled onto the erect penis before any contact with the vulva is made, leaving the tip of the condom empty to accommodate the ejaculate (not necessary if the nipple-ended condom is being used).
3. Uncircumcised men should pull back the foreskin before rolling on the condom.

4. During withdrawal, the condom should be held firmly at the base of the penis so that it remains in place until after the penis has been withdrawn.

5. The condom must be checked for holes or breakage.

6. The condom should be wrapped in tissue and discarded in a bin, not flushed down the toilet.

7. Condoms should not be carried in a hip pocket or car glove compartment as trauma/heat may damage the product.

8. Oil-based lubricants such as Vaseline, baby oil and petroleum jelly drastically reduce the tensile strength of condoms. Other vaginal creams and pessaries such as antifungal and estrogen preparations can be oil-based and could theoretically also affect the strength of latex condoms.

9. Condom users should always be informed about the availability of emergency contraception and STI testing should the condom burst or slip off.

SPERMICIDES

These contraceptive agents comprise a chemical capable of destroying sperm, incorporated into an inert base. The commonly used spermicides contain non-ionic surfactants which alter sperm surface cell membrane permeability, thus causing osmotic changes which result in sperm death.

Nonoxinol '9' is the non-ionic detergent commonly used in most products. It is a surfactant that disrupts cell membranes and when used alone is moderately effective as a contraceptive. It is not known whether the contraceptive efficacy of nonoxinol '9' is affected by formulation or dose. It has been shown to be an irritant in animal and human models causing epithelial disruption in the vagina and rectum. This increases in proportion to the frequency of use of the spermicides.[8]

Products available in the United Kingdom are a cream formulation of nonoxinol '9' 2%, and pessaries containing nonoxinol '9' 5%, but gels, suppositories and foams are available in North America.

• Creams and gels

The chemical is incorporated into a stearate soap base, into a cream, or into a water-soluble base in a gel. Both liquefy at body temperature and disperse rapidly throughout the vagina.

• Vaginal pessaries

The base consists of gelatin, glycerine or wax. The pessaries are foil-packed and easy to handle. Since they spread less easily throughout the vagina, weight for weight, they are probably less effective than creams and gels but women often find them more convenient. A cool place (8–15°C) is recommended for storage.

Mode of action

1. The base material of the preparation physically blocks sperm progression.
2. An active chemical kills sperm.

Effectiveness

Nonoxinol '9' and its derivatives are unable to diffuse into cervical mucus. Sperm, which enter the cervical mucus before being immobilized by spermicide within the vagina, can survive and ascend the genital tract. Failure rates range from 18 to 28 per HWY.

Nonoxinol '9' has not been shown to reduce the risk of STIs and may increase the risk of HIV among sex workers. It should not be used rectally.[8]

Indications

1. Spermicides are used in conjunction with diaphragms and caps.

Contraindications

1. Allergy in either partner.
2. Not to be used to prevent STIs (HIV).
3. Absence of vaginal sensation.
4. Not to be used rectally.

Advantages

1. Provide extra lubrication if vaginal dryness is a problem.
2. Readily available without a prescription.
3. No evidence of topical vaginal toxicity.
4. Possible protection against carcinoma of the cervix (transmission of HPV).

Disadvantages

1. Unacceptably high failure rate when used alone.
2. Requires premeditation prior to intercourse.
3. Varying degrees of 'messiness' according to the preparation.
4. Pessaries unsuitable for use in tropical countries, as they melt. However, melted pessaries will solidify if cooled in the pack, and still retain their activity.
5. Occasional complaints of an unpleasant odour, stinging or discomfort in the vagina. A few individuals are allergic to nonoxynol-9.

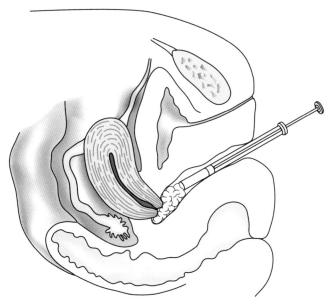

Figure 9.21 Foam insertion

6. Usage of spermicides in excess of normal dosages can cause irritation and ulceration in the vaginal mucosa and the effect appears to be dose related. The damaged vaginal epithelium may potentially enhance the entry of sexually transmittable organisms such as HIV.

7. There is no apparent increase in spontaneous abortion or fetal abnormality associated with using spermicides in the periconceptional phase.

Instructions to users

1. Creams may be inserted into the vagina with an applicator 2 to 3 minutes before intercourse.

2. Pessaries are inserted 15 minutes before intercourse.

3. One full applicator of cream should be inserted into the vagina just before intercourse and emptied (**Fig. 9.21**).

4. If spermicide is inserted more than 2 hours before intercourse takes place, a second application of spermicide should be used.

• The vaginal contraceptive sponge

The 'Today' sponge is an 'over-the-counter' method which has achieved some popularity in the UK and North America. It is currently available in the USA and Canada and awaiting a relaunch in the UK and Europe in 2007.

Figure 9.22 Today vaginal contraceptive sponge

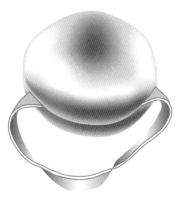

It consists of a soft, white circular sponge 5.5 cm in diameter, made of polyurethane foam and impregnated with 1 g nonoxinol '9' which releases 125 mg over 24 hours of use. A polyester loop is attached to facilitate removal (**Fig. 9.22**). The sponge should be inserted high into the vagina, with the indented surface positioned over the cervix. The spermicide is activated when the sponge is moistened prior to insertion.

Mode of action

The sponge is a delivery method which prevents pregnancy in three ways: as a barrier, as a mechanism for absorbing semen and as a carrier for spermicide.

Effectiveness

A systematic review comparing the sponge and diaphragm found the sponge to be much less reliable than the diaphragm.[10] The sponge, if used correctly for every act of intercourse, is 89–99% effective. Women have found it a very acceptable addition to the currently available range of barrier methods of contraception.

Indications

1. Women who want to use a vaginal method of contraception but do not wish to seek a health professional's instruction on fitting.
2. Women of lower fertility, such as lactating mothers or perimenopausal women, and those spacing pregnancies.

Advantages

1. One size is suitable for most women, although it has been suggested that a larger size of sponge may further reduce the risk of pregnancy in parous women.

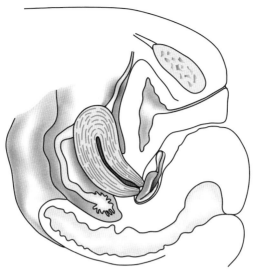

Figure 9.23 Today sponge in situ

2. It can be purchased over the counter.
3. Women find it convenient and simple to use, and particularly like the absence of messiness, or when travelling under unhygienic conditions.
4. There is no need for additional spermicide before each act of intercourse.

Disadvantages

1. The relatively high failure rate.
2. A small number of cases of toxic shock syndrome has been reported, but the overall risk appears to be in the region of 1 case per 2 million sponges used, which is reassuring. Traumatic manipulation, lengthy periods of insertion and use during menstruation or in the immediate postpartum period increase the risk of toxic shock syndrome.
3. A very small number of women or their partners may be sensitive to the spermicide.
4. Expensive.

Instructions for use

1. The sponge must be moistened thoroughly and inserted high into the vagina (Fig. 9.23).

2. It may be left in situ for up to 24 hours.
3. Intercourse may be repeated as often as desired during this time.
4. The sponge should be kept in place for at least 6 hours after the last intercourse, removed and then thrown away.
5. Use during menstruation should be avoided.
6. It may be kept in place during swimming or bathing.

• Spermicides of the future

There is currently widespread global interest and investment in developing 'microbicides' (see Chapter 23 for further details).

OTHER BARRIERS AND LUBRICANTS

• Dental dams

Dental dams are available to reduce the transmission of STIs during oral or anal sex. They consist of small, thin-gauge latex squares, individually wrapped. A range of flavours and sizes are available. Water-based lubricant should be applied before placing the dam over the vagina or anus. The partner should hold the dam in place during oral sex. Only one side is for use and they are not reusable.

• Lubricants

Oil-based or water-based gels increases sexual pleasure by ensuring the contact surfaces are slippery and moist, which can reduce friction and possible irritation. Lubricants are colourless, odourless, non-sticky and tasteless. They have no contraceptive effect. Only water-based lubricants should be used with latex condoms (KY Jelly®, Aquagel®, Durex Play®).

ADAPTATIONS OF COITAL TECHNIQUE

• Coitus interruptus

This is the oldest method of birth control, widely used in Christian and Muslim communities but less so in Oriental countries. It was first described in the Bible (Genesis 38, verse 9), when Onan spilled his seed on the ground to prevent conception when forced to have sexual intercourse with his brother's widow. St Augustine based his condemnation of contraception on this, leading eventually to the doctrine set out in the Papal encyclical Humanae Vitae which still today condemns the practice of coitus interruptus.

Description

Coitus interruptus is the withdrawal of the erect penis from the vagina before ejaculation. It is described by users as 'being careful', 'withdrawal' and by local euphemisms implying stopping before the effective 'end of the line'. When questioned, users often claim not to use contraception and, unless asked specifically about coitus interruptus, a false history of infertility may be assumed. The method requires discipline on the part of the male and is practised most successfully by men able to recognize the imminence of orgasm and to withdraw quickly prior to ejaculation. Unfortunately, it is often the method practised unsuccessfully by young inexperienced men.

This method is used by 4% of the sexually active population in the UK.[2]

Mode of action

Since ejaculation occurs outside the vagina, semen is not deposited within the vagina and therefore pregnancy should not occur. However, pre-ejaculatory secretions containing thousands of sperm may escape from the urethra during penetration, resulting in pregnancy.

Effectiveness

Failure rates vary with the age and experience of the couples.

Advantages

1. No supplies, preparation or health professional required.
2. Costs nothing.
3. No serious side effects.
4. Allows total privacy in the couple's sexual relationship.

Disadvantages

1. High failure rate.
2. No protection from STIs and HIV.
3. Limits full enjoyment of sexual intercourse.

• Coitus outwith the vagina

Oral and anal sex are now widespread sexual practices. Individuals may request specific advice on them particularly in relation to STIs and there is evidence that oral sex has become a more widespread practice since concern over risk of HIV.

REFERENCES

1. Smith L (2006) Contraception in the 16th century. Journal Family Planning Reproductive Health Care 32(1): 59–60.
2. Taylor T, Keyse L, Bryant A (2006) Contraception and Sexual Health 2005/06 Office for National Statistics. Department of Health.

3. Smith C, Farr G, Feldblum PJ, Spence A (1995). Effectiveness of the non-spermicidal fit-free diaphragm. Contraception 51: 289–291.

4. Mauck C, Glover LH, Miller E, et al. (1996) Lea's Shield.
A Study of the Safety and Efficacy of a New Vaginal Barrier Contraceptive used with and without spermicide.

5. Mauck C, Callahan M, Weiner DH, Dominik R, The FemCap Investigators' group (1999) A comparative study of the safety and efficacy of FemCap, a new vaginal barrier contraceptive, and the Ortho All-Flex diaphragm. Contraception 60: 71–80.

6. Shihata AA (1998) The FemCap: a new contraceptive choice. The European Journal of Contraception and Reproductive Health Care 3: 160–166.

7. Eduoard L (2006) In condoms we trust: to, one's own. Journal Family Planning and Reproductive Health Care 32(4): 262–264.

8. World Health Organization (2002) WHO/Conrad Technical Consultation on Nonoxynol-9. 2001. Report Reprod. Health Matters 10: 175–181.

9. Weller S, Davis AR (2006) Condom effectiveness in reducing heterosexual HIV transmission. (Review) The Cochrane Library.

10. Kuyoh MA, Toroitich-Ruto C, Grimes DA, Schulz KF, Gallio MF, Lopez LM (2002) Sponge versus diaphragm for contraception. Cochrane Database of Systematic Reviews 2002, Issue 3: CD003172.

FURTHER READING

Trussell J (2004) Contraceptive efficacy. In: Hatcher RA Trussell J, Stewart F, et al. (eds) Contraceptive Technology, New York: Ardent Media.

10 Fertility awareness methods and postpartum contraception

Jane Smith

Chapter contents

FERTILITY AWARENESS CONTRACEPTION

Family planning based on fertility awareness (FA), formerly and more colloquially known as natural family planning, has been defined by the World Health Organization as 'the voluntary avoidance of intercourse by a couple during the fertile phase of the menstrual cycle in order to avoid a pregnancy' (WHO 9th Annual Report, 1980). For decades now, effective artificial methods of contraception have not only enabled couples to plan their pregnancies and limit the size of their families but have also allowed sexual behaviour to be largely released from reproductive consequences. In societies where contraceptive services are freely available, voluntary periodic abstinence can therefore seem a curious choice today. Moreover, FA methods are also associated with higher failure rates than other available methods of contraception. However, efficacy and sexual freedom are not the only considerations taken into account by men and women when they are choosing their contraceptive method. Natural methods are often perceived as being better for women's health than hormonal or intrauterine methods. The ability to manage family planning without dependence on healthcare providers is another attraction. Some choose natural methods on moral or religious grounds; others because they have experienced, or have concerns about, the side effects of artificial methods or because they have medical conditions which limit their contraceptive choice. Even with the wide range of contraceptive choices available today, methods of family planning based on periodic abstinence continue to be an important option and are attractive to many couples at least at some time during their reproductive lives.

• Fertility cycle

Family planning based on FA involves a continual awareness of fertility status and can therefore be used equally effectively to achieve or prevent pregnancy. The essential event which determines the time of the fertile phase in the cycle is, of course, ovulation. The ovum survives for not more than 24 hours after release from the ovary and is capable of being fertilized for probably only about 12 hours of its life span. It is more difficult to be precise about sperm survival because this depends upon environmental factors. The average survival time is probably about 3 days but there is evidence that in some circumstances sperm may survive for up to 7 days. This means that a woman is potentially fertile for no more than 6–8 days of the cycle and probably less in most cases. On most of the fertile days, moreover, the chance of conception is considerably below 20%. FA contraceptive methods depend on various ways of identifying the time of ovulation and the likely fertile days in the cycle and then confining intercourse to the infertile days.

• How can the fertile phase of the cycle be detected?

The reproductive cycle in a woman is controlled by the pituitary hormones follicle stimulating hormone (FSH) and luteinizing hormone (LH). These two hormones in turn control the production of the ovarian hormones, estrogen and progesterone. Conventionally, the cycle starts on the first day of menstruation (day 1). In the early preovulatory phase of the cycle (follicular phase), FSH acts on the ovary to stimulate the development of follicles. The ripening follicle produces increasing amounts of estrogen which stimulates proliferation of the endometrium to prepare for implantation of a fertilized ovum. Estrogen levels reach a peak approximately 24 hours before ovulation stimulating a surge of LH which triggers ovulation. During the postovulatory phase of the cycle (luteal phase), the dominant hormone is progesterone produced by the corpus luteum which develops from the ruptured follicle. Progesterone levels reach a peak about 7 days after ovulation. The main function of progesterone is to stimulate the development of secretory phase endometrium to ensure successful implantation of the ovum should fertilization occur. If fertilization and implantation do not occur, progesterone levels drop as the corpus luteum disintegrates. Estrogen levels also decline. The endometrium can no longer be maintained and menstruation occurs.

The length of the follicular phase of the cycle and therefore the day of ovulation may vary both between individuals and between cycles in any one woman. Cycle length is particularly prone to variation in the later reproductive years. The duration of the luteal phase from ovulation until the next menstruation is, in contrast, fairly constant at 14 ± 2 days but the exact day of ovulation can vary even in regular cycles (i.e. it will not always be day 14 in a 28-day cycle).

The cyclical changes in estrogen and progesterone concentrations are associated with a number of important signs and symptoms which women are naturally aware of, or can be taught to be so. Figure 10.1 shows a composite picture of the main events of the menstrual cycle. During the follicular phase, rising estrogen levels cause changes in the quality and quantity of mucus produced at the cervix and in the appearance and position of the cervix itself. Following menstruation, the mucus forms a viscid plug in the cervix and the vaginal entrance feels dry. Under the influence of estrogen, the mucus increases in amount and becomes clear and slippery as ovulation approaches. The vulva feels moist or even wet. The physical changes in the mucus together with alterations in the amount of sugars and trace elements facilitate survival and transport of sperm. The cervix itself rises up in the pelvic cavity under the influence of estrogen and becomes soft and more open at the os.

After ovulation, the first secretion of progesterone reverses abruptly the estrogen effect on mucus, causing it to become thick, viscid and scant in amount and form a plug in the cervix. The cervix in turn closes, becomes firmer and descends in the pelvis. Progesterone is also thermogenic and produces a rise in basal body temperature (BBT) after ovulation which is maintained until around the onset of the next menstruation.

There are a variety of other symptoms associated with ovulation and with the changes in ovarian hormone concentration. Some women experience periovulatory pain (mittelschmerz) and bleeding. Some are aware of cyclical changes in breasts, skin and hair and also in mood and libido.

• Methods of fertility awareness contraception

The limited life span of both ovum and sperm together with the signs and symptoms associated with the cyclical changes in hormone concentration provide women with the means to identify when fertility is beginning, the day of maximum fertility in the cycle and the onset of the postovulatory infertile phase. The various methods of FA contraception depend on the use of one or more of the indicators of fertility and infertility to enable sexual behaviour to be appropriately adjusted to either prevent or achieve a pregnancy.

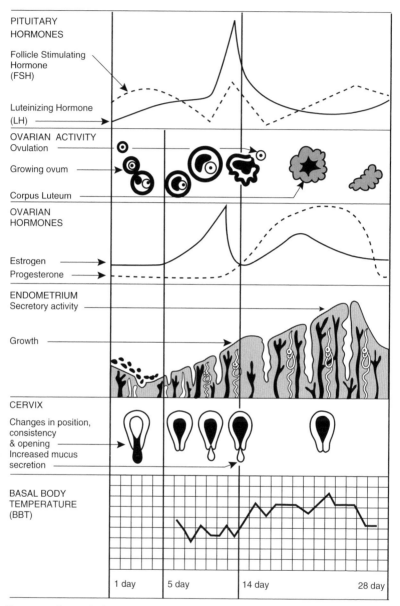

Figure 10.1 Changes in pituitary and ovarian hormones, follicle growth, endometrial development, position and characteristics of the cervix and mucus and changes in basal body temperature during the ovarian cycle

• Calendar or rhythm method

This method of FA contraception is widely used worldwide but is the least effective of the fertility awareness techniques. In the United Kingdom, it is used largely to provide background information about when ovulation may be expected in regular cycles. Cycle length is recorded for a minimum of six cycles. Likely fertile days are then calculated on the basis of the cycle length, allowing for the survival time of sperm and ova, using the following formula:

First fertile day = shortest cycle minus 20
Last fertile day = longest cycle minus 10.

For example, if a woman's cycle length varies from 28 to 35 days, her fertile phase begins on day 8 (28 – 20) and ends on day 25 (35 – 10). It is immediately clear that this method of FA contraception demands a significant period of sexual abstinence for women with even minor variations in cycle length. For women with a very regular 28-day cycle, the calendar method still requires sexual abstinence for 10 days in each cycle.

• Temperature method

This method depends upon the increase in BBT of 0.2–0.4°C produced by the rise in progesterone levels after ovulation. It is quite widely used but suffers from the disadvantage that ovulation is identified retrospectively and intercourse is therefore only allowed in the latter part of the cycle if the method is to be followed correctly. For this reason, the temperature method is usually used together with other fertility indicators in a combination approach to FA contraception.

Practical instructions

1. Temperature must be recorded daily immediately after >3 hours rest and before undertaking any physical activity. A special ovulation or fertility thermometer is helpful because the markings are widely spaced at 0.1°C intervals making it easy to read.

2. Temperature can be taken orally, vaginally or rectally but the same route must be used throughout the cycle. The thermometer must be left in place for a minimum of 3–5 minutes.

3. Temperature should be recorded on a specially designed chart to make the postovulatory phase easy to recognize.

4. The fertile phase ends after three consecutive high temperatures are recorded (>0.2°C above the six preceding recordings). This is known as the '3 over 6' rule (Figure 10.2).

5. Intercourse must be avoided from the onset of menstruation until the day on which the third higher level temperature has been recorded. Intercourse is then allowed until the onset of the next menstruation.

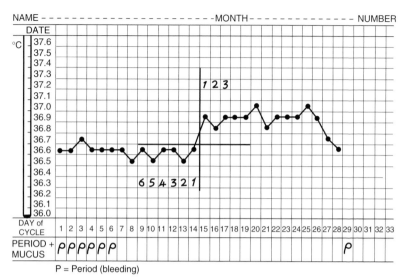

Figure 10.2 Basal body temperature chart demonstrating the acute rise due to ovulation and the '3 over 6' rule

Advantages and disadvantages

If rigorously applied, the temperature method offers a high degree of reliability. However, since intercourse is only allowed after ovulation, it requires a long period of abstinence in each cycle. This is a particular drawback for women with very irregular cycles. Even for women with a regular 28-day cycle, abstinence is required for about 18 days in each cycle. The necessary adherence to the daily routine of temperature recording is another disadvantage. In addition, infection, illness and certain forms of medication can affect body temperature and interfere with the method.

• Cervical mucus method

This method, sometimes called the 'ovulation' or Billings[1] method relies upon recognition of the changes in cervical mucus during the menstrual cycle. About 95% of women, regardless of cultural or educational background, can learn to use cervical mucus observation to recognize when they ovulate.[2] As with the temperature method, the cervical mucus method can be used alone or in a combination approach to FA contraception.

Practical instructions

1. Observation includes both sensation of dryness or wetness and visual inspection of the mucus which appears at the introitus. These observations can be made at a convenient time such as going

													X	1	2	3	4											
DAY	1	2	3	4	5	6	7	8	9	10	11	12	13	14	15	16	17	18	19	20	21	22	23	24	25	26	27	28
PERIOD/ SPOTTING																												
SENSATION						DRY	DRY	MOIST	MOIST	MOIST	MOIST	WET	WET	MOIST	DRY	DRY	DRY	DRY	DRY	DRY	DRY	DRY	DRY			MOIST	MOIST	
APPEARANCE									THICK	THICK	THICK	STRETCHY	STRETCHY													THICK	THICK	

Figure 10.3 Charting the cervical mucus method. The couple must abstain from intercourse from the first sign of moist sensation and mucus to the fourth day after peak mucus

to the toilet. Before micturition, the vulva is wiped with toilet tissue and examined for mucus.

2. The thick, sticky, opaque mucus following menstruation changes some days before ovulation to a clear, watery, slippery appearance rather like raw egg white. It can be stretched between the finger and thumb or between two pieces of tissue for several centimetres without breaking (a characteristic called spinnbarkheit). After ovulation, the mucus becomes thick and minimal again.

3. Observations should be recorded each evening on a special chart. Menstrual bleeding, dry days and mucus days are recorded using sticky labels or coloured pens. The day of peak mucus – the last day when mucus is clear and slippery – is marked with a cross on the chart (Figure 10.3).

4. Intercourse can take place on the dry days following menstruation, though couples are advised to have intercourse only on alternate days since the presence of residual semen in the vagina may make it difficult to recognize the first appearance of fertile mucus.

5. At the first sign of mucus, intercourse must be avoided and can only be resumed on the fourth day after the peak mucus. It can then continue as desired until the next menstrual period.

Advantages and disadvantages

For women who experience definite dry days after menstruation, the cervical mucus method has the advantage of allowing intercourse at this time, thus reducing the degree of abstinence required. The method also has the advantage of requiring no equipment other than a chart for daily recordings. However, it takes time for women to learn to recognize the mucus changes, to interpret the charted recordings and to apply the rules of the method.

• Cervical palpation method

The position and texture of the cervix can also be used as a fertility indicator. After menstruation, the cervix feels lower in the vagina and is firm and dry to the touch. As ovulation approaches, the cervix rises up 1–2 cm in the pelvic cavity and feels softer and more moist. The first sign of softening and upward shift of the cervix marks the onset of the fertile phase. The end is the fourth day after reversal of these changes in the cervix. This indicator is seldom used alone but can be part of a combination or multiple approach to FA contraception.

• The double check method

This is the most efficient of the natural methods and combines calendar calculations with cervical mucus observation and BBT shifts. The first day of fertile mucus is cross-checked with the shortest cycle length minus 20 to determine the first fertile day in the cycle. The indicator which comes first is taken as marking the beginning of the fertile phase. To determine the end of the fertile phase, the fourth day after the peak mucus day is cross-checked with the morning of the third day after the BBT shift and the indicator which comes last marks the end.

• Multiple index or symptothermal methods

Various combination methods of FA contraception exist, the aim being to increase the accuracy of identification of the fertile period. Essentially, these involve using BBT and cervical mucus observations in combination with secondary signs or symptoms such as periovulatory pain or bleeding, breast changes, mood swings or bloatedness (Figure 10.4). Teaching women to recognize a variety of cyclical changes enables them to be more in tune with their bodies and allows them to focus on the particular indicators of fertility and infertility which best suit their individual needs and circumstances.

• Personal fertility monitor

The signs and symptoms associated with cyclical changes in hormone levels are not always easy to recognize and FA methods relying on these indicators often demand excessive sexual abstinence to ensure adequate safety margins. A more direct and potentially more accurate approach to identifying the fertile phase is to monitor directly the concentrations of hormones which accompany ovulation. Such a personal hormone monitoring device (Persona, Unipath UK) has been available in the United Kingdom for the past decade. Persona consists of a hand-held monitor with disposal urine test sticks which measure the concentrations of estrone 3 glucuronide (E3G, the principal urinary metabolite of estrogen) and LH in the urine. It is designed to detect concentrations of E3G at a level reached 5–6 days before ovulation and concentrations of LH that identify the ovulatory LH peak so that both the beginning and the end of the fertile phase can be identified.[3]

The monitor indicates the fertile and infertile days by displaying a red or a green light respectively. The woman starts the monitor on the first day of menstruation. The day of the cycle is indicated on a liquid crystal display

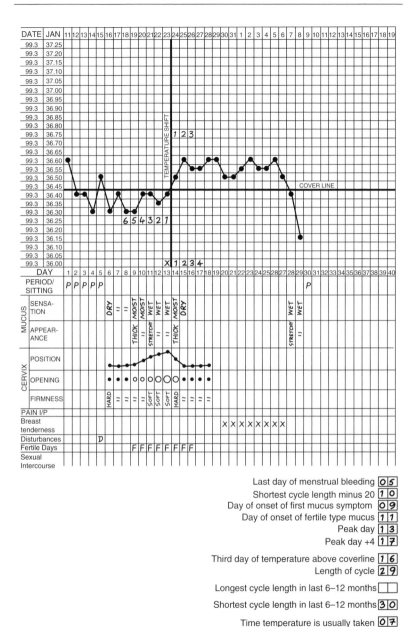

Figure 10.4 Chart for recording the multiple cyclical symptoms and signs for the symptothermal method

Figure 10.5 Hormone monitoring device (Persona, Unipath, UK)

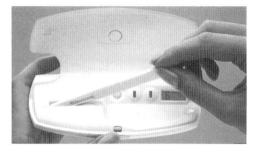

and the monitor also indicates with a yellow light the days on which a test is required (Figure 10.5). The dipstick should be used on an early morning sample of urine and the monitor takes about 5 minutes to read the test before displaying either a green light or a red one which signifies that there is a risk of conception. The computer in the monitor has rules built into its software which enable it to make decisions on fertility status based on background data obtained from large numbers of women. Once a woman starts to use Persona, the computer stores information from her last six cycles so that the data adapt to her cycle pattern and fewer urine tests are required. In the first cycle, the monitor requires 16 tests but as more information about the individual user is stored, the number of tests required comes down to about 8 per cycle. A red light is generally shown for 6–10 days in each cycle.

In the United Kingdom, the persona fertility monitor is available from pharmacies at a cost of £64.95. A packet of dipsticks costing £9.95 is required for each cycle. Persona is not available on the NHS and is therefore an expensive method of contraception. Its proper use is also quite exacting as the urine must be tested within 3 hours of the time when the monitor is first switched on at the start of the cycle. If the monitor is started at 7 a.m. on the first day of the cycle, urine tests must be done no later than 10 a.m. on each test day. If the test is late, it will not be read and the accuracy of the monitor is reduced because it depends on cumulative biochemical information. According to the manufacturers, Persona is 93–95% reliable if used correctly. Media-based publicity suggests a higher failure rate but it is not clear whether this is due to inaccuracies in the monitoring system, inadequate testing or failure to modify sexual behaviour appropriately. There is evidence from one study using Persona that women do fail to perform the required urine tests even when carefully instructed on the rationale for and the importance of regular, accurate testing.[4] Persona is quite widely used by women planning a pregnancy and wishing to identify the fertile phase in order to achieve conception.

• Effectiveness of fertility awareness contraception

It is very difficult to make a simple assessment of the effectiveness of FA methods. FA provides couples with information not contraception. The contraceptive efficacy of the methods depends on how carefully and correctly that information is applied as well as on the accuracy of the techniques used to assess fertility. Reported failure rates vary enormously between studies though many pregnancies are due to acknowledged failure to comply with the rules of the methods.

1. The temperature method used by itself is very effective when perfectly used because intercourse is only allowed in the postovulatory part of the cycle. A failure rate of 1.2 per hundred women years (100WY) has been reported.[5]

2. The cervical mucus method was tested in a large multicentre study involving three developing and two developed countries.[6] A total of 725 women were involved and there was a 3-month teaching period. The failure rate when the method was perfectly used was 2.8 per 100WY and an average of 15.4 days of abstinence was required per cycle. The actual failure rate for typical use, which includes acknowledged failure to comply with the method rules, was 22.3 per 100WY.

3. Similar efficacy patterns exist for other FA methods. The European multicentre study for FA contraception[7] found failure rates for perfect use of the double check method to be 2.3 per 100WY and for the symptothermal method 3.6 per 100WY but with typical use, the rates were much higher.

• Teaching fertility awareness

FA methods can be highly effective but only if adhered to rigorously. The success of FA contraception requires thorough teaching by well-trained individuals. A list of qualified FA teachers is held by Fertility UK (Clitherow House, 1 Blythe Mews, London W14 0NW) and information about FA contraception is available on their website (http://www.fertilityUK.org). Ideally, FA should be taught to couples so that both partners can share the responsibility for family planning and adjust their sexual behaviour accordingly.

• Advantages of fertility awareness contraception

1. An effective method of contraception when properly taught and adhered to.

2. Non-hormonal and non-invasive and therefore free from side effects.

3. Independent of healthcare providers once methods are taught. Can therefore be used where artificial methods are unavailable or high in cost.

4. No interference with lactation.

5. Enhances a woman's awareness of her body and her fertility.

6. Can be used to achieve as well as prevent pregnancy.
7. Involves both partners in the responsibility for family planning.
8. Is acceptable to the Roman Catholic Church and to those whose religious or moral beliefs prohibit artificial contraception.

- ## Disadvantages of fertility awareness contraception

1. Requires long periods of sexual abstinence.
2. Requires good teaching and a long learning period (3–6 months).
3. Fertility indicators must be monitored daily.
4. Requires a stable and committed relationship as both partners must be involved in appropriate adjustment of sexual behaviour.
5. Not suitable for women who are uncomfortable about exploring their bodies.
6. Offers no protection against sexually transmitted infections.
7. Failures of FA methods are most likely to occur at the extremes of the fertile period when sperm and/or ova are ageing. However, there is no evidence that this affects the outcome of the pregnancy or the sex of the offspring.
8. Fertility indicators are difficult to identify during times when cycles are abnormal (for example, in the perimenopause and during breast-feeding).

POSTPARTUM CONTRACEPTION

The choice of a contraceptive method after childbirth will depend on a number of factors including the timing of the return of fertility, when sexual activity is resumed, the pattern of infant feeding, medical issues (such as hypertension, venous thromboembolism and puerperal sepsis), social factors and, of course, the woman's personal preferences. It is important to plan and commence a suitable method of contraception before the woman is at risk of pregnancy. In practice, however, the delivery of contraceptive advice for the postpartum period is often rather haphazard. It is rarely addressed antenatally and is given only cursory attention on the post-natal ward. In the United Kingdom, the routine post-natal check traditionally takes place at 6 weeks postpartum. Whilst contraception is usually discussed at this time, ideally it should have been addressed earlier. In non-breast-feeding women, gonadotrophin levels begin to rise within 30 days after delivery and the first ovulation occurs on average at 45 days postpartum. It is therefore advised that women who bottle-feed their babies should start using contraception by 4 weeks after delivery. The resumption of ovulation and the return of fertility, whatever the method of feeding, can often only be identified retrospectively by the occurrence of menstruation.

• Lactation and contraception

Breast-feeding delays the return of fertility after childbirth. The FA contraceptive methods described in the first section of this chapter are difficult, if not impossible, to use postpartum but the effect of breast-feeding on ovulation provides the basis for a method of natural fertility control which is extremely important world-wide.

Effect of breast–feeding on fertility

The high circulating levels of estrogen, progesterone and prolactin associated with pregnancy fall abruptly after delivery. In the absence of breast-feeding, prolactin concentrations return to pre-pregnant levels within about 4 weeks, gonadotrophin levels increase rapidly and by the 8th week postpartum most women will show evidence of follicular development. In breast-feeding women, prolactin concentrations remain high as long as frequent suckling occurs and there are acute episodes of prolactin secretion stimulated by each feed. It is not known whether prolactin is directly involved in the suppression of ovarian activity or whether suckling itself acts through some neuroendocrine mechanism to alter gonadotrophin releasing hormone (GnRH) secretion patterns. FSH levels return to normal within a few weeks of delivery even in the presence of breast-feeding but LH levels remain suppressed throughout the period of regular lactation. In particular, the pulsatile release of LH is disturbed reflecting a block of the pulsatile release of GnRH from the hypothalamus.

As the frequency and duration of breast-feeding episodes declines over time and with the introduction of foods other than breast milk, the effect on the hypothalamo-pituitary-ovarian axis diminishes and ovarian activity resumes. The duration of lactational infertility is therefore dependent on infant feeding patterns and the age of the baby. The resumption of menstruation may be preceded by ovulation or there may be follicular development with sufficient estrogen production to stimulate endometrial proliferation followed by shedding when estrogen levels fall without the occurrence of ovulation. In any case, the return of menstruation is a sign of present or impending fertility.

Lactational amenorrhoea method of family planning (LAM)

In 1988, a conference was held in Bellagio, Italy at which clinical and endocrine data were pooled to produce guidelines relating to the link between lactation and fertility.[8] A consensus statement was issued to the effect that a woman who is fully or nearly fully breast-feeding and who remains amenorrhoeic has less than a 2% chance of conceiving during the first 6 months after childbirth. When put into practice, this statement formed the basis of a natural method of family planning known as the lactational amenorrhoea method or LAM.[9] This method is illustrated by the decision tree shown in Figure 10.6. It enables a woman to determine her fertility status

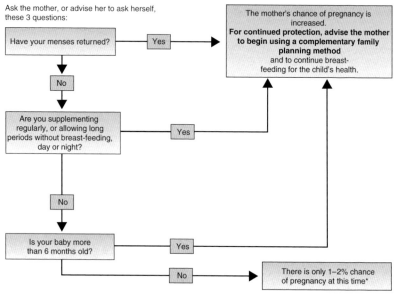

Ask the mother, or advise her to ask herself, these 3 questions:

Have your menses returned? — Yes → The mother's chance of pregnancy is increased. **For continued protection, advise the mother to begin using a complementary family planning method** and to continue breast-feeding for the child's health.

↓ No

Are you supplementing regularly, or allowing long periods without breast-feeding, day or night? — Yes →

↓ No

Is your baby more than 6 months old? — Yes →

— No → There is only 1–2% chance of pregnancy at this time*

*However, the mother may choose to use a complementary method at any time

Figure 10.6 The lactational amenorrhoea method (LAM) (after Labbok et al. 1994[9])

according to the age of her child, her pattern of breast-feeding and the return of her menses.

The effectiveness of LAM has been confirmed in a number of prospective studies. A cumulative pregnancy rate of 0.45% over the first 6 months postpartum was demonstrated by Perez et al.[10] In another study, amongst women who remained amenorrhoeic for 1 year (whether or not fully or nearly fully breast-feeding), the pregnancy rate was only 1.12%.[11] It is likely therefore that in societies where prolonged breast-feeding is the norm, LAM will be an important method of fertility control for much longer than the 6 months recommended in the Bellagio guidelines.

In developed countries, the average duration of breast-feeding is short and few women are fully or nearly fully breast-feeding their babies beyond 4 months. In the United Kingdom, despite efforts to encourage breast-feeding, in 1990 65% of mothers in England and 50% in Scotland breast-fed their babies and 39% of them were giving supplement bottle feeds by 6 weeks.[12] With these infant feeding patterns, LAM is of limited use. However, in developing countries – and particularly in rural areas – women breast-feed for much longer and the potential to use LAM is much greater. In societies where services for contraceptive delivery are limited, LAM is a very important natural method of fertility control.

• Artificial methods of postpartum contraception

As discussed above, women who do not breast-feed their babies are advised to start using contraception from 4 weeks postpartum. For women who breast-feed and rely on lactational amenorrhoea for contraception, the rules of LAM should be followed. In developed countries, supplement feeds are often introduced by breast-feeding mothers well before 6 months postpartum and a complementary method of family planning is therefore required. Whilst breast-feeding is continued, all contraceptive methods have low failure rates when used consistently and carefully.

Combined hormonal contraception

The use of combined hormonal contraception is contraindicated in breast-feeding women in the first 6 weeks postpartum because the estrogen component of the pill or patch reduces the production of breast milk (WHOMEC category 4 condition). From 6 weeks to 6 months, the evidence for a detrimental effect on milk production is not clear-cut and if breast-feeding is fully established, the use of a combined hormonal method may be considered if alternative methods are unacceptable (WHOMEC category 3).

For women who do not breast-feed, the combined pill or patch can be used from 21 days postpartum. Prior to this, it is unnecessary as fertility will not have returned and there is also an increased risk of venous thromboembolism during the puerperium. If the start is delayed beyond 21 days and does not coincide with the onset of menstruation, additional contraception (e.g. condoms) should be used for the first 7 days.

Progestogen–only methods

Progestogen-only methods of contraception do not have an adverse effect on breast milk volume. There is a theoretical concern about the effect sex steroids may have on the neonate and it is generally recommended for this reason that progestogen-only methods should not be used by breast-feeding women before 6 weeks postpartum. There is no significant evidence for such concerns, however, and if a complementary method is required during the first 6 weeks by a breast-feeding woman, a progestogen-only method may be used if other contraceptive methods are unacceptable. Implanon is not licensed for use by breast-feeding women but this is largely because of the expense and difficulty involved in undertaking the research required for regulatory approval of a new method. The arguments above apply for all progestogen-only methods.

For non-breast-feeding women, progestogen-only methods of contraception can be started at 21 days postpartum or thereafter with additional precautions for a week if not coinciding with the onset of menstruation.

Intrauterine methods

An intrauterine device (IUD) may be safely inserted within the first 48 hours of delivery. There is a higher rate of expulsion under these circumstances, but no increase in the rate of infection or perforation. Immediate insertion of an IUD after delivery of the placenta is rare in developed countries but common in societies where access to contraceptive services are limited and of necessity opportunistic. Unless an IUD can be inserted within 48 hours postpartum, insertion should be delayed until 4 weeks after delivery by which time the risks of expulsion and perforation are no different from those associated with insertion at any other time. For women who have a caesarean section, an IUD insertion should be delayed until 6 weeks postpartum to allow time for healing. The levonorgestrel-releasing intrauterine system can also be inserted from 4 weeks postpartum regardless of whether or not a woman is breast-feeding since the amount of progestogen which gets into the systemic circulation (and therefore to the neonate) is extremely small.

Barrier methods and spermicides

Barrier methods are often particularly acceptable to women in the postpartum period because they wish to avoid hormonal or intrauterine methods whilst their bodies return to normal after pregnancy and because sexual activity is usually quite limited at this time. Condoms and spermicides can be used as soon as sexual activity is resumed after delivery. Recent recognition of the link between the use of spermicides containing nonoxynol-9 and damage to the vaginal and cervical epithelium which might increase the risk of sexually transmitted infections (STIs), including HIV, underlies the advice that women at high risk of STIs should not use these spermicides. The use of diaphragms and caps should be postponed until involution of the uterus is complete at about 6 weeks postpartum. The fit should be checked as a different size of diaphragm or cap may be required for women who have used this method previously.

Emergency contraception

Unprotected intercourse before day 21 postpartum is not an indication for emergency contraception regardless of the method of infant feeding. Otherwise, emergency contraception should be prescribed as necessary on the basis of assessed risk of pregnancy. Women who are breast-feeding can use progestogen-only emergency contraception without restriction as there is no effect on breast milk production and no evidence of harm to the baby. If emergency contraception is indicated and the woman is over 4 weeks postpartum, an IUD may be considered, particularly if the woman wishes to use this as an ongoing method of contraception.

Sterilization

Female sterilization can be done within the first 3 days postpartum by mini-laparotomy or at the time of caesarean section. However, it may be associated with a higher failure rate than interval sterilization, perhaps because the fallopian tubes are very vascular and somewhat oedematous at the time of delivery so the clips, rings or ties may become loose when the tubes return to their non-pregnant state. There is also an increased incidence of regret if sterilization is performed immediately after childbirth and careful antenatal counselling is required.

Vasectomy is an effective method of contraception which some couples may choose after the birth of the baby which completes their family. Again, however, choosing an irreversible method of contraception at this time may leave scope for regret and it is advisable in most cases to delay the decision for sterilization.

REFERENCES

1. Billings EL, Billings JJ (1973) The idea of the ovulation method. Australian Family Physician 2: 81–85.

2. World Health Organization (1981) A prospective multi-centre trial of the ovulation method of natural family planning. I. The teaching phase. Fertility and Sterility 36: 152–158.

3. Bonnar J, Flynn AM, Freundl G, Kirkman R, Royston R, Snowden R (1999) Personal hormone monitoring for contraception. British Journal of Family Planning 24: 128–134.

4. Hapangama DK, Glasier AF, Baird DT (2001) Noncompliance among a group of women using a novel method of contraception. Fertility and Sterility 76: 1196–1201.

5. Marshall J (1985) A prospective trial of muco thermic method of natural family planning. International Review of Natural Family Planning 9: 139–143.

6. World Health Organization (1981) A prospective multi-centre trial of the ovulation method of natural family planning. II. The effectiveness phase. Fertility and Sterility 36: 591–598.

7. Freundl G (1993) The European Natural Family Planning Study Groups. Prospective European multi-centre study of natural family planning (1989–1992). Advances in Contraception 9: 269–283.

8. Kennedy KI, Rivera R, McNeilly AS (1989) Consensus statement on the use of breast-feeding as a family planning method. Contraception 39: 477–496.

9. Labbok MH, Perez A, Valdez V, et al. (1994) The lactational amenorrhoea method (LAM): a postpartum introductory family planning method with policy and program implications. Advances in Contraception 10: 93–109.

10. Perez A, Labbok MH, Queenan TJ (1992) Clinical study of the lactational amenorrhoea method of family planning. Lancet 339: 968–970.

11. Kazi A, Kennedy K, Visness CM, Khan T (1995) Effectiveness of the lactational amenorrhoea method in Pakistan. Fertility and Sterility 64: 717–723.

12. Office of Population, Census and Surveys (1992) Infant Feeding 1990. HMSO: London, p. 127.

11 Emergency contraception

Susan Brechin

Chapter contents

Emergency contraception can provide a safe and effective choice for women at risk of pregnancy when other methods of contraception have not been used or have been used incorrectly. Methods of emergency contraception licensed for use in the UK are hormonal (containing levonorgestrel) or non-hormonal (copper intrauterine device). Access to emergency contraception has increased with emergency hormonal contraception available free of charge from family planning clinics, sexual health clinics, general practice, walk-in centres (England), some pharmacies and some accident and emergency departments. Nurses can supply hormonal emergency contraception using a Patient Group Directive. In addition, emergency hormonal contraception can be given to women in advance of need. Measuring the impact of this advanced supply has suggested increased use but has not shown a reduction in unintended pregnancies.[1] Evidence-based guidance for clinicians on the use of emergency contraception was published in 2006.[2]

INDICATIONS FOR USE

There are many situations where emergency contraception is indicated (Table 11.1). Use should be considered on an individual basis and after discussion with the woman about her risk of pregnancy. A pragmatic approach is often required.

Table 11.1 Indications for use of emergency contraception (EC)

Clinical scenario	Indication for EC use
When there has been a potential risk of pregnancy	Sex where no contraception is used Ejaculation onto the external genitalia When relying on withdrawal method Following rape or sexual assault
Following a potential contraceptive failure:	
Missed combined oral contraceptive pills	If three or more 30 microgram pills are missed (or two or more 20 microgram pills) in the first week of pill taking (days 1 to 7) and unprotected sex has occurred in week 1 or in the pill free week
Missed progestogen-only pills	If one or more pill is missed or taken > 3 hours late (>10 hours for desogestrel-only pills) and unprotected sex has occurred in the two days following this
Late progestogen-only injectable	If the contraceptive injection is late (>14 weeks since the last injection of depot medroxyprogesterone acetate or >12 weeks for norethisterone enanthate) and unprotected sex has occurred since the injection was late
Intrauterine contraception	If compete or partial expulsion is identified or mid-cycle removal is required and unprotected sex has occurred in the previous 7 days
Barrier methods	Following a burst or displaced condom. When removal of a diaphragm or cervical cap within 6 hours of sex or dislodgement during sex has occurred
Use of liver enzyme inducing drugs with combined contraception, progestogen-only pill or progestogen-only implant	If an additional method of contraception is not used or there is a condom accident during this time or in the 4 weeks following cessation of liver enzyme inducing drugs
Use of non-liver enzyme inducing antibiotics with combined hormonal contraceptive pills or patch	If an additional method of contraception such as condoms is not used during antibiotic use or in the 7 days after cessation or if there is a condom accident during this time

BACKGROUND RISK OF PREGNANCY

Many factors may influence the risk of pregnancy such as frequency or timing of intercourse in relation to the menstrual cycle, background fertility and whether another method of contraception is being used. Women may be unreliable about their menstrual history and therefore clinicians cannot be certain there is no risk of pregnancy following unprotected sex. Sperm can survive around 5 days in the upper reproductive tract and rarely up to a maximum of 7 days. The ovum itself can survive around 24 hours if not fertilized. There is a low risk of pregnancy following unprotected sex in the first few days of the menstrual cycle and more than 24 hours after ovulation. It has been estimated that following a single episode of unprotected sex the risk of pregnancy in regular 28-day cycle for women not using another method of contraception is estimated to be 2–3% on days 1–9 or days 18–28; and 20–30% on days 10–17.

When women are using other methods of contraception (such as a combined oral contraceptive pill or a progestogen-only pill) the risk of pregnancy will depend on how many pills were missed and when they were missed.

TYPES OF EMERGENCY CONTRACEPTION

• Levonorgestrel

Levonorgestrel-only emergency contraception (marketed by Schering Health Care Limited) is the only hormonal method now available in the UK.[3] The standard formulation contains 1.5 milligrams of levonorgestrel as a single tablet (Levonelle One Step for pharmacy supply and Levonelle 1500 available on prescription). The previous regimen Levonelle-2 (comprised two 0.75 milligram tablets) may still be available in some areas.

A 1.5 milligram regimen is licensed to be used as soon as possible and within 72 hours of unprotected sex. Although this regimen can be used between 73 and 120 hours of unprotected sex if other methods (such as a copper intrauterine device) are unacceptable this is outside the terms of the product licence.[2] Emergency hormonal contraception can be used more than once in a cycle if there has been further risk of pregnancy. If however, further unprotected sex occurs within 12 hours of taking a 1.5 milligram dose of levonorgestrel current advice is that a further dose is not required. If a woman is already pregnant emergency hormonal contraception will not induce an abortion. Use of levonorgestrel emergency contraception is not associated with an increased risk of fetal abnormalities.

• A copper intrauterine device

A copper intrauterine device (Cu-IUD) containing at least 300 mm² of copper is effective as emergency contraception. Some women may opt to continue with the Cu-IUD as an ongoing method therefore, where possible, a banded Cu-IUD with at least $380\,mm^2$ of copper on the stem on the horizontal arms should be used. If it is not possible to insert this device another Cu-IUD can be used. Of note, a levonorgestrel-releasing intrauterine system is ineffective as emergency contraception and should not be used.

A Cu-IUD can be inserted up to 5 days after the first episode of unprotected sex regardless of the number of episodes of sex. Alternatively, a Cu-IUD can be inserted within 5 days of the earliest expected date of ovulation (for example up to day 19 in a regular 28-day cycle).[2]

MODE OF ACTION

• Levonorgestrel

The mechanism of action of levonorgestrel emergency contraception is not completely known.[4] It is likely that ovulation is inhibited by levonorgestrel rather than having any effect on implantation. If taken prior to ovulation this can be inhibited for between 5 and 7 days by which time most sperm in the reproductive tract will have lost their ability to fertilize an ovum.[5] It may be less effective in the 48 hours immediately preceding ovulation when the risk of pregnancy is greatest.

• Copper intrauterine device

A Cu-IUD works primarily by preventing fertilization due to the toxic effects of copper on sperm and ovum and may also prevent implantation (see Chapter 7). A Cu-IUD is not an abortifacient if used within current clinical guidelines.

EFFECTIVENESS

The effectiveness of emergency contraception is difficult to accurately measure as many factors previously noted may influence this. Estimates of efficacy are measured in clinical studies and data are presented as the number of expected pregnancies prevented which may otherwise have occurred if emergency contraception had not been used.

• Levonorgestrel

A large randomized trial showed that a single 1.5 milligram dose of levonorgestrel taken within 72 hours of unprotected sex can prevent 84% of expected pregnancies.[6] The use of this regimen between 73 and 120 hours of unprotected sex may prevent 63% of expected pregnancies although data are limited. No data are available on efficacy if used more than 120 hours after unprotected sex.

The contraceptive efficacy of levonorgestrel emergency contraception may be reduced by medical conditions or concurrent drug use. For women with malabsorption syndromes (for example due to Crohn's disease or small bowel resection) the absorption and efficacy of levonorgestrel may be reduced. Liver enzyme inducing drugs (such as some anti-epileptics, rifampicin, some antiretrovirals and St John's Wort) may increase the rate of metabolism of levonorgestrel and may reduce efficacy. Ideally a Cu-IUD, which is unaffected by concurrent drug use, should be used. If use of a Cu-IUD is unacceptable to the woman and she chooses to use levonorgestrel emergency contraception the dose should be increased. The use of an increased dose is outside the terms of the product licence but is based on clinical judgement and on the type of product available. Where Levonelle-2 is used then three tablets (a 50% increase in dose to 2.25 milligrams) should be taken at first presentation. When Levonelle 1500 or One-Step is used two tablets (a 100% increase in dose to 3 milligrams) should be taken at first presentation.

The use of a non-liver enzyme inducing antibiotic does not affect absorption or metabolism of levonorgestrel and the usual regimen can be used.

The effect of anticoagulant drugs (warfarin and phenindione) may be increased with hormonal emergency contraceptive use and monitoring may be required.

- Copper intrauterine device

If used as emergency contraception a Cu-IUD is very effective regardless of the time of the cycle or the time since intercourse. At least 99% of expected pregnancies can be prevented. A Cu-IUD is more effective than levonorgestrel emergency contraception and ideally this option should be discussed with all women who attend for emergency contraception even if presenting within 72 hours of unprotected sex. There are no medical conditions or drugs known to reduce the effectiveness of a Cu-IUD.

CLINICAL ASSESSMENT

- Assessing the risk of pregnancy

In all women attending for emergency contraception, clinicians should assess the most likely date of ovulation (based on the last menstrual period and the usual cycle length) and when the first episode of unprotected sex occurred.

- Considering the risk of sexually transmitted infections

A medical history (including a sexual history) should be taken from all women attending for emergency contraception to assess the risk of sexually transmitted infections (STIs). Women at higher risk for STIs (aged <25 years; >25 years with a new partner or with more than one partner in the last year)[7] can be offered testing for *Chlamydia trachomatis* (as a minimum) and for *Neisseria gonorrhoea* (if prevalence is high locally). An STI screen can be offered at initial presentation but this may only identify pre-existing infection. It can take 2 weeks for swabs to be positive and therefore testing may need to be postponed until this time. Nevertheless, a study investigating the value of delaying testing in women attending a family planning clinic for emergency contraception found that testing at presentation will detect the majority of infected women.[8] Serological tests for HIV, hepatitis B and syphilis can be offered with counselling 12 weeks after sexual contact. Post-exposure prophylaxis for HIV after sexual exposure (PEPSE) can be considered on an individual basis. The use of PEPSE is only recommended if women present within 72 hours of a potential exposure.[9]

When women at higher risk for STI opt for an emergency Cu-IUD, screening for STIs should be performed at insertion. Results are unlikely to be available before insertion and therefore antibiotic prophylaxis at least to cover *Chlamydia* should be considered.

• Assessing medical eligibility criteria

There are few strong medical contraindications to the use of emergency contraception (Table 11.2). Use in these circumstances can be considered on an individual basis. The summary of product characteristics advise caution for use of levonorgestrel emergency contraception by women with hepatic dysfunction, hereditary problems of galactose intolerance, the Lapp lactose

Table 11.2 UK Medical Eligibility Criteria (UKMEC) categories for emergency contraceptive use where there is a contraindication to use (adapted from UKMEC)[11]

Emergency contraception	UKMEC 3 (risks outweigh benefits)	UKMEC 4 (unacceptable health risk)
Levonorgestrel	Gestational trophoblastic neoplasia when serum hCG concentration is abnormal*	
Cu-IUD	Current venous thromboembolism using anti-coagulants†	Use within 4 weeks postpartum‡ Gestational trophoblastic neoplasia when serum concentrations of hCG remain abnormal

* Effect of levonorgestrel on disease progression is not clear but risk of a further pregnancy is greater.
† Due to potential risk of bleeding or haematoma formation at insertion due to concurrent anticoagulant use.
‡ Due to potential risk of perforation or increased risk of expulsion.

deficiency or glucose–galactose malabsorption or known hypersensitivity to components of the tablet.

The use of a Cu-IUD as emergency contraception has the same contraindications as for use as a regular method of contraception. A history of a previous ectopic pregnancy, young age, nulliparity and risk of STI are not contraindications to use of an emergency Cu-IUD.

SIDE EFFECTS

• Levonorgestrel

Nausea occurs in up to 14% of women following levonorgestrel use but vomiting is rare (1%). If a woman vomits within 2 hours of taking levonorgestrel a further dose is required.

Unscheduled bleeding is common following levonorgestrel use but most women (95%) will have a normal menstruation within 7 days of their expected date. If bleeding patterns are abnormal pregnancy (including ectopic pregnancy) should be considered.

• A copper intrauterine device

There can be a 6-fold increase in the risk of pelvic infection in the 3 weeks following Cu-IUD insertion (see Chapter 7). Other side effects associated with Cu-IUD use are similar to that seen with longer-term use.

AFTER CARE AND FOLLOW-UP

• Levonorgestrel

Women should be advised to return for a pregnancy test if menstrual bleeding is more than 7 days late or abnormal. Women should be advised that levonorgestrel does not provide effective contraception for the remainder of the cycle and another method or abstinence is advised. If women are currently using a method of hormonal contraception they may continue with use (Table 11.3). Ideally, women should be advised to wait until their next menses before starting a new method of contraception. However, if abstinence or condom use is unlikely, a new method can be started before the next menses and follow-up for a pregnancy test arranged (Table 11.3).

• A copper intrauterine device

Following Cu-IUD insertion, women should be advised to return if abnormal bleeding, pain or discharge occurs. A Cu-IUD will provide immediate contraceptive protection and can be continued as an ongoing method of contraception. A follow-up 3–4 weeks after insertion or after

Table 11.3 Advice regarding contraception following emergency contraceptive use

Contraception	Wishes to start	When to start following use of emergency hormonal contraception
When no regular method of contraception is used	Combined hormonal contraception	Start up to and including day 5 of the next menstrual cycle and no additional contraception is required
		Can start immediately but will require condoms for 7 days and follow-up pregnancy test after 3 weeks
	Progestogen-only pill	Start up to and including day 5 of the next menstrual cycle and no additional contraception is required
		Can start immediately but will require condoms for 2 days and follow-up pregnancy test after 3 weeks
	Progestogen-only injectable	Start up to and including day 5 of the next menstrual cycle and no additional contraception is required
		Can be started immediately if women would not continue with a pregnancy should emergency contraception fail
		Condoms required for 7 days and pregnancy test after 3 weeks
	Progestogen-only implant	Start up to and including day 5 of the next menstrual cycle and no additional contraception is required
		Can be started immediately but condoms required for 7 days and pregnancy test after 3 weeks
	Intrauterine contraception	Insert Cu-IUD after next menses if reasonably certain she is not pregnant. Insert LNG-IUS after next menses if reasonably certain she is not pregnant nor had unprotected sex. Condoms required for 7 days following insertion
Already using a regular method of contraceptive	Combined hormonal contraception	Continue as usual with condoms for 7 days
	Progestogen-only pill	Continue as usual with condoms for 2 days
	Progestogen-only injectable	The next injection can be given with condoms advised for the next 7 days and pregnancy test after 3 weeks

menstruation is recommended. If a Cu-IUD is not to be continued as an ongoing method it can be removed after the next menses if no unprotected sex has occurred since menses or if hormonal contraception has been started within the first 5 days of that cycle.

THE FUTURE FOR EMERGENCY CONTRACEPTION

Anti-progestogens have been compared to levonorgestrel and found to be safe and effective methods of emergency contraception.[10] Currently however, this type of emergency contraception method is not available but may be in the next few years.

REFERENCES

1. Glasier A (2006) Emergency contraception. British Medical Journal 333: 560–561.

2. Faculty of Family Planning and Reproductive Health Care Clinical Effectiveness Unit (2006) Emergency contraception. Journal of Family Planning and Reproductive Health Care 32(2): 121–128.

3. Schering Health Care Limited (2005) Levonelle 1500 – Summary of Product Characteristics. http://www.emedicines.org.uk.

4. International Planned Parenthood Federation (2002) IPPF Medical Bulletin. Emergency contraception pills: how do they work? 36[6].

5. Croxatto HB, Brache V, Pavez M, et al. (2004) Pituitary-ovarian function following the standard levonorgestrel emergency contraceptive dose or a single 0.75-mg dose given on the days preceding ovulation. Contraception 70: 442–450.

6. von Hertzen H, Piaggio G, Ding J, et al. (2002) Low dose mifepristone and two regimens of levonorgestrel for emergency contraception: a WHO multicentre randomised trial. The Lancet 360: 1803–1810.

7. SIGN Guideline (2002) SIGN Guidelines – Management of genital *Chlamydia trachomatis* Infection: United Kingdom.

8. Kettle H, Cay S, Brown A, Glasier A (2002) Screening for *Chlamydia trachomatis* infection is indicated for women under 30 using emergency contraception. Contraception 66(4): 251–253.

9. BASHH (2006) 2001 National Guidelines on the Managment of Adult victims of Sexual Assault.

10. Creinin MD, Schlaff WD, Archer DF, Wan L, Frezieres R, Thomas MR, Rosenberg M, Higgins J (2006) Progesterone receptor modulator for emergency contraception: a randomized controlled trial. Obstetrics & Gynaecology 108: 1089–1097.

11. Faculty of Family Planning and Reproductive Health Care Clinical Effectiveness Unit (2006) UK Medical Eligibility Criteria for Contraceptive Use. http://www.ffprhc.org.uk/admin/uploads/UKMEC200506.pdf.

12 Female sterilization

Mary W Rodger

Around 180 million women worldwide use female sterilization to prevent unwanted pregnancy with over three-quarters of sterilization users living in China and India.[1] In the UK in 2001, prevalence of sterilization as a contraceptive method was high amongst older women, with an estimated 44% of women aged between 45 and 49 years of age either sterilized or with a sterilized partner.[2] Popularity of female sterilization, however, now appears to be declining in the UK with a 30% decrease in the incidence of tubal occlusion and, since 1996, sterilization incidence in men has exceeded that in women in the UK as a whole.[3]

When the term female sterilization is used, in most cases it describes some method of blocking or occluding the fallopian tubes.

APPROACHES TO THE FALLOPIAN TUBES

• Abdominal

Laparoscopy

Laparoscopic tubal occlusion is the commonest method of female sterilization in the UK and the US. It is quicker than open surgical approaches and causes significantly less minor morbidity. It requires suitable surgical training and equipment to be carried out safely. Where possible it should be carried out as a daycase procedure.[3]

Minilaparotomy

Minilaparotomy is any open, surgical, abdominal entry with an incision of less than 5 cm. The incision is usually suprapubic for interval procedures and subumbilical for postpartum procedures. Although it is rarely used as a tubal approach in the UK, globally it is popular and can be carried out safely by suitably trained nurse-midwives or non-specialized medical staff. It does not require specialized equipment and can be performed as a daycase procedure.

Laparotomy

Laparotomy is open, abdominal entry with a planned incision of greater than 5 cm. It is rarely used as a primary procedure to access the fallopian tubes.

• Transcervical

Blind

Quinacrine hydrochloride pellets placed in the uterine cavity using an intrauterine device (IUD) inserter, were first used to cause occlusion of the fallopian tubes in Chile in the 1970s. Insertions cause tubal blockage by creating inflammation and fibrosis. This sterilization method has been used in many countries following the publication of a large Vietnamese study in 1993 which suggested a low failure rate after 1 year's use.[4] While the method is cheap and accessible to non-surgically trained personnel, longer-term assessment of its efficacy and safety is required.

Hysteroscopic

Although various devices are under development, Essure® (Conceptus Europe) is the only licensed product available currently in the UK for hysteroscopic tubal occlusion. A 4 cm inert, nickel-titanium coil containing polyester fibres is inserted through each tubal ostium, under direct hysteroscopic vision (see Figure 12.1). These generate fibrosis around the device and cause tubal occlusion by 3 months after the procedure. Worldwide efficacy studies carried out over 5 years suggest a success rate of greater than 99% following correct insertion. While experience with the device is more extensive in the US and Australia, a recent UK-conducted cohort controlled study is the first to directly compare Essure®, an office-based, hysteroscopic procedure, with laparoscopic sterilization performed under general anaesthesia and suggests a high level of patient satisfaction with Essure® when compared with standard laparoscopic tubal occlusion[5]. Larger numbers and longer assessment of efficacy and safety are still required.

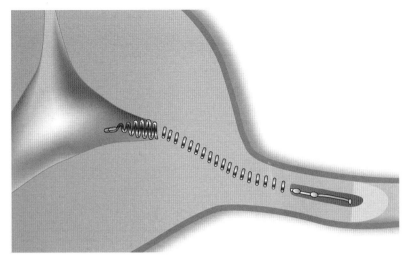

Figure 12.1 Essure®, redrawn with permission of Conceptus

• Vaginal

Colpotomy/endoscopy

Both major and minor morbidity are higher using vaginal approaches to the fallopian tubes. These techniques have been largely abandoned and are contraindicated in UK best practice.[3]

TUBAL OCCLUSION TECHNIQUES

• Mechanical devices

These are designed for laparoscopic use but can be used for open procedures performed at a suitable interval after pregnancy. It is recommended that local anaesthetic, usually in gel form, be applied with the device to reduce the incidence of postoperative pain.

Clips

Inert clips can be applied at right angles across the isthmic or narrowest portion of the tube approximately 1–2 cm from the uterine cornu (Figure 12.2). Specially designed and appropriately maintained applicators are required. Correct placement of the clip leads to compression and subsequent occlusion of a small portion of tube. Spring-loaded Hulka-Clemens clips appear to have a higher failure rate over 2 years than titanium and silicon Filshie clips and the RCOG guidelines recommend use of the latter device.[3]

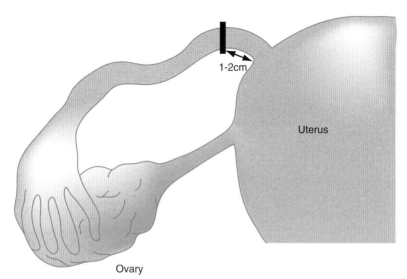

Figure 12.2 Tubal occlusion with clip

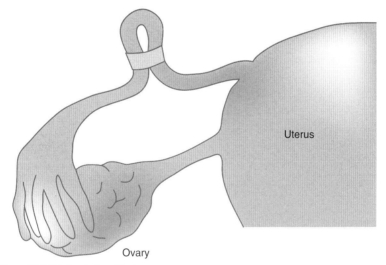

Figure 12.3 Tubal occlusion with ring

Rings

Silastic bands such as the Falope or Yoon ring are placed over a loop of tube using a specially designed and maintained applicator (**Figure 12.3**). These devices are harder to use than clips and have a higher intra-operative failure

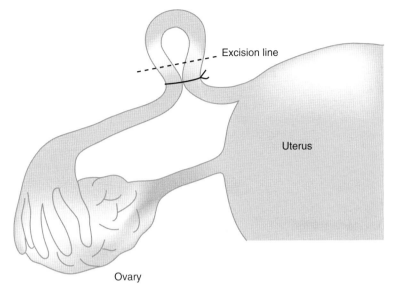

Figure 12.4 Pomeroy technique

rate.[3] A larger segment of tube is destroyed than with clip application. Short-term efficacy is comparable with the Filshie clip.

• Electrocautery (diathermy)

Bipolar diathermy administered between the jaws of grasping forceps applied across the tube should be considered only as a second-line sterilization method when other methods are not possible or have failed. This is because of the risk of thermal bowel injury, extensive tubal trauma and a significantly increased risk of post-procedure ectopic in comparison with other mechanical techniques.[3]

• Ligation and excision (partial salpingectomy)

A variety of surgical techniques have been described but the most commonly used are the Pomeroy technique and the Parkland technique. These techniques are cheap, easily taught and require no specialist equipment. They offer the lowest risk of failure in women under the age of 34 and in women in the postpartum or post abortion period. They cause extensive tubal damage and limited prospect of reversal of sterilization.

Pomeroy technique

A minimum 2 cm loop from the mid portion of the tube is ligated with absorbable suture material at its base. The tube lying above the ligature is excised. As the suture material is absorbed the tubal ends pull apart (Figure 12.4).

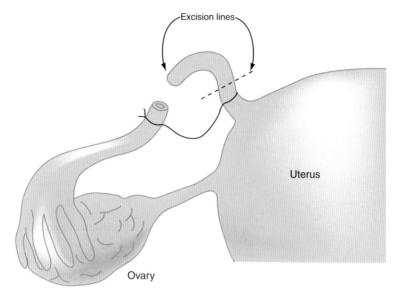

Figure 12.5 Parkland technique

Parkland technique

A length of tube is separated from the mesosalpinx. This is most safely achieved using a cheese-wiring technique with two lengths of suture. The tube is then tied in two places and a minimum 2 cm segment of tube is excised from between the ligatures. Absorbable suture material is used to reduce the risk of inflammation as this can lead to tubal fistula formation

ANAESTHESIA

General anaesthesia is most commonly used for laparoscopic tubal occlusion in the UK and the US where there is easy access to skilled medical personnel. Regional anaesthesia may also be used for laparoscopic or open surgical approaches. The majority of tubal occlusions worldwide are however performed under local anaesthetic.

TIMING OF THE PROCEDURE

• Postpartum

Immediate postpartum tubal occlusion following vaginal delivery is rare in the UK but can be safely performed by subumbilical minilaparotomy, ideally within 48 hours of delivery and, with care, up to 7 days postpartum. Tubal occlusion can also be performed at the time of caesarean section. It is recommended that ligation and excision of the tubes (partial salpingectomy) is used in the postpartum period as the tubes are bigger and more vascular at this time and more difficult to occlude using mechanical methods such as clips or rings. There is evidence that the failure rate of partial salpingectomy is lower. RCOG guidelines recommend that postpartum sterilization or tubal occlusion at the time of caesarean section should only be carried out if the decision has been made at least 1 week prior to delivery as there is evidence of an increased incidence of regret and dissatisfaction in this group of women.[3]

• Post abortion

Current best practice in the UK is to perform sterilization if requested as an interval procedure and not at the same time as a therapeutic abortion. Data regarding efficacy and safety of concurrent tubal occlusion are mixed, but the evidence, with particular reference to feelings of regret afterwards, is weighted against sterilization at the same time as termination of pregnancy.[3]

• Interval

Whenever possible, tubal occlusion should be carried out as an interval procedure, at least 6 weeks following pregnancy. Ideally, the procedure should take place within the first 10 days of the menstrual cycle to avoid failure due to 'luteal phase pregnancy' where conception has occurred during the same cycle as surgery. From an organizational point of view it would be difficult to deliver such a service and pragmatically women should be advised to use effective contraception until their operation date. A pregnancy test should be performed immediately preoperatively although this does not entirely exclude the possibility of luteal phase pregnancy.

Women using the combined oral contraceptive pill, progestogen-only pill or contraceptive patch should continue this until the end of the packet or cycle. Women with a copper intrauterine device or levonorgestrel-releasing intrauterine system in place should defer removal of this until their next period or at least 7 days after tubal occlusion.[3]

CONTRAINDICATIONS

There are no absolute contraindications to female sterilization apart from a continuing pregnancy or an incomplete family. The UK Medical Eligibility Criteria lists four categories relating to male and female sterilisation – accept, caution, delay and special (Table 12.1). Conditions for which caution is recommended imply that the procedure may be conducted in a routine setting but with extra preparation, precautions and counselling. Young age is such a condition. The risk of failure of the procedure and the incidence of ectopic pregnancy and experience of regret after the procedure are highest in women under the age of 30[6,7]. In one study up to 40% of women sterilized before the age of 25 years sought advice regarding reversal.[8]

Table 12.1 UK Medical Eligibility Criteria for female sterilisation. Conditions which indicate the need for caution or delay

Caution
Young age (<30)
Nulliparity
At time of caesarean section
Obesity
Hypertension
History of ischaemic heart disease or stroke
Uncomplicated valvular heart disease
Epilepsy
Depressive disorders
Current breast cancer
Uterine fibroids
Past pelvic inflammatory disease
Fibrosis of the liver, mild cirrhosis and liver tumours
Diabetes
Anaemia, thalassaemia and sickle cell disease
Diaphragmatic hernia
Kidney disease
Severe nutritional deficiencies
Sterilisation concurrent with elective abdominal surgery

Delay
Pregnancy
Recent childbirth of abortion <6 weeks
Current VTE on anticoagulants or immobility which may risk VTE
Unexplained vaginal bleeding
Trophoblastic disease while hCG raised
Cervical cancer awaiting treatment
Endometrial and ovarian cancer
Current PID
Current purulent cervicitis, Chlamydia or gonorrhoea
Current gall bladder disease
Active viral hepatitis
Iron deficiency anaemia
Local abdominal skin infection
Acute respiratory disease, systemic infection or gastroenteritis
Sterilisation with concurrent emergency abdominal surgery

With some conditions, such as anaemia or current Chlamydia infection for example, there is no reason not to perform male or female sterilisation but the procedure should be delayed until the condition has been investigated and/or treated. A few conditions may dictate that the procedure should be undertaken in a setting with experienced surgeon or equipment or anaesthesia. In the UK all female sterilisation is undertaken in specialist settings with full facilities but this is not always the case with vasectomy which is often done in community family planning clinics or GP surgeries.

FAILURE

The main causes of failure of laparoscopic sterilization are unidentified luteal phase pregnancy, incorrect placement of clips or rings and development of a tubo-peritoneal fistula. The lifetime failure rate of tubal occlusion is 1:200 when all methods and women are considered.[3]

The US Collaborative Review of Sterilization (CREST) followed up 10 685 women and found that risk of failure was related both to the method used and age of the patient. Failure rates were highest with Hulka-Clemens clips and diathermy and also in women under the age of 34 unless partial salpingectomy was used.[6] The CREST study did not assess the efficacy of the Filshie clip, which is currently the most commonly used mechanical occlusive device in the UK.[3] A retrospective survey of 30 000 Filshie clip applications suggests an approximate failure rate of 2–3/1000 applications. While the absolute risk of pregnancy following tubal occlusions is low, a high percentage of these pregnancies are ectopic with reported rates as much as 76%. The risk[3] of ectopic pregnancy is highest following tubal diathermy and amongst women under the age of 30. Women must be clearly advised to seek medical advice if pregnancy is suspected or symptoms of ectopic pregnancy such as abdominal pain and abnormal vaginal bleeding are experienced following sterilization.

RISKS

• Immediate complications

The major complications of laparoscopy are damage to bowel, bladder or blood vessels which requires laparotomy. These complications occur in approximately 2/1000 women with a risk of death of 1/12 000 women.

Minor complications such as wound infection or haematoma occur more frequently but overall affect less than 1% of women.

Factors such as obesity and previous abdominal or pelvic surgery or sepsis significantly increase the risk of all complications and these women must be fully informed of the possible requirement for remedial laparotomy. Minilaparotomy entails a similar risk with around 1% of women experiencing a major or minor complication of surgery.

• Long-term complications

While there is an association, particularly amongst women sterilized at younger age, between tubal occlusion and subsequent hysterectomy, there is no evidence to suggest that the procedure plays a causative role in subsequent menstrual disorder or uterine problems. Women using hormonal methods of contraception prior to sterilization must be made aware that they may experience heavier or more painful periods when these are stopped.[3]

Women with symptoms of menstrual disorder at the time of sterilization counselling should have this investigated as a levonorgestrel-releasing intrauterine system (Chapter 8), or in some cases, hysterectomy, may be the most appropriate treatment.

Regret is a commonly experienced complication and is estimated to affect at least 14% of women.[8] Those at greatest risk of regret are young women (<30 years), women of low or nulliparity, women in an unstable relationship, women sterilized immediately postpartum or post abortion, women subsequently bereaved of a child and women who make a sudden decision to undergo the procedure.[3] The commonest prompt for feelings of regret in the UK is the formation of a new sexual relationship.

OUTPATIENT CONSULTATION

• History and discussion

A full current and past medical, surgical, gynaecological and obstetric history must be taken. This should include details of menstrual cycle, past and present contraceptive use and smear history. Issues such as age, relationships and parity should be explored. Particular care should be taken when counselling women under the age of 30 and women with no living children. All suitable methods of reversible contraception should be discussed with reference to their advantages, disadvantages and relative failure rates. Recent audits suggest that, following informed counselling, approximately one-third of women will choose a reversible method of contraception, in particular long-acting methods, instead of tubal occlusion and that they will still be successfully using this method 2 years later.[9]

Possible changes to menstrual patterns on stopping hormonal contraception must be explained and the benefits of long-acting reversible contraceptives such as the levonorgestrel intrauterine system for menstrual disorder discussed. Clear advice on interim contraceptive use should be given. Vasectomy should also be discussed and women fully informed regarding its lower relative risk and failure rate. The irreversibility of sterilization must be emphasized. In the UK, access to reversal of sterilization and assisted conception is not available on the National Health Service for the vast majority of women.

The proposed method of tubal occlusion must be described and full surgical consent obtained following discussion of risks and failure rates.

Suggested consent advice is available on RCOG website (see under Further reading).

All information should be available in written form. A suitable information leaflet is also available on RCOG website (see under Further reading).

• Examination

Women should have their body mass index (BMI) assessed. Many day surgery protocols include strict rules for upper limits of BMI. An abdominal and pelvic examination should be performed to exclude pathology or previously undisclosed surgery.

• Immediate preoperative assessment

The date of the last menstrual period should be ascertained. Preoperative contraceptive use must be determined and a urinary hCG pregnancy test checked. It remains the responsibility of the operating doctor to ensure that there has been appropriate preoperative counselling and investigation.

• Postoperative advice

Appropriate advice regarding hormonal contraception and intrauterine devices should be given (see under 'timing'). Women must be advised about immediate complications such as wound infection or bruising and know where to seek help should these arise. An explanation about expected work absence is necessary, with most women needing 5 working days off work. The woman and her GP should be advised of the method of tubal occlusion and should know to seek re-referral if any signs of bowel or visceral trauma, such as malaise, pyrexia or abdominal pain become apparent during the first postoperative week following discharge.

Women should be reminded of the importance of reporting any subsequent symptoms of pregnancy with reiteration of failure rates and ectopic pregnancy rates. This information should be available in written form and given to the woman prior to discharge.

A patient record standard for tubal occlusion procedures in women is available in Appendix 2 of the RCOG guidelines.[3]

REVERSAL OF STERILIZATION

Reversal of female sterilization involves laparotomy (to access the occluded fallopian tubes) with all the surgical and anaesthetic risks associated with major abdominal surgery. Approximately 50% of women will achieve pregnancy following surgery to reconnect the tubes with around 10% of pregnancies being ectopic. Efficacy of the procedure is dependent on the original method of tubal occlusion used. The best rates occur in women who were sterilized with clips with lower rates achieved in women sterilized with rings. The lowest rates occur following partial salpingectomy or electrodiathermy, where a much larger section of tube is destroyed at the time of the primary surgery. Pregnancy rates are highest in the first year following reversal and higher in younger women. The procedure is rarely available within the NHS and few private medical policies provide cover for it. Current UK costs to the patient for the procedure are in the region of £3000 and in some cases, particularly where clips have not been used, in vitro fertilization (IVF) may provide a more cost-effective option.

REFERENCES

1. United Nations (2002) World population monitoring. New York: United Nations.

2. Taylor T, Keyse L, Bryant A (2006) Contraception and sexual health 2005/06. London: Office for National Statistics.

3. Royal College of Obstetricians and Gynaecologists (RCOG) (2004) Male and female sterilisation. Evidence based clinical Guideline Number 4. RCOG: London.

4. Hieu DT, Tran TT, Tan DN, et al. (1993) 31781 cases of non surgical female sterilization with Quinacrine pellets in Vietnam. Lancet 342: 213–217.

5. Duffy S, Marsh F, Rogerson L, et al. (2005) Female sterilisation: a cohort controlled comparative study of ESSURE versus laparoscopic sterilisation. BSOG 112(11): 1522–1528.

6. Peterson HB, Xia Z, Hughes JM, et al. (1996) The risk of pregnancy after tubal sterilization: findings from the US Collaborative Review of Sterilisation. Am J Obstet Gynecol 174: 1161–1170.

7. Peterson HB, Xia Z, Hughes JM, et al. (1997) The risk of ectopic pregnancy after tubal sterilization. New England Journal of Medicine 336(11): 762–767.

8. Schmidt JE, Hillis SD, Marchbanks EA, et al. (2000) Requesting information about and obtaining reversal after tubal sterilization: findings from the US Collaborative Review of Sterilization. Fertil Steril 74(5): 892–898.

9. Mattinson A, Mansour D (2006) Female sterilisation: is it what women really want or are alternative contraceptives acceptable? J Fam Plann Reprod Health Care 32(3): 181–183.

FURTHER READING

RCOG (2004) Consent advice for diagnostic laparoscopy. RCOG. http://www.rcog.org.uk

RCOG (2004) Sterilisation for women and men: what you need to know. RCOG. http://www.rcog.org.uk

13 Vasectomy

Richard A Anderson

Chapter contents

In Britain, almost 30% of all couples, and almost 50% of those over 40, are using either female or male sterilization as their method of contraception, with approximately 64000 vasectomies performed in England in 1999, compared to 47000 tubal ligations.[1] The number of vasectomies in the UK is however falling, as is the number of female sterilizations. While this may reflect the increased use of long-acting contraceptive methods changes in service provision are likely to be at least as important.

TECHNIQUES

Vasectomy involves the division or occlusion of the vas deferens to prevent the passage of sperm. It can be performed under local anaesthetic (LA, the preferred procedure) or general anaesthetic (GA) if there is a specific reason to avoid LA. A variety of techniques for vas division are available but the principle is the same in all of them. New techniques for occlusion are being developed, one aim being to make reversal easy and effective, thus perhaps in the future vasectomy may change from being a method of permanent sterilization to being one of the long-acting reversible methods.

Figure 13.1 Vas ligated

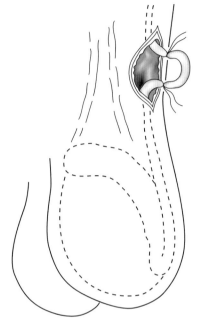

• Division and ligation

The vas is palpated through the skin of the upper scrotum and fixed either instrumentally or between the fingers and thumb. The vas within its fascial sheath is exposed through a small single midline skin incision or by two incisions, one on each side. The fascia is opened longitudinally and the vas ligated and divided (Figs 13.1 and 13.2). The evidence base for different techniques is not predominantly derived from randomized controlled trials but it is now established that interposing the fascial sheath between the cut ends of the vas (fascial interposition) increases the effectiveness of the procedure and should be routinely performed, and that clips may be less effective.[2,3] The sheath and scrotal skin are closed separately. Variations in technique include:

1. *The 'no-scalpel vasectomy' (NSV)*, developed in China in the 1970s is now regarded as the method of choice.[1] Specially designed instruments are used to isolate and deliver the vas through the scrotal skin after making a small puncture instead of an incision in the skin. It is claimed that NSV is quicker, and has a lower incidence of infection and haematoma: of the two studies addressing this, supportive evidence was provided by one (the larger) but not the other.[4]

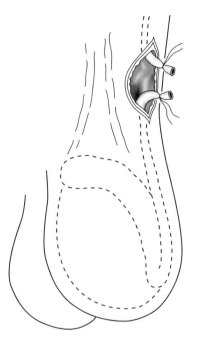

Figure 13.2 Vas divided

2. *Occlusion using unipolar diathermy* with a specifically designed needle probe which is passed 1 cm proximally and distally down the divided vas, coagulating the tissue for 3 to 4 seconds until the muscle becomes opaque. This technique may be more effective than excision with fascial interposition.[5]

3. *Excising a small portion of vas.* It is unlikely that this increases effectiveness unless at least 4 cm of vas is excised. Excision makes reversal more difficult but allows the portion of vas to be examined histologically. This may help in subsequent cases of litigation but it increases the cost and is not recommended in routine practice.

4. *Looping* each cut end of vas back on itself.

5. *Occlusion using a small clip.* Probably less effective and no longer recommended.

6. *Open-ended vasectomy* – the vas can simply be divided and the cut ends left open. This technique is seldom used as it is associated with higher failure rates but it does facilitate reversal.

Irrigation of the vas is not recommended as it does not increase success rates or time to clearance of sperm. Several studies have demonstrated that fascial interposition increases the success rate (azoospermia), and cautery of the vas lumen increases this still further.[2,3,5] However fascial interposition is also technically more difficult. Undoubtedly efficacy is partly dependent on the experience of the surgeon. Current guidance from the Faculty of Family Planning & Reproductive Healthcare (FFPRHC) states that trainees without relevant experience should perform 10 operating sessions or 40 procedures under supervision, and those with relevant prior surgical experience eight supervised procedures.[1]

• Vas occlusion

Percutaneous injection of sclerosing agents or occlusive intravas devices (IVDs) have been investigated. These techniques avoid skin incision and the plugs may be removable. A recent randomized trial compared a urethane intravas device (IVD) with NSV in nearly 300 men in China. The IVD was slightly less effective and took a little longer to insert, but postoperative recovery was quicker and satisfaction was scored higher.[6] Long-term failure rates remain to be established. Pressure within the proximal vas is lower than following vasectomy because the IVD acts as a filter rather than a complete plug which may account for the reduction in complications.

Yet a further possibility is the injection into the vas of substances that damage the sperm as they pass.[7] This has the advantage of being rapidly effective, but although effectiveness for at least 1 year has been demonstrated, the duration of action is unknown. Reversal may be possible by injection of a solvent into the vas, which dissolves the contraceptive chemical.

COUNSELLING

Most couples seeking sterilization have been thinking about the operation for some time. The counselling session should provide opportunities for information, explanation, discussion and advice and should enable a couple to decide what is in their own best interests. Whenever possible the couple should be seen together. The couple should be prepared to provide details about themselves, their circumstances and the reason for requesting sterilization. The counsellor should cover:

a. description of operation and associated myths/misconceptions
b. failure rates (1 in 2000 **after** clearance has been given)
c. risks/side effects
d. which partner should be sterilized
e. the alternative of using long-acting reversible methods as they are at least as effective as female sterilization and allow a change of heart
f. reversibility
g. possibility of wanting more children.

Information sought from the couple should include:

a. reason for the request
b. relevant medical history
c. age, occupation and social circumstances
d. numbers, ages and health of their children
e. previous and current contraception and any problems experienced
f. stability of the marriage and the possibility of its breakdown
g. quality of their sexual life.

Vasectomy is often done under LA in a clinic setting or in the general practitioner's surgery. Specially trained nurses may do the counselling and only seek a medical opinion if there are contraindications, doubts or clinical problems. Sessionally employed surgeons operate on men who have been counselled by someone else. Locally agreed protocols should protect the surgeon from being faced with a patient he/she would prefer not to sterilize for whatever reason.

ASSESSMENT

A history should be taken to exclude anything which may complicate the operation and which may determine whether LA or GA should be used. These should include:

1. A history of previous genital or inguinal surgery, e.g. orchidopexy.
2. A history of reaction to LA or contraindications to GA (including fear or extreme anxiety).

EXAMINATION

Where the man is not seen by the surgeon until the actual operation, it is good practice to examine the man prior to recommending him for vasectomy. It is annoying for the patient and a waste of operating time if a problem which precludes vasectomy under LA is not discovered until the patient is being prepared for surgery.

TIMING OF OPERATION

Some couples see pregnancy as a convenient time during which the vasectomy can become effective but surgeons may insist on delay until the safe delivery of a healthy baby. Each couple should be considered individually in respect of timing of the operation.

PREOPERATIVE AND POSTOPERATIVE ADVICE

1. The patient is usually asked to shave the upper scrotum himself before he attends for operation – this saves both time and embarrassment.

2. He is advised to wear underpants which give good scrotal support for a few days after the procedure.

3. Most men return to work the following day but the risk of haematoma formation is probably reduced if strenuous physical exercise is avoided for 3 or 4 days.

4. It **must** be made clear that it takes some time for remaining sperm to disappear from the distal vas and that an alternative method of contraception **must** be used until there is azoospermia. The rate at which azoospermia is achieved depends on the frequency of ejaculation, but age is also a factor independent of ejaculation frequency. Older men take longer to achieve azoospermia. In developing countries without facilities for semen analysis, couples are advised to use other contraception until after 20 ejaculations. In the UK, seminal fluid is examined after 12 and 16 weeks and, if sperm are still present, usually monthly thereafter. Not until two consecutive negative samples have been confirmed can the vasectomy be considered complete. Clear instructions for the collection of specimens and their delivery to the laboratory should be given to the patient who should be informed once the vasectomy is complete. Despite this, approximately 10% of men will not complete follow-up.

5. Men who experience complications or in whom vasectomy fails seem particularly ready to sue. It is imperative that counselling for vasectomy is clear and detailed and covers every eventuality. A checklist which counsellors tick as they cover all the points in discussion with the couple may help (see Appendix 13.1). In Edinburgh, a detailed information leaflet (Appendix 13.2) is sent out with the first appointment informing the couple about complications and the failure rate before they attend for counselling. They are asked to sign a form stating that they have read and understood the information sheet in addition to the standard operation consent form.

COMPLICATIONS

• Early

1. *Bruising and haematoma.* Some scrotal bruising is very common but in 1–2% of men postoperative bleeding will be sufficient to cause a haematoma. Local scrotal support and analgesia are usually

adequate treatment but admission to hospital for drainage of the haematoma may be required.

2. *Wound infection* occurs in up to 5% of men, and can occasionally be serious.

3. *Immediate failure* – up to 2% of men fail to achieve azoospermia. If many sperm are present, the possibility of repeating the vasectomy can be discussed. Rarely, if very few *non-motile* sperm persist in the ejaculate the surgeon and patient may agree that this indicates that the operation has been successful but this decision should be made cautiously. Recanalization can also occur over the initial months following operation, and may result in the first sample being azoospermic yet sperm being present in the second.

• Late

1. *Sperm granulomas* – small lumps may form at the cut ends of the vas as a result of a local inflammatory response to leaked sperm. These may be painful and persistent. Excision usually solves the problem.

2. *Chronic intrascrotal pain and discomfort* (post-vasectomy syndrome) – some men complain of a dull ache in the scrotum which may be exacerbated by sexual excitement and ejaculation. The symptoms are probably due to distension and granuloma formation in the epididymis and vas deferens. Pain may also result from scar tissue forming around small nerves. Chronic pain may require excision of the epididymis and obstructed vas deferens.

3. *Late recanalization* – failure can occur up to 10 years after vasectomy despite two negative samples following the procedure. It is rare (1 in 2000) but pregnancy as a result of late recanalization is always a sensitive issue. Seminal analysis can be offered but the presence of small numbers of sperm in the ejaculate can be intermittent and if no sperm are seen in the ejaculate this may cause major problems for the couple. Every case must be handled individually but it is sometimes best simply to offer a re-do without semen analysis.

4. *Antisperm antibodies* – after vasectomy, most men develop detectable concentrations of autoantibodies presumably in response to backpressure and leakage of sperm. Their presence may compromise fertility if reversal is sought.

5. *Cardiovascular disease* – There is no evidence that vasectomy increases atherosclerosis in men. Several large studies have suggested that vasectomy is associated with a lower death rate.[8] In an analysis of the husbands of women who took part in the Nurses Health Study, vasectomy was associated with reductions

in mortality from cardiovascular disease (relative risk, 0.76; 95% confidence interval, 0.63–0.92), and was unrelated to mortality from all forms of cancer.[9]

6. *Cancer* –Testicular cancer is no more common in men who have been vasectomized than in other men.[10] A recent analysis of over 20 studies concluded that while men with a vasectomy may be at a small increased risk of prostate cancer, bias could not be excluded.[11]

INDICATIONS

1. Couples who are absolutely certain that their family is complete.
2. Individuals or couples who choose to have no children.
3. When one partner:
   a. carries a significant risk of transmitting an inherited disorder
   b. suffers from chronic ill-health which would (in the case of the woman) contraindicate pregnancy or affect the couple's ability to bring up children.

In the last two instances, it is sensible to sterilize the affected partner.

CONTRAINDICATIONS

Unless couples are absolutely certain that, for whatever reason, they want no, or no more, children, sterilization should not be performed. Up to 10% of couples regret the decision to undergo sterilization and 1% will seek reversal. Factors which are known to increase the risk of regret include:

1. Marital/relationship problems.
2. Young age.
3. Timing of sterilization – women who are sterilized immediately postpartum or post-abortion are more likely to seek reversal, and the same is likely to be true for men.
4. Psychiatric illness in either partner.

ADVANTAGES

The advantages of *male as opposed to female sterilization* are:

1. It is a simpler, cheaper, more effective procedure.
2. It can be performed under local anaesthetic as an outpatient.
3. Mortality and significant operative morbidity are virtually non-existent.

The advantages of *female as opposed to male sterilization* are:

1. It is immediately effective.
2. A woman's reproductive life is finite; a man retains his fertility for many years and has potentially more opportunity to regret the decision to be sterilized.

DISADVANTAGES OF VASECTOMY

The disadvantages of vasectomy *as opposed to other reversible methods of contraception:*

1. It cannot always be reversed.
2. It is more complicated than alternative methods of contraception requiring the provision of specialized facilities and trained personnel.
3. It is not effective immediately, and lab testing is required to ensure effectiveness.

EFFECTIVENESS

Vasectomy is generally accepted as being more effective than female sterilization. The Oxford/FPA study found a failure rate of 0.02 per HWY after vasectomy (1 in 2000).[12]

REVERSIBILITY

Despite careful counselling that vasectomy is intended to be permanent, it is inevitable that a few couples will request reversal. This is most likely to happen when the marriage breaks down and one or other partner starts a new relationship, and is much more common when vasectomy has been performed at a young age.[13] Counselling for sterilization should include information on the success rates associated with reversal.

Sperm patency rates of up to 90% are reported with the use of micro-surgical vasovasostomy but pregnancy rates are lower (approximately 60%). While this is often attributed to the presence of anti-sperm antibodies their functional significance is unclear. The time interval between vasectomy and attempted reversal is an important predictor, with much lower success rates after 10 years. Alternatives include surgical sperm retrieval with sperm aspirated from the epididymis or extracted from a testicular biopsy for use in IVF/intracytoplasmic sperm injection. While widely available, this will generally be outwith the NHS and will also involve significant intervention for the female partner. Sperm may also be cryopreserved at the time of vasectomy reversal for potential use in ICSI if spontaneous pregnancy does not occur.[14]

Some laboratories now offer a sperm banking service prior to vasectomy. The availability of such services complicates counselling since this seems to contradict the advice that a couple should not consider vasectomy unless they are absolutely certain they want no more children. Very few men return to use stored sperm.[15]

REFERENCES

1. Royal College of Obstetricians and Gynaecologists (2004) Male and female sterilisation. Evidence-Based Clinical Guideline No 4. London: RCOG Press.

2. Cook LA, Van Vliet HA, Pun A, Gallo MF (2004) Vasectomy techniques for male sterilization: systematic Cochrane review of randomized controlled trials and controlled clinical trials. Hum Reprod 19: 2431–2438.

3. Labrecque M, Dufresne C, Barone MA, St-Hilaire K (2004) Vasectomy surgical techniques: a systematic review. BMC Med 2: 21.

4. Cook LA, Pun A, van Vliet H, Gallo MF, Lopez LM (2006) Scalpel versus no-scalpel incision for vasectomy. Cochrane Database Syst Rev CD004112.

5. Sokal D, Irsula B, Chen-Mok M, Labrecque M, Barone MA (2004) A comparison of vas occlusion techniques: cautery more effective than ligation and excision with fascial interposition. BMC Urol 4: 12.

6. Song L, Gu Y, Lu W, Liang X, Chen Z (2006) A phase II randomized controlled trial of a novel male contraception, an intra-vas device. Int J Androl 29: 489–495.

7. Chaudhury K, Bhattacharyya AK, Guha SK (2004) Studies on the membrane integrity of human sperm treated with a new injectable male contraceptive. Hum Reprod 19: 1826–1830.

8. Massey FJ, Jr., Bernstein GS, O'Fallon WM, et al. (1984) Vasectomy and health. Results from a large cohort study. JAMA 252: 1023–1029.

9. Giovannucci E, Tor D, Tosteson SD, Speizer FE, Martin P, Vessey MP, Colditz GA (1992) A long-term study of mortality in men who have undergone vasectomy. New England Journal of Medicine 326: 1392–1398.

10. Moller H, Knudsen LB, Lynge E (1994) Risk of testicular cancer after vasectomy: cohort study of over 73,000 men. BMJ 309: 295–299.

11. Dennis LK, Dawson DV, Resnick MI (2002) Vasectomy and the risk of prostate cancer: a meta-analysis examining vasectomy status, age at vasectomy, and time since vasectomy. Prostate Cancer Prostatic Dis 5: 193–203.

12. Vessey M, Lawless M, Yeates D (1982) Efficacy of different contraceptive methods. Lancet 1: 841–842.

13. Potts JM, Pasqualotto FF, Nelson D, Thomas AJ, Jr., Agarwal A (1999) Patient characteristics associated with vasectomy reversal. J Urol 161: 1835–1839.

14. Glazier DB, Marmar JL, Mayer E, Gibbs M, Corson SL (1999) The fate of cryopreserved sperm acquired during vasectomy reversals. J Urol 161: 463–466.

15. Audrins P, Holden CA, McLachlan RI, Kovacs GT (1999) Semen storage for special purposes at Monash IVF from 1977 to 1997. Fertil Steril 72: 179–181.

Appendix 13.1

Family Planning & Well Woman Services	PATIENTS NAME:
	CLINIC NO:
Partner's name:	No of children in current relationship:
Partner's age:	Ages of children:
Length of relationship:	Health of children:
Partner present at counselling YES/NO	No of other children:
Reason for vasectomy:	Consideration of female sterilization:
Failure rate:	Failure rate: Other long term methods:

Relationships/sexual relationships

Partner's medical and gynaecological history

CHECK LIST: Please tick

Loss of child ....
Loss of partner ....
Breakdown of relationship ....
Irreversibility ....

EFFECTS OF OPERATION
Testes ....
Sperm ....
Seminal fluid ....

EFFICACY
Short term failure rate ...
Long term failure rate ....
Recanalization 1 in 2000 ....
Reversal requests ....

DETAILS OF OPERATION
Anatomy ....
Technique ....
Local anaesthetic ....
Sutures ....

PROBLEMS OF OPERATION
Pain ....
Haematoma 1 in 100 ....
Infection ....

LONG TERM EFFECTS
Antibodies ....
Prostate cancer ....
Testicular cancer ....
Sperm granuloma ....
Testicular pain ....

PRACTICAL ADVICE
Pre Op shaving ....
Post Op tests for fertility
  (12 & 16 weeks) ....
Continued ejaculation req ...
Post Op contraception ....

CONSENT ....

Recommendations

NAME: SIGNATURE: DATE:

SEMINAL ANALYSIS			
No.	Date sent	Date Report recd.	Result

Final Notification of Completion:

G.P. notified..

patient notified...

Appendix 13.2

VASECTOMY INFORMATION

You have expressed an interest in vasectomy and have been given an assessment appointment to come and discuss the procedure before a date is arranged for your operation. It may be useful for your partner to come along too, but this is not essential.

This leaflet tells you about the operation, its reliability and possible problems. In preparing this leaflet, we have used information from medical studies as well as feedback and comments from men who have had a vasectomy. It is designed to give you the facts and to help you decide if vasectomy is right for you. It is not meant to sound off-putting but it is important we tell you about the rare complications as well as the many advantages of vasectomy. This first appointment gives you a chance to discuss any questions or concerns and it allows us to find out if there are any reasons the procedure cannot be performed for example under local anaesthetic.

You might find it helpful to keep this leaflet until after your operation, as it also tells you what to expect after a vasectomy.

- ### What is vasectomy?

A tube called the vas deferens carries sperm from each testis into the penis. Vasectomy involves cutting or blocking both these tubes to prevent the passage of sperm. The tubes are cut just above the testis. Vasectomy does not otherwise interfere with the production of seminal fluid so you will not notice any difference in the fluid you produce when you ejaculate. The fluid simply will not contain sperm and may not look quite as milky in colour. It may look slightly bloody in the first few weeks after your operation. There should be no difference in your sexual function.

The operation is done under local anaesthetic in this clinic (similar to the injection used at the dentist). We do not 'put you to sleep' with a general anaesthetic, so there is no need to avoid eating beforehand. In fact it is probably better to make sure you have eaten a meal or snack before you come in. Vasectomy takes around 10 to 20 minutes. A very small cut is made in the skin on each side of the scrotum, or sometimes just one cut is made in the middle. The tubes, which lie just beneath the skin, are blocked or cut on both sides. The small skin cuts are closed with a dissolvable stitch. These do not need to be removed but if they become tight or uncomfortable

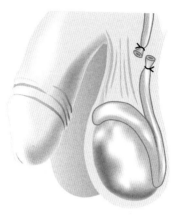

they can be removed. Some men worry that their stitches gape a little or even come out, but this does not usually matter.

• How effective is vasectomy? What is meant by short-term failure?

After the operation, you and your partner must continue to use another method of contraception until you receive the 'all clear' from us. It takes 16 weeks or longer for remaining sperm in your tubes to clear away. The time that this takes depends on how often you have sex. On average the sperm will not be completely cleared until you have ejaculated 20+ times. You will be asked to send 2 semen samples, obtained during ejaculation, at 12 and 16 weeks after the operation. Staff at the laboratory will check to make sure there are no sperm. If both samples are free of sperm we will inform you that you can stop using your previous method of contraception. If your samples continue to contain sperm, we will ask you to continue to use another method of contraception and to send in further samples at 3-week intervals, until two consecutive samples are free of sperm.

Around 2% of men still continue to produce samples containing large numbers of sperm. This can indicate that the operation has failed. This is very disappointing; the only compensation is that you find out from a lab report, rather than an unexpected pregnancy, as when other methods of contraception fail. If this happens you would be invited to speak to the surgeon about the possibility of repeating the operation, which sometimes needs to be done under general anaesthetic in hospital.

• What is meant by long-term failure?

This is much rarer than short-term failure and only happens to 1 in 2000 men. The vasectomy is initially successful, there are two semen samples free of sperm and the all clear is given. At a later stage, even years later, the ends of the tubes join back together and allow sperm to pass again, which may result in pregnancy.

• Rare non-motile sperm

Up to a third of men may produce a positive result at the 12-week sample. This shows a small number of sperm only. This very often clears to become negative in subsequent samples, with some men it takes a long time to clear the samples, again this is very disappointing. If this situation persists, discussion with the surgeon follows to decide on further options which may include a re-do operation.

• What are the advantages of vasectomy?

Vasectomy is more reliable than most of the other methods of contraception. Even female sterilization has a failure rate of 1 in 200. Once you have been given the all clear the chance of failure is only 1 in 2000. Vasectomy is a quicker, safer operation than female sterilization and does not generally require hospital visits or general anaesthetic.

Unlike the contraceptive pill or injection, there is no possibility of hormonal side-effects like headache or mood swings. Your own hormones are unaffected. There is no need to remember to take a pill every day, or an injection every few months. Unlike the condom, or cap, there is no interference with sexual intercourse.

• Are there any problems?

For most men, there are no significant problems after vasectomy. The complications that can be experienced occur either immediately or much later.

• Short-term problems

Up to 10% of men experience minor local problems after the operation. Once the local anaesthetic wears off, after about 2 hours, you probably feel some discomfort. You are unlikely to need anything stronger than paracetamol. If you will have a long journey back home, remember to ask for painkillers before you leave the clinic, or bring some with you.

Most men notice some bruising and swelling around the operation site which lasts just a few days. Sometimes the site can become infected and persistent pain, swelling, redness or discharge from the stitch line are signs to see your GP in case you need antibiotics for an infection. Occasionally the infection involves the testis itself this presents as a red hot swollen testicle which sometimes requires intravenous antibiotics in hospital.

Rarely, a small amount of bleeding continues after the operation and blood collects as a large swelling or 'haematoma' at the base of the scrotum. If this happens, it usually clears up spontaneously but a small minority of men (1:100) with a haematoma need hospital treatment or an operation.

Even then, it does not cause any long-term problems. If you think you have a problem after the vasectomy, we are very happy to speak to you over the phone to discuss things and may well be able to reassure you. However, if it seems that you need to be seen by a doctor, much the quickest way to get an appointment is to see your GP. The surgeons who perform vasectomy here only come in to operate and are not generally available for the post-operative consultations. Your GP should be happy to examine you and give you advice.

AFTER THE OPERATION

• How much time should I take off work?

This really depends on what type of job you do. If your job involves a lot of physical activity, you will need to take things easy and avoid anything which causes discomfort at the operation site. Most men only take a couple of days off work but if your job is very heavy, or you still feel uncomfortable, you may need a week or so. If you take a lot of physical exercise in the first few days after the operation you may be more likely to develop a haematoma.

• When can I resume sexual intercourse?

You can start having sex when you feel comfortable to do so, but don't be alarmed if you notice a small amount of blood in the seminal fluid. This should clear quickly. Remember that it is repeated sexual intercourse (or ejaculation) which clears all the sperm out of your tubes after the vasectomy.

• Long-term problems

1. Chronic scrotal pain

   In postal surveys, up to 3 in 10 men say that they experience some testicular pain 3 months after the operation. The cause of this pain is unknown. Most settle down with no treatment. At the end of 1 year 6–8% of men are still complaining of some scrotal discomfort. There are operations that can be performed which can relieve this pain. Very few of them do require such an operation. Some men do say they wish they had not had the operation for this reason.

2. Sperm granuloma

   In some 10–15% of men, leakage of sperm from the cut ends of the tube causes some inflammation and discomfort. In less that 1% of men, small painful lumps called 'sperm granulomas' may appear. This problem rarely persists and only very rarely requires further surgery.

3. Testicular and prostate cancer

   Having a vasectomy does not increase your risk of testicular cancer.

   There is still some debate with regards to increased risk of prostate cancer. However, there is increasing evidence that there is in fact no increased risk of prostate cancer following vasectomy operations.

In conclusion most experts now believe that vasectomy does not increase the risk of any serious diseases.

• Can vasectomy be reversed?

Vasectomy is intended to be irreversible. If you have any doubt at all about your plans to have more children, it is better not to have a vasectomy at this point in your life. Sometimes feelings or circumstances change after a vasectomy. Reversal operations are not routinely available on the NHS and cost the patient over £2000. The chances of achieving pregnancy after reversal of vasectomy may be as low as 1 in 5 or as high as 4 in 5, depending on the length of time since vasectomy and the age and fertility of your partner. Fifty percent of men may eventually produce antibodies against their own sperm and this may make reversal less likely to be successful.

It is possible to make arrangements for you to store your sperm as an insurance policy against changing your mind. There is a charge for banking sperm and you should bear in mind that if you and your partner ever wanted to use the stored sperm that the procedures involved (artificial insemination) are complicated and time consuming and success is not guaranteed. If you would like to know more about sperm banking please ask for information but bear in mind that vasectomy is meant to be irreversible and if you seriously wonder whether you might change your mind perhaps you are not ready for a vasectomy.

14 Sexual health services for young people

Paula Baraitser

Chapter contents

INTRODUCTION

The World Health Organization (WHO) defines young people as aged between 10 and 24 years and adolescents as those aged 10–19 years. More than 1 billion young people are in their second decade of life and 85% of these live in developing countries.[1] Young people are not a homogeneous group and their sexual health needs vary according to age, sex, individual experience and social context. Worldwide they carry a disproportionate burden of sexual ill health; limited access to sexual health services and information exacerbates this.

Interventions to improve sexual health among young people should acknowledge the internationally agreed rights of adolescents to gender equality, education and health including reproductive and sexual health information and to services appropriate to their age, capacities and circumstances.[2]

This chapter reviews the burden of sexual ill health experienced by young people worldwide and relates this to sexual behaviour and the causes of sexual ill health, particularly among vulnerable groups. Following this review it describes strategies to improve sexual ill health among young people including young-people-friendly services, education and outreach. The chapter focuses on sexual health in the United Kingdom but provides an international context for this discussion.

SEXUAL HEALTH AMONG YOUNG PEOPLE: AN INTERNATIONAL PERSPECTIVE

Young people experience high rates of sexual and reproductive ill health including sexually transmitted infections, unintended pregnancy, the consequences of poor access to obstetric care, unsafe abortion and coerced sexual relationships. The levels and types of morbidity and mortality vary between countries but across all continents young people are at higher risk of sexual ill health than their older peers. This section summarizes current data on sexual ill health among young people.

• Sexually transmitted infections

In the United Kingdom rates of diagnoses of sexually transmitted infections (STIs) continue to rise among those aged 16–24. In 2004 young women and men in this age group accounted for 74% and 56% of all chlamydia diagnoses and 70% and 41% of gonorrhoea diagnoses respectively. Among sexually active adolescents the prevalence of chlamydia infection is 10% in most settings. In the United States there are approximately 19 million STIs diagnosed each year and almost half of these are among young people aged 15–24.[3] These infections increase the risk of ectopic pregnancy and tubal infertility.

• Teenage pregnancy

Since the early 1980s birth rates among young people under 20 have been consistently higher in the UK than those in comparable Western European countries.[4] Although some pregnancies may be intended, many are not and 39% of pregnancies among girls under 20 years and 54% among under-16-year-olds end in abortion.[5] Early child bearing in the UK is associated with limited educational and employment opportunities.

In Eastern and Central Europe teenage pregnancy rates are three to four times higher and in the United States up to ten times higher than those

Table 14.1 Rate of births per 1000 women aged 15–19. Data are from 1998. Data from: UNICEF[6]

Country	Births
Korea	2.9
Japan	4.6
Switzerland	5.5
Netherlands	6.2
Sweden	6.5
Italy	6.6
Spain	7.9
Denmark	8.1
Greece	11.8
Germany	13.1
Czech Republic	16.4
Australia	18.4
Canada	20.2
New Zealand	29.8
USA	52.1

in Western Europe. The Netherlands and Switzerland have some of the lowest rates in Europe and Korea and Japan among the lowest in the world (Table 14.1).

• HIV infection

In the United Kingdom young people aged 16–24 account for about 11% of the HIV diagnoses each year. This figure has remained relatively constant over time. Between 1981 and 2005 10396 young people were diagnosed with HIV infection, 938 were diagnosed with AIDS and 481 had died.[7]

Worldwide, it is estimated that 50% of all new HIV infections are among young people (about 7000 young people become infected every day), and that 30% of the 40 million people living with HIV/AIDS are in the 15–24-year age group. The vast majority of young people who are HIV positive do not know that they are infected, and few sexually active young people know the HIV status of their partners (see 'Useful Websites').

Patterns of HIV infection among young people vary. In Eastern Europe and Central Asia nearly all reported HIV infections are linked to drug injection. In parts of Latin America and Asia and in many industrialized countries small epidemics exist among men who have sex with men. In much of sub-Saharan Africa the majority of new infections are among young people aged 15–24; young women are up to five times more likely to be infected as young men.[6]

• Those particularly vulnerable to sexual ill health

Poverty and female sex are consistently associated with sexual ill health among young people. Those who are poor often lack educational or livelihood opportunities, are less informed about sexual ill health and more vulnerable to abuse.

Gender inequalities contribute to sexual ill health. Young women in many cultures suffer severe restrictions on their freedom of movement, educational and personal development, security and life choices after puberty. In many societies gender inequalities mean that women find it difficult or impossible to choose their sexual partners or control their sexual activity. For many young women (married and unmarried) adolescence is a time of high risk of violence including sexual abuse. Nearly 50% of all sexual assaults worldwide involve girls aged 15 or younger.[1]

Unmarried sexually active young women suffer the consequences of unsafe abortion and lack of access to contraceptive and obstetric care. They are also more vulnerable to sexually transmitted infections, biologically, culturally and socio-economically than young men. Although the majority of STIs in women are asymptomatic their consequences, such as ectopic pregnancy and pelvic sepsis, may be life threatening. Unmarried young women suffer more stigma in seeking treatment for sexual ill health than young men who are often expected and encouraged to be sexually active during adolescence.

Gay, lesbian, bisexual and transgender young people suffer discrimination and therefore have very restricted access to relevant information on sexual health. This increases their risks of STIs including HIV. Few HIV prevention programmes target this group in developing countries.

Married adolescent women (see Table 14.2) are a group whose risk of sexual and reproductive ill health, particularly HIV infection, is often forgotten. Early marriage is strongly associated with poverty and few

Table 14.2 Percentage of women married before the age of 18 by region. Data from: UNICEF[9]

Region	% women married before the age of 18
Southern Asia	48
Latin America & the Caribbean	29
Africa	42

educational opportunities. Young married women are often socially isolated with limited autonomy and freedom of movement leading to a lack of access to reproductive health services. Girls aged 15–19 are twice as likely, and girls under 15 five times as likely, to die in childbirth as those in their twenties because of lack of access to obstetric care.[8]

SEXUAL BEHAVIOUR AMONG YOUNG PEOPLE

Sexual behaviour among young people changes with time and context. Across Western Europe mean age at first intercourse among women decreased after the 1960s by 2–3 years. It then remained stable until the early 1990s when there was a further small decrease.[10]

The behaviour of young people in Britain makes them vulnerable to sexually transmitted infection because they have more sexual partners, more concurrent partners and a higher frequency of partner change than their older peers.[11] The second British National Survey of Sexual Attitudes and Lifestyles (NATSAL2) reported a median age for first heterosexual intercourse of 16 years and 30% of men and 26% of women interviewed reported first heterosexual intercourse before 16 years.[12] Age at first intercourse is a useful measure of the potential demand for sexual health services among young people but tells us little about whether that demand is being met. Rates of contraceptive and/or condom use at first intercourse are often low; 7.4% of men and 9.8% of women aged 16–19 reported having used no contraception at first intercourse.[12]

In the United States in 2005, 47% of high school students had never had sexual intercourse.[13] Sexual behaviour among young people in the US is similar to that in Western Europe but rates of contraceptive use are lower leading to higher rates of teenage pregnancy.[14] More sophisticated numerical measures of early sexual experience have been developed to incorporate variations in individual development and the idea that first intercourse should be a positive and healthy experience.[12] Sexual competence is one such measure (see Box 14.1).

Box 14.1 Sexual competence incorporates the following variables:

- Regret – the extent to which a young person wished they had waited longer
- Willingness – extent to which partners were not equally willing
- Autonomy – reason for intercourse, e.g. the idea that intercourse was a natural progression of relationship is defined as high on a scale of autonomy and being drunk as the reason for intercourse is defined as low
- Whether effective contraception was used

(Adapted from Wellings et al.[12])

> **Box 14.2 Factors associated with increased risk of teenage pregnancy in the UK**
>
> - Poor educational attainment or employment aspirations
> - Risky sexual behaviour, for example non use of contraception at first intercourse or evidence of other risk-taking behaviours, for example involvement in crime or alcohol and substance misuse
> - Lack of accurate sexual health information
> - Problems accessing sexual health services
> - Difficulties in negotiating safer sex – particularly for young women
> - Lack of a supportive environment for personal development at home or at school, for example violence and bullying at school or lack of parental support

In the United Kingdom sexual non-competence increases with declining age, with 91% of girls and 67% of boys aged 13–14 identified as sexually non-competent at first intercourse.[12]

THE CAUSES OF SEXUAL ILL HEALTH AMONG YOUNG PEOPLE

Poor sexual health among young people reflects a complex combination of personal, social, economic and environmental factors. Socio-economic deprivation, poor opportunities for education and employment, inadequate sexual health information and services and pressures of gender and culture that promote high-risk sexual behaviours all contribute.

Learning from other countries suggests that cultural openness about sexuality, equitable income distribution across the population, good access to sexual health services and gender equality are associated with better sexual health indicators among young people.[14,15] In the Netherlands, for example, parents, health professionals and schools work together to promote positive attitudes to the needs of young people to learn about sex while avoiding the potential risks.[16] Similarly, in Sweden, teenage fertility rates decreased rapidly after 1975 as a result of improvements in the compulsory school sex education programme and contraceptive services reflecting an open and positive attitude to sexual activity among young people.[17]

Worldwide access to education for young women is associated with delayed childbearing, reduced poverty and increased autonomy and security for young women and girls and improved sexual health.

IMPROVING SEXUAL HEALTH AMONG YOUNG PEOPLE

Since sexual health is the product of personal, social, economic and environmental factors, interventions to improve the sexual health of young people should impact on all of these. The World Health Organization (WHO)[18] recommends that strategies to improve sexual health among young people should include four elements:

- Creating a safe and supportive environment through promoting delayed marriage and childbearing, expanding access to education and training, and providing income-earning opportunities.
- Providing information and skills (life and livelihood) so that adolescents are better equipped to make good decisions.
- Expanding access to health services that are affordable, accessible, confidential, and non-judgemental.
- Providing counselling for adolescents.

Improving social support for young people from family, schools and other relevant social institutions and the provision of counselling for adolescents is beyond the scope of this chapter. Sexual health services and sexual health information for young people are considered below.

SEXUAL HEALTH SERVICES FOR YOUNG PEOPLE

All sexual health services should be easy to get to and easy to find. They should provide a confidential service that is non-judgemental and friendly, with short waiting environments. Staff should be well trained and should provide the full range of contraceptive service in a pleasant environment.[19-21] These fundamentals apply to service provision for all age groups, however, young people's access to clinical service and sexual health information is often restricted and improving this is a priority. This section describes the features of young-people-friendly services.

• The setting for young-people-friendly services

High-quality sexual health services can be provided within a wide range of contexts. The setting for service provision will vary between health systems but the basic attributes of a high-quality service remain constant. In the United Kingdom sexual health services are provided by general practitioners and community pharmacists, and by specialist providers in sexual and reproductive health clinics, genito-urinary medicine departments and dedicated young people's services. In addition satellite services may be run in schools, youth clubs or from mobile units.

An holistic approach where all sexual-health-related services are provided together would potentially benefit users but there is no consensus on how to combine services for contraception, STIs, abortion counselling and sexual health promotion. In many developing countries, HIV prevention for young people and contraceptive services have taken priority and efforts to expand young people friendly services for the management of STIs have lagged behind.[22]

• The essential features of young-people-friendly services

To ensure that they are accessible and acceptable to young people sexual health services should:

- Be easy and inexpensive to get to with excellent public transport links
- Be easy to find with highly visible and clear signposting
- Have long opening times that are simple to understand, easy to remember and convenient for young people including evenings, weekends and after school
- Be well advertised in a form that is attractive and visible to this age group
- Require no fee for service or medication
- Have short waiting times and provide a pleasant environment to wait in
- Have friendly, welcoming and non-judgemental staff who understand and support the rights of young people to access sexual health services
- Display a clear and visible confidentiality policy
- Involve young people in regular evaluation of quality of care and have a commitment to act on the results of this evaluation.

• Confidentiality

Health professionals have a duty of care to all people, regardless of age, and young people's access to information and services should not be restricted.

Young people in the United Kingdom have the same rights to confidentiality during consultations with health professionals as adults except where there is a risk of harm to the young person or their peers. Where a health professional believes that there is a risk to the health, safety or welfare of a young person or others which is so serious as to outweigh the young person's right to privacy, they should follow locally agreed child protection protocols (Appendix 14.1). In these circumstances, the over-riding objective must be to safeguard the young person. Concern about a lack of confidentiality is an important barrier to the use of sexual health services by young people and information about local confidentiality policies should be clearly displayed including the circumstances in which confidentiality may be breached.

• Staff attitudes

A friendly, welcoming and non-judgemental approach is valued by all sexual health service users but is particularly important where negative social attitudes to sexual activity by young people exist. Staff support, training and ongoing evaluation of user experience is important to identify and change inappropriate staff attitudes. Young people's views on staff attitudes should be actively sought in an environment where they feel comfortable and confident to relate their experiences.

• Involving young people in the development and evaluation of services

Young people, like all service users, have an essential contribution to make to service development. Strategies for involvement may range from recording young people's requirements for a high-quality service to involvement in service planning, development and evaluation. A wide range of methodologies may be used from formal focus groups or interviews or mystery shopper programmes to less formal methods such as waiting room graffiti boards or comments card schemes. Each will deliver different types of data and different experiences of involvement. In all cases the contribution of young people to the process should be formally valued and acknowledged.

Many of the attributes of high-quality services for young people are the same as those of high-quality services for all age groups. Young people have provided a wealth of information on their expectations. Implementing their recommendations would improve the quality of sexual health services in general.

PREVENTING HIV INFECTION AMONG YOUNG PEOPLE

Every day between 5000 and 6000 young people aged 15–24 become newly infected with HIV. Sexual health services have an important role to play in preventing HIV infection and the WHO recommends the following key strategies:[18]

- Develop young people's knowledge about the transmission of HIV, and their personal skills in daily life to avoid the risks of infection
- Increase access to services and supplies to avoid or treat infections
- Create a safe and supportive social environment that, for example, reduces levels of sexual violence
- Provide opportunities for young people to participate and contribute.

Interventions to implement these strategies might include sexual health information programmes in schools and young-people-friendly sexual health services. In addition media campaigns to promote safer sexual behaviour and community outreach to ensure that those most at risk have access to the information and services that they need are important.

SEX EDUCATION/SEXUAL HEALTH INFORMATION FOR YOUNG PEOPLE

Good sex education programmes provide accurate and relevant information about sex, sexual identity and sexual relationships. They support the development of the skills that young people need to make informed decisions about their sexual behaviour and to implement these choices.

Education on sexual health and relationships should start before puberty with an age-appropriate primary school sex education programme. Teacher-delivered school sex education programmes should have clear learning outcomes and be provided by well-trained staff who are comfortable with the subject. Teacher-delivered programmes may be supplemented by educational outreach programmes from clinical services. These could provide practical information on service use and an opportunity to meet clinic staff. Parents may also benefit from support to help them discuss sexual health issues with their children and young people may value peer education programmes delivered by and for young people. Sex education programmes should include discussion of sexuality and health information for gay, lesbian and bisexual young people. They should include specific information on contraceptive methods, sexually transmitted infections and how to avoid them and how to access clinical services.[23]

Early provision of sexual health information is not associated with early onset of sexual activity. On the contrary it is likely to delay sexual activity and reduce unintended pregnancy and sexually transmitted infection.[24] There is no high-quality scientific evidence to support the effectiveness of education programmes that aim only to delay sexual activity among young people without providing information on the topics listed above.[25]

SEXUAL HEALTH INFORMATION SERVICES FOR YOUNG MEN

Young men may perceive contraceptive services to be exclusively for women and feel excluded from them. They often lack access to sexual health information and may feel social pressure to conform to cultural stereotypes of masculinity that encourage high-risk sexual behaviour. Young gay men may feel particularly isolated and in need of support and information.

Young men need opportunities to discuss sexual health in a supportive environment and they need services where they feel welcome. They often value carefully facilitated, small group discussion in informal environments such as sports facilities or youth clubs with the opportunity to discuss in confidence, with an appropriately trained and trusted adult, any concerns raised by the group session.

CONTRACEPTIVE METHODS FOR YOUNG PEOPLE

The indications and contraindications for most methods of contraception apply to young people and readers are referred to the chapters on individual methods. The UK Medical Eligibility Criteria for Contraceptive Use among young people are summarized in Table 14.3.

Table 14.3 UK Medical Eligibility Criteria for women under 20 years

	Contraceptive method				
	Combined hormonal contraception; 1 progestogen-only pill; 1 emergency contraception; 1 barrier methods 1	Fertility awareness based methods[c]	Sterilization[c]	Cu IUD/ LNG IUD 2	Long acting progestogen-only methods Implanon 1 Depo-Provera 2
Guidance in relation to young age	No restriction on medical grounds in relation to age	Menstrual irregularities are common post-menarche and may render these methods more difficult to learn and use	Up to 20% of women sterilized at a younger age later regret this decision. Young age is one of the strongest identifiable predictors of regret	Risk of sexually transmitted infection relates to sexual behaviour LNG IUD may be difficult to insert due to its wider diameter	Evidence shows decreased bone mineral density over time among adolescent DMPA users but not among levonorgestrel implant users. No evidence for increased risk of fracture

[c]Caution

Young people should be given complete and accurate information on all methods of contraception and be supported to make a decision based on their personal preferences and circumstances. No contraceptive method should be recommended or withheld on the basis of age alone, but in each case the risks and benefits of a particular method should be discussed in relation to the individual's preferences, requirements and circumstances. Young people should be advised against the use of regular hormonal contraception before menarche and if sexually active should be advised to use condoms.[20]

Since fertility during adolescence is high there is little margin for error in contraceptive use and young people should be aware of this when considering less-effective methods such as the diaphragm, methods which require regular action such as oral contraceptives or those that are intercourse-related such as condoms. Young people who are new to a particular contraceptive method will require clear instructions reinforced by written information and an opportunity to ask questions. All contraceptive consultations should include information about emergency contraception and how to access it in case of contraceptive error.

As in all contraceptive consultations risk of sexually transmitted infection as well as pregnancy should be assessed and information about strategies for prevention and treatment provided.

• Barrier methods

Condoms are often the first method of contraception that a young person uses. Most young people in the UK are aware of condoms as a contraceptive option but may require clear and detailed information on how to use them. Condoms in the UK are available without the need to visit a health professional but accessing them from any source may be perceived as embarrassing. Negotiation of consistent condom use may be a challenge for young people who are worried that this may imply that they have a history of high-risk sexual behaviour or a lack of trust in their partner. The disadvantage of the relatively low contraceptive effectiveness of condoms compared with hormonal contraceptives is arguably outweighed by their effectiveness in preventing infection including HIV. Diaphragms and caps are seldom used by teenagers. Although they are as effective as male condoms for pregnancy prevention they have little benefit in terms of STI prevention.

• Oral contraception

Young people may change their method of contraception from condom use to oral contraceptives once they feel that a relationship is established. This transition may put them at risk of sexually transmitted infections that are carried asymptomatically by one of the partners and continued condom use or infection screening should be recommended. Classical progestogen-only pills (POP) which must be taken at the same time each day demand rigorous adherence to this routine if they are to provide effective contraception. The desogestrel-containing POP (Cerazette®) has a 12-hour window for taking missed pills and so is no more demanding than the combined pill. However, both types of oral contraceptives rely heavily on consistent and correct use for their effectiveness and failure rates are relatively high among young people. The commonest reason for discontinuation of hormonal contraception is perceived weight gain; the lack of an effect of oral contraceptives on weight and the potential beneficial effect of combined hormonal contraception on acne should be discussed with all young people.

See Table 14.4 for types of contraception used by different age groups.

• Long-acting contraception

Long-acting contraceptive methods have lower failure rates than those that require daily pill taken or intercourse-related activity. Increasing numbers of young people use Depo-Provera® (Table 14.3). Unlike other hormonal contraceptives, weight gain does appear to be causally related to the use of Depo-Provera® and its effect on bone mineral density should be considered (see Chapter 5). The UK Committee on Safety of Medicine (CSM) in 2005 advised that Depo-Provera® could be used by adolescents provided other contraceptive methods had been found to be unacceptable or inappropriate. Their advice that use of Depo-Provera® should be reviewed after 2 years is commonly misinterpreted to mean that women, particularly young women, can use the method for *only* 2 years, which is not the case. The UK Medical Eligibility Criteria state that the benefits of using Depo-Provera®

Table 14.4 Current use of contraception (%) by age. Data from the Omnibus ONS Survey on Contraception and Sexual Health 2005/06

Method	16–17	18–19	20–24
Pill	69	60	63
Male condom	78	50	43
Withdrawal	6	–	4
IUD	–	2	–
Injection	4	17	6
Implant	8	4	7
Fertility awareness	–	–	–
Cap/diaphragm	–	–	2
Spermicide	4	–	–
IUS	–	–	–
Female condom	–	6	0
Emergency contraception	12	–	1

outweigh the theoretical risks for women under 18 years of age (category 2). The risks of unintended pregnancy (which also reduces bone mineral density) outweigh the concerns about the effect of Depo-Provera® on risk of fracture. The effect on bone mineral density plateaus after 2 years but risk of unintended pregnancy continues.

Low-dose long-acting progestogen-only contraception in the form of contraceptive implants requires no action by the user during the 3 years between fitting and removal. The risk of unpredictable bleeding should be carefully discussed prior to insertion. There appears to be no clinically significant effect of progestogen-only contraceptive implants on bone mineral density.

In a study of 400 teenage mothers in California[26] given the choice of condoms, pills or implants for contraception there were no pregnancies among the 64% of girls who continued using Norplant for 2 years. One-third of girls using the pill and one-third of those using condoms were pregnant again within 2 years and only 34% and 42% respectively were continuing to use the method.

• Intrauterine contraception

Intrauterine contraception is rarely used by young people under 20. Young people are more likely to be at risk of sexually transmitted infection and insertion may be difficult if the uterus is small (particularly the intrauterine system). Nonetheless, these methods are not contraindicated for young people at low risk of sexually transmitted infection who choose to use this method. Difficulties with insertion may be overcome by the use of local anaesthetic.

CONCLUSION

Young people are a vulnerable group often with limited power to demand services or information. They suffer significant morbidity and mortality from sexually transmitted infections and the consequences of unintended pregnancy, unsafe abortion and childbirth. Much of this burden of ill health is preventable through high-quality sex and relationship education (starting before puberty) and good access to excellent clinical services. Sexual health service providers could improve the situation of young people still further by lobbying for universal access to education particularly for young girls, gender equality and promoting sexual health service use by young men.

REFERENCES

1. UNICEF (2003) Adolescents: Profiles in Empowerment. New York.
2. UNFPA (2003) State of the Worlds Population: Investing in Adolescents Health and Rights, New York.

3. Weinstock H, Berman S, Cates W (2004) Sexually transmitted diseases among American youth: Incidence and prevalence estimates, 2000. Perspectives on Sexual and Reproductive Health 36(1): 6–10.

4. Department of Education and Skills (2006) Teenage Pregnancy Next Steps: Guidance for Local Authorities and Primary Care Trusts on Effective Delivery of Local Strategies.

5. Office of National Statistics (2001) Abortion Statistics, Series AB 28, TSO: London.

6. UNICEF (2002) Young people and HIV/AIDS Opportunity in Crisis. New York.

7. Health Protection Agency (2006) A Complex Picture. HIV and Other Sexually Transmitted Infections in the United Kingdom. London.

8. United Nations (2001) We the Children: End-Decade Review of the Follow-up to the World Summit for Children: Report of the Secretary-General (A/S-27/3). New York: United Nations.

9. UNICEF (2005) Early Marriage: A Harmful Traditional Practice. New York: United Nations.

10. Bajos N, Guillaume A, Kontula O (2003) Reproductive health behaviour of young Europeans. Population Studies 42.

11. Johnson A, Mercer C, Erens B, et al. (2001) Sexual behaviour in Britain: Partnerships, practices and HIV risk behaviours. Lancet 358: 1835–1842.

12. Wellings K, Nanchahal K, Macdowall W, et al. (2001) Sexual behavour in Britian: early heterosexual experience. Lancet 358: 1843–1850.

13. CDC (2006) Youth Risk Behavior Surveillance—United States, 2005 [pdf 300K]. Morbidity & Mortality Weekly Report 55(SS-5): 1–10.

14. Alan Guttmacher Institute (2001) Can More Progress Be Made? Teenage Sexual and Reproductive Behavior in Developed Countries, New York.

15. Cheesbrough S, Ingham R, Massey D (1999) A review of the international evidence on preventing and reducing teenage conceptions: The United States, Canada, Australia and New Zealand. Health Education Authority, London.

16. Thompson E (1993) Personal services. Health Service Journal, 29th April, 30–31.

17. Santow G, Bracher M (1999) Explaining trends in teenage childbearing in Sweden. Studies in Family Planning 30: 169–182.

18. WHO (2004) Protecting young people from HIV and AIDS: The role of health services. WHO: Geneva.

19. Teenage Pregnancy Unit (2001) Best practice advice on the delivery of contraceptive services and advice for young people. www.doh.gov.uk/tpu

20. FFPRHC (2004) Guidance on contraceptive choices for young people. Journal of Family Planning and Reproductive Health Care 30: 237–251.

21. Baraitser P, Pearce V, Blake G, Collander-Brown K, Ridley A (2005) Involving service users in sexual health service development. Journal of Family Planning and Reproductive Health Care 31(4): 281–284.

22. Dehne K, Riedner G (2005) Sexually Transmitted Infections among Adolescents: The need for adequate health services. WHO: Geneva.

23. Satelli et al. (2006) Abstinence only education policies and programs: A position paper of the Society for Adolescent Medicine. Journal for Adolescent Health 38: 83–87.

24. Baldo M (1994) Does sex education lead to earlier or increased sexual activity in youth? World Health Organization Global Programme on AIDS, Geneva.

25. Manlove J, Romana-Papillo A, Ikramullah E (2004) Not Yet: Programs to Delay First Sex among Teens. Washington DC. National Campaign to Prevent Teenage Pregnancy.

26. Darney PD, Callegari LS, Swift A, Atkinson ES, Robert AM (1998) Condom practices of urban teens using Norplant contraceptive implants, oral contraceptives and condoms for contraception. Am J Obstet Gynecol 180: 929–937.

FURTHER READING

Baraitser P., Fettiplace R., Dolan F., Massil H. and Cowley S (2002) Quality mainstream services with proactive targeted outreach: a model of contraceptive service provision for young people. Journal of Family Planning and Reproductive Health Care 28(2): 90–94.

Population Council (2004) Adverse Health and Social Outcomes of Coerced Sex: Experiences of women in developing countries. Population Council:

USEFUL WEBSITES

www.who.int/child-adolescent-health/asrh.htm

http://www.hpa.org.uk/publications/2006/hiv_sti_2006

www.who.int/child-adolescent-health/OVERVIEW/AHD/adh_sheer.htm

Appendix 14.1

DEPARTMENT OF HEALTH BEST PRACTICE GUIDANCE FOR DOCTORS AND OTHER HEALTH PROFESSIONALS ON THE PROVISION OF ADVICE AND TREATMENT TO YOUNG PEOPLE UNDER 16 ON CONTRACEPTION, SEXUAL AND REPRODUCTIVE HEALTH

The following matters summarize the Department of Health for England and Wales guidance on confidentiality. This guidance covers England and Wales and is described below but not reproduced in full. Readers are referred to the full document on the Department of Health Website and to the document Working Together to Safeguard Children which sets out how individuals and organizations should work together to safeguard and promote the welfare of children. www.everychildmatters.gov.uk/workingtogether

Young people have the same rights to confidentiality as adults and every sexual health service should have an explicit policy on confidentiality which is prominently displayed. All staff should be trained in the implementation of this policy and deliberate breaches of confidentiality should be serious disciplinary matters.

The duty of confidentiality is not, however, absolute. Where a health professional believes that there is a risk to the health, safety or welfare of a young person or others which is so serious as to outweigh the young person's right to privacy, they should follow locally agreed child protection protocols. In these circumstances, the over-riding objective must be to safeguard the young person. If considering any disclosure of information to other agencies, including the police, staff should weigh up against the young person's right to privacy the degree of current or likely harm, what any such disclosure is intended to achieve and what the potential benefits are to the young person's well-being. Except in exceptional circumstances serious disclosure should only take place after consulting the young person involved.

In England and Wales a doctor or health professional is able to provide contraception, sexual and reproductive health advice and treatment without parental knowledge to a young person under 16 provided that:

- She/he understands the advice provided and its implications
- Her/his physical or mental health would otherwise be likely to suffer and so provision of advice/treatment is in their best interest.

It is considered good practice for doctors and other health professionals to ensure that the criteria commonly known as the Fraser Guidelines are met. These are listed below:

- The young person understands the health professional's advice
- The health professional cannot persuade the young person to inform his or her parents or allow the doctor to inform the parents that he or she is seeking contraceptive advice
- The young person is very likely to begin or continue having intercourse with or without contraceptive treatment
- Unless he or she receives contraceptive advice or treatment, the young person's physical or mental health or both are likely to suffer;
- The young person's best interests require the health professional to give contraceptive advice, treatment or both without parental consent.

Under English and Welsh Law the age of consent is 16. Children under the age of 13 are considered of insufficient age to give consent to sexual activity and separate guidance applies in this circumstance. If a child who is sexually active under the age of 13 presents to a sexual health service in England and Wales a full assessment should be undertaken including a decision on a child protection referral made in conjunction with the lead for child protection within the professionals employing authority. The police must be notified as soon as possible when a criminal offence has been committed or is suspected of having been committed against a child unless there are exceptional reasons not to do so. The obligations of health professionals in this circumstance are set out in the document Working Together to Safeguard Children.

15 Legal aspects of family planning

Susan Jones

Chapter contents

INTRODUCTION

When it comes to the potential for things to go wrong, sexual and reproductive health is no different from any other area of medicine. The aim of this chapter is to draw attention to legal and ethical issues that may affect those working in this field.

A healthcare professional may be on the receiving end of a complaint either to their employer or their regulatory body. Their actions might be the subject of a claim in clinical negligence. They might be asked to give evidence at an inquest – for example, the woman who dies from a pulmonary embolism after being prescribed the pill in the presence of contraindications. An intimate examination may result in allegations of indecent assault. If very young patients are involved, there may be conflicts between the duty of confidentiality on the one hand and the responsibility to notify possible abuse on the other.

However, it is important to remember that most consultations do not result in complaints, claims or other medicolegal problems. Applying the advice offered throughout this chapter may help to reduce the risk that such a situation will arise.

RULES FOR AVOIDING LITIGATION

• Pay attention to record keeping

The General Medical Council (GMC) advises that the professional must 'keep clear, accurate and legible records, reporting the relevant clinical findings, the decisions made, the information given to patients, and any drugs prescribed or other investigation or treatment'.[1] Similar advice is given by the Nursing and Midwifery Council (NMC).[2] For detailed guidance on keeping clinical records, see the NMC's A–Z of Advice.[3]

Medical records are the account of a consultation. They exist for the benefit of the patient, to inform healthcare professionals involved in their care. When things go wrong it can be some time after the event that an explanation is sought, so it is essential to be able to rely on the notes. For example, a thorough examination prior to fitting of an intrauterine device (IUD) may have taken place, but if the position and sounding of the uterus are not documented, it may be difficult to refute a complaint that the insertion was carried out without due care.

The GMC also advises that the professional must 'make records at the same time as the events you are recording or as soon as possible afterwards'.[1] If a non-contemporaneous entry is made, the date or timing of the entry should be recorded. There are many examples of healthcare professionals, tempted to add to the notes after a complaint has arisen, who have found themselves in more serious trouble, facing allegations of attempting to mislead.

It is important to remember that patients have a right to access their records and to seek explanations of the information contained in them.

• Keep training and skills up to date

Clinicians should attend appropriate professional courses and refresh their knowledge periodically. If they intend to insert IUDs, they should get a letter of competence and do enough insertions to maintain their skills. Similarly, healthcare professionals should receive instruction in the relevant techniques before undertaking the insertion and removal of implants. Claims have been successfully pursued against doctors attempting implant removal without adequate training. Although the doctor was usually acting to minimize inconvenience for the woman, liability for consequent pain, suffering and scarring could not be denied.

- ## Always obtain appropriate consent for any procedure or treatment

See the section on consent below.

- ## Respect patient confidentiality

See the section on confidentiality below.

- ## Offer explanations or an apology if appropriate

The GMC advises that 'If a patient under your care has suffered harm or distress, you must act immediately to put matters right, if that is possible. You should offer an apology and explain fully and promptly to the patient what has happened, and the likely short-term and long-term effects.'[1] An apology is not necessarily an admission of liability and should not be withheld because it might result in litigation. An explanation or apology given early can help to avoid a subsequent complaint.

- ## Know your limitations

Clinicians should always seek assistance if inexperienced or unfamiliar with a procedure or technique.

- ## Follow appropriate local or national procedures and protocols

In family planning this may include policies for dealing with children and young people.

- ## Develop and maintain good relationships with patients and colleagues

Most people work with others and should remember they are part of a team. Being a good team-player is considered an essential component of professional practice.[1]

CONSENT AND COMPETENCE

Consent is not just about asking patients to sign a consent form before an operation. No consultation, examination, treatment or other action or intervention can take place legitimately unless consent is obtained.

Each healthcare institution should have a consent policy, and staff should familiarize themselves with it.

Consent may be express or implied.

• Implied consent

Although it is not routine to seek consent from patients before recording details of their history, the fact that they voluntarily provide information and witness it being recorded infers that they have consented.

Similarly, it is not routine practice to record that consent has been obtained for a basic clinical examination. All doctors and nurses know that they cannot begin to examine patients without permission and would normally first explain what they intend to do. If the patient, understanding what is proposed, raises no objection and follows instructions, consent is implied. However, you should take care to ensure that explanations are appropriate. You should also be sensitive to religious or cultural customs and practice so that patients have an opportunity to express their consent or dissent at an early stage.

It is not uncommon for a patient to misunderstand a perfectly proper examination because it has not been explained adequately. Unfortunately, in some circumstances this gives rise to the serious allegation of indecent assault.

• Intimate examinations

The regulatory bodies all publish similar guidance regarding intimate examinations. The GMC,[4] for example, advises that before conducting an intimate examination the healthcare professional should:

1. Explain to the patient why an examination is necessary and give the patient an opportunity to ask questions.
2. Explain what the examination will involve, in a way the patient can understand, so that the patient has a clear idea of what to expect, including any potential pain or discomfort.
3. Obtain the patient's permission before the examination and record that permission has been obtained.
4. Give the patient privacy to undress and dress and keep the patient covered as much as possible to maintain their dignity. Do not assist the patient in removing clothing unless you have clarified with them that your assistance is required.

Chaperones

If an intimate examination is proposed, good practice dictates that a chaperone should be offered. This guidance applies regardless of whether the patient and doctor are of the same sex – the patient should still be given a choice. The GMC has published recent guidance,[4] which states, 'You should record any discussion about chaperones and its outcome. If a chaperone is present, you should record that fact and make a note of their identity. If the patient does not want a chaperone, you should record that the offer was made and declined.'

The GMC also offers guidance on who can act as a chaperone. It states that, whilst a chaperone 'does not have to be medically qualified' and may in some circumstances be 'a member of practice staff, or a relative or friend of the patient', a chaperone will ideally 'be familiar with the procedures involved in a routine intimate examination'.[4] Your employer may well have a policy on chaperones, which you should follow. See also the NMC's guidance on chaperoning.[3]

• Express consent

Express consent is a formal expression of consent, although it may not involve signing a consent form. Verbal consent for most routine and low-risk procedures does not usually need to be documented, however, if you think that the consent might be disputed in the future, or the patient has expressed particular concerns, you should record the verbal consent in the notes. It is also advisable to document the substance of discussions held with the patient during the consent process, even when written consent has been obtained by the signing of a consent form.

Consent forms

Each country in the UK has a standardized consent form for NHS organizations. These may have been adapted by individual organizations to provide procedure-specific consent forms listing the main areas which should have been discussed. Such forms are in common usage in family planning, for example when consent for a sterilization is taken.

Employing organizations should have clear guidelines for when written consent is needed and be able to provide appropriate forms. If consent forms are provided, they should be used.

Completed consent forms are retained in the clinical records. They are not legal documents, but in medicolegal situations can provide additional evidence that the process of obtaining valid consent has been undertaken.

• Who should take consent?

Consent should be taken by the person undertaking the procedure or delegated to an appropriate healthcare professional. The person taking consent must be familiar with the procedure, the risks, benefits and alternatives and be able to answer the patient's questions. If not, they must be able to give the patient access to someone who can.

• From whom should consent be sought?

If patients are competent adults, no one else can consent on their behalf. In certain circumstances, which might include sterilization, it is customary to consult with both partners. Whilst this may be good practice, it is not a legal requirement.

• Valid consent

In general, the validity of consent is not dependent upon whether a written consent form is completed or not. For consent to be valid:

- the patient should have the capacity to consent
- consent should be informed
- consent should be given freely, without undue pressure.

• Capacity to consent

The patient must be able to understand, at a level suitable for them, the nature and purpose of the proposed examination or procedure. As a general rule most adults would be deemed competent to consent to or refuse treatment unless they had a learning difficulty or mental impairment. However, in family planning, many consultations take place with patients under the age of majority.

Young patients

In England, Wales and Northern Ireland a child is legally considered a minor until they are 18, but once they reach the age of 16 they may consent to treatment in the same way as an adult.[5]

In Scotland, 16-year-olds have legal capacity to enter into any transaction. Children under 16 years of age 'have the legal capacity to consent' if they understand 'the nature and possible consequences of the procedure or treatment.[6]

The situation is the same in the rest of the UK, but the right of children under the age of 16 to consent to treatment rests on case law rather than legislation. The significant case in this area is the Gillick case (see Box 15.1).

Box 15.1 The Gillick Case[7]

In 1980 the Department of Health and Social Security published a circular to reassure doctors that they would not be acting unlawfully in prescribing contraceptives to girls under 16 years old, as long as they were acting in good faith to protect patients against the harmful effects of sexual intercourse.

On learning this, Mrs Gillick sought an assurance from her local area health authority that her daughters would not be given advice or contraception without her consent. When this was refused, she challenged the legality of the guidance.

This case went to the House of Lords for a final decision, which established that parents' rights to consent on behalf of their children ends when the child is able fully to comprehend the proposed treatment.

A number of factors, named after Lord Fraser who set them out in his judgment in the Gillick case, should be taken into consideration when medical practitioners are considering offering contraceptive services to under-16s without parental knowledge or permission (see **Box 15.2**).

Although competent minors may *give* consent, they cannot withhold consent for treatment that would be in their best interests; if necessary, the courts can override their refusal.[8] Neither are parents entitled to withhold consent to treatment that would be in the child's best interests.

The Gillick judgment and the main principles arising from it are now widely applied to all cases where a patient under 16 consults unaccompanied by an adult relative. Good documentation in such cases is essential; in its 2004 Guidance, the Faculty of Family Planning gives the following advice:[9]

> *'If a young person is assessed competent this should be documented in case notes as her being 'Fraser ruling competent' (advice understood, will have or continue to have sex, advised to inform her parents, in her best interest).'*

Assessing capacity

'A person is unable to make a decision for himself if he is unable

1. to understand the information relevant to the decision
2. to retain that information
3. to use or weigh that information as part of the process of making the decision, or
4. to communicate his decision (whether by talking, using sign language or any other means).'[10]

Adults are presumed to have capacity, but if there is any doubt, their capacity to consent to the treatment in question should be assessed. 'This assessment and the conclusions drawn from it should be recorded within the patient's notes.'[11]

Box 15.2 The Fraser Guidelines

- The young person understands the advice being given.
- The young person cannot be convinced to involve parents/carers or allow the medical practitioner to do so.
- It is likely that the young person will begin or continue having intercourse with or without treatment/contraception.
- If the treatment/contraception is not given, the young person's physical or mental health (or both) is likely to suffer.
- The young person's best interests require contraceptive advice, treatment or supplies to be given without parental consent.

Capacity is not an all-or-nothing concept, but will depend on what is being proposed. Capacity may also fluctuate, so timing an assessment can be crucial.

Assessing mental capacity is not always easy, but the Department of Health suggests the following techniques:[12]

- Ask patients to repeat or rephrase what you have said.
- Ask patients to compare alternatives or think of consequences other than those you have told them about.
- Check whether they can apply the information you have given them to their own case.

It is important that the information is expressed in a way, and in a format, that patients can understand, according to their individual abilities. Photographs, drawings, or other aids may need to be used; or the help of a translator, speech therapist or a person close to the patient may be required.

Patients with learning difficulties

Health professionals sometimes wrongly assume that patients with learning disabilities are unable to reach informed decisions about their own health care. In fact, depending on the complexity of what is being proposed, they may be perfectly capable of understanding the implications and consequences of a proposed treatment.

When patients are unable to consent to medical examination or treatment, it is usually up to healthcare professionals to decide what is in their best interests. If there is uncertainty about whether a proposed course of action is in a patient's interests, an application should be made to the courts to adjudicate on the matter (see Box 15.3).

Box 15.3 Lack of capacity to consent to sterilization[13]

F was aged 36 and had been in residential care since she was 14 years old. She had the mental capacity of a 5-year-old and there was no prospect of her mental capacity improving.

When F formed a sexual relationship with another resident, it was feared she might become pregnant and doctors considered it in her best interests to carry out a sterilization. Her mother applied for a declaration from the court that sterilization would not be unlawful because of her daughter's lack of consent. The House of Lords decided that sterilization would be in F's best interests.

This case established that:

- Someone with appropriate qualifications must decide, in line with a responsible body of medical opinion, what is in the best interests of a patient who lacks the capacity to consent.
- In cases of sterilization, the involvement of the court is thought desirable but not necessary.

In Scotland, the patient may have a continuing or welfare attorney who is empowered to consent on the patient's behalf. Alternatively, the court may appoint a guardian to fulfil the same function. Similar provisions will be available in England and Wales once the Mental Capacity Act comes into force.

A decision to involve the courts depends on what treatment is being proposed. Sterilization, being an invasive and permanent solution, for example, may not receive widespread support, whereas the use of depot preparations may be more readily agreed to be in the patient's best interests. Such decisions should be made in discussion with the patient (as far as is possible), the patient's carers and healthcare professionals.

• Informed consent – How much information do you need to give?

There is no legislation governing 'informed consent', so guidance is derived from case law. The two most relevant cases are Sidaway[14] and Chester v Afshar.[15] Sidaway confirmed that it is for clinicians to decide how much information they should give a patient, but their decision may be challenged by the courts if there is a conflict of medical opinion about what constitutes appropriate disclosure. Chester v Afshar confirms that even remote risks, if the potential injury is severe enough, should be discussed with the patient during the consent process.

When discussing a proposed treatment or intervention, the patient should be given details of all the risks and benefits a reasonable person would wish to know about all the treatment options. This includes relatively minor – but likely – complications and severe – but unlikely – complications. There is no such thing as a 'one per cent rule'. If the incidence of a complication is below 1%, but it would have a serious impact on the patient, the patient should be told about it. Patients' lifestyles, aspirations and means of making a living should also be taken into account when determining what they need to know. Patients who have yet to start a family, for example, will probably be more concerned about a slight risk to their fertility than those who feel their families are complete.

Where good practice guidance is available, whether local or national, on the points that should be discussed with a patient prior to a particular treatment or procedure, it is always wise to follow this. Leaflets and other material can be a useful adjunct but beware that sometimes patients will not use them – they cannot be regarded as a substitute for discussion.

• Consent should be freely given

Healthcare professionals may not necessarily agree with a patient's choice but this does not automatically mean the patient is unreasonable (see Box 15.4). Everyone is entitled to make decisions, which may or may not conform to another person's view. Some patients are so frightened about undertaking

> **Box 15.4 The case of Re C[16]**
>
> C suffered from paranoid schizophrenia and was confined in a secure hospital when he developed a gangrenous foot. Doctors concluded he had only a 15% chance of survival unless he had an amputation. C refused to consent to this, so his foot was managed conservatively. However, the hospital refused to give an undertaking not to amputate in the future.
>
> C sought an injunction to stop the hospital carrying out an amputation of his leg without his express consent. The hospital contended that C was not competent to withhold consent, on the grounds that his mental illness did not allow him to appreciate the risk of death if the operation was not performed.
>
> The court decided that although C's mental abilities were to some extent impaired, he was still able to comprehend, believe and weigh the information about his treatment options in the balance. The injunction was granted.

a procedure that they are unable to think logically. They may just need an opportunity to take stock and consider the information.

When a patient has made a decision that seems peculiar (maybe by opting out of the recommended treatment), the healthcare professional must be sure that they have provided sufficient information and presented it in a way that the patient can understand. There must then be adequate time for reflection, ensuring that the patient is not suffering from undue pressure or coercion (from staff or friends and relatives).

Once competence has been established, individuals can apply their personal beliefs in making decisions about treatment – even where it may seem irrational or likely to cause permanent injury or even death.

CONFIDENTIALITY

• The principle

In their ethical guidelines, the GMC[17] and the NMC[2] both place a strong emphasis on the importance of confidentiality. It is central to the trust between clinicians and patients, and registered practitioners are responsible for protecting patients' personal information.

• Avoiding inadvertent breaches

Breaches of confidentiality can be unintentional, although invariably avoidable. It is easy to forget, for example, that others may overhear discussions with colleagues in a corridor or lift. Similarly, patients or non-medical staff may be able to view confidential information left on a computer screen or on an unattended desk.

Written records should be kept securely, and this includes anything containing patients' names, addresses or birthdates. Care should be taken with appointment books or lists, and with telephone enquiries about patients, as the fact that they are attending your clinic or surgery is confidential information.

• Sharing information with healthcare professionals

Patients have a right to know how the information they give will be used and that they can refuse to allow information-sharing within and across organizations. Leaflets explaining 'how and why' patient information is shared and what patients can do if they object, should be easily available.

However, it is important to recognize that the presence of leaflets and notices is not sufficient, in itself; the NHS Code of Practice[18] is very clear on this point. It specifies that staff must 'Check that patients have seen the available information leaflets' and suggests various ways in which this might be achieved within the context of care. Furthermore, the NHS Code stresses that it cannot be assumed that a patient has either read or understood the literature available to them and 'Difficulty in communicating does not remove the obligation to help people understand'.

Many young patients prefer the relative anonymity of a family planning clinic to attending their GP and they may ask clinic staff not to pass information on to their GP. It is good practice to explain to patients why communication with their GP is important – e.g. reducing the risk of drug interactions because GP and clinic are unaware of what the other is prescribing – and encourage them to keep the GP informed.

It is recognized that 'Young people under 16 are the group least likely to use contraception and their concern about confidentiality remains the biggest deterrent to seeking advice. Publicity about the right to confidentiality is an essential element of an effective contraception and sexual health service.'[19]

• Non-patient care

Occasionally, information is disclosed for reasons other than treatment, and this will usually take place with the patient's informed consent. When clinical information is used for clinical audit or administration and planning, it should be kept to a minimum necessary for the purpose of the audit. As a rule, use of identifiable information for anything other than the direct delivery of patient care requires the patient's express consent. Anonymised information, however, can generally be used without the patient's consent.

• Disclosure in the public interest or the patient's best interests

There may be occasions when it is considered necessary to disclose information without consent in the public interest. These will be situations where all the available means of obtaining consent have been considered but they are not practical, or the patient is not competent to give consent. Exceptionally, the patient may have withheld consent.

It is essential to weigh up the possible harm, both to the patient and the doctor–patient relationship, against the benefits to an individual, a group in the community or society as a whole that are likely to arise from the release of information.

It is usually considered justifiable to release patient information without a patient's consent – or sometimes even in the face of a patient's refusal to consent – if failure to do so would expose the patient or others to risk of death or serious harm. In most circumstances, such a decision would not be made in isolation – it is always best to discuss the issues first with a senior colleague, seek advice from the Trust's Caldicott Guardian or take legal advice if necessary. It is important that the decision-making process is documented in the patient's medical record, making clear the justifications for disclosing.

• Children and mentally incapacitated adults

Children who have the maturity and intelligence to understand the pros and cons of disclosure after you have explained them can be deemed 'Fraser-ruling, competent' (see **Box 15.2**) and their wishes should be respected unless there is a good reason for overriding them. An example would be where there is concern that a child is being abused.

If abuse or exploitation is suspected, concerns should be voiced to the patient if this is possible, and an explanation given of why it is necessary to involve a parent and/or another body. You may then be in a position to support a voluntary disclosure of information. Even if you need to make a disclosure without consent, at the very least the patient is prepared for this.

If the child is too young to consent and the person with parental responsibility is withholding consent to such information sharing, it is possible to override the parent's refusal if you believe the child's welfare is at stake. The golden rule is that the child's best interests are paramount.

Trusts will have information-sharing protocols which give guidance through the process of decision-making and direct staff to the appropriate agencies for disclosure, depending on the circumstances. Any trust should have locally agreed child protection protocols as outlined in *Working Together to Safeguard Children*.[20] As part of its 'Every Child Matters' programme, the UK government has produced a practitioners' guide to information sharing.[21]

There may also be situations where you are concerned that an incompetent adult is a victim of neglect or abuse. In such circumstances the same principles apply, namely that there may be occasions where it is important for the protection of a patient to disclose information – to social services, for example.

THE SEXUAL OFFENCES ACT 2003

Amongst its provisions, this Act makes it a statutory offence to engage in sexual activity with a child under the age of 13 years. This could be one reason why some local protocols require the reporting of any sexually active children under 13 either to the police or to social services. This has been the source of much debate and concern that it will discourage young people from seeking medical advice.

The Act is fully in force in England and Wales and only limited provisions extend to Northern Ireland and Scotland. The position in Northern Ireland differs in that sexual activity with a child under 14 years of age is a statutory offence. Moreover, as the law there currently stands, in principle it is a criminal offence to conceal knowledge of sexual activity in a child of this age.

Some practitioners in England and Wales may also have concerns about their actions being interpreted as contributing to a criminal act, but the 2003 Act makes it clear that in these jurisdictions a person acting for the protection of a child in one of the following ways is not committing an offence:

(a) *'protecting the child from sexually transmitted infection*
(b) *protecting the physical safety of the child*
(c) *preventing the child from becoming pregnant, or*
(d) *promoting the child's emotional well-being by the giving of advice,*

....and that person is not acting for the purpose of obtaining sexual gratification or for the purpose of causing or encouraging the activity constituting the offence.'[22]

The above subsections would clearly apply to family planning consultations with young patients, where the principal aim is to provide appropriate advice on sexual health and not to encourage under-age intercourse.

Guidance from the Department of Health also confirms that 'The Sexual Offences Act 2003 does not affect the duty of care and confidentiality of health professionals to young people under 16.'[23]

CLINICAL NEGLIGENCE

Although a case before a regulatory body or a complaint can be daunting, what concerns many healthcare professionals most is the prospect of a claim in negligence. This may be because being deemed negligent seems to imply some sort of neglect. There may also be the fear of a trial and all the associated consequences of the publicity that might surround it. In fact, few cases go to trial because it usually becomes clear beforehand whether or not there is a case to be answered. It is important also to be aware that negligence is not necessarily associated with a lack of care and can quite easily arise in circumstances where there has been genuine concern for the welfare of the patient.

• How negligence is established

Three hurdles need to be overcome:

1. **A duty of care has to be established** – in the clinical setting, simply engaging in a consultation is enough to establish this.
2. **The duty of care has to be breached** – something has to go wrong. This does not necessarily mean a deliberate act or omission.
3. **There has to be harm** to the patient as a consequence of the breach of duty.

• What is the expected standard of care?

The test of the standard of care has been set by two significant cases in English case law (see Boxes 15.5 and 15.6).

Box 15.5 The Bolam case[24]

Mr Bolam was a patient advised to undergo electro-convulsive therapy. He signed a consent form but was not informed of the small risk of fracture.

During treatment, the patient suffered injuries and subsequently brought a claim in negligence in respect of these.

The use of relaxant drugs would have avoided the risk of fracture. However, in the court case that followed, there were two competent bodies of medical opinion: one favoured their use as standard practice and the other favoured confining their use to cases where there was a particular indication because of risks associated with the drugs. There was no particular reason to use the drugs in Mr Bolam's case.

There were also two differing, yet competent, bodies of opinion about whether patients should be warned beforehand of the small risk of fracture.

The judge found the hospital had not been negligent, establishing these principles, amongst others:

- The standard of care provided by a doctor has to be the standard of the ordinary skilled practitioner in the specialty: a consultant anaesthetist must meet the standard of a competent consultant anaesthetist; a family planning specialist must meet the standards of a competent family planning specialist.
- Practitioners are not negligent if they are acting in accordance with a practice supported by a responsible body of practitioners experienced in the relevant specialty, even if there is another body of opinion that takes a contrary view.

Box 15.6 The Bolitho case[25]

A 2-year-old boy with a history of croup was re-admitted to hospital.

The following day there were two short episodes in which the patient had obvious breathing difficulties.

The senior paediatric registrar was called both times, but did not attend, delegating a junior colleague to attend at the second incident. The patient suffered total respiratory failure and a cardiac arrest shortly after the second incident, resulting in severe brain damage.

In the legal action that followed, it was accepted that the registrar was in breach of her duty of care by not attending. But it was contended that the cardiac arrest would not have been avoided even if she or another suitable deputy, had attended.

The child might not have suffered a cardiac arrest if he had been intubated before the final episode of respiratory failure. However the registrar stated that even if she had attended, she would not have intubated at that time because of the associated risks to the child.

In this case, argument revolved around whether intubation would have been indicated. Expert views were diametrically opposed – but both represented a responsible body of opinion. The case went to the House of Lords for a decision.

Qualifying Bolam, this case established that doctors can be negligent in their diagnosis and treatment, despite there being a body of professional opinion to support it, if the judge is not satisfied that the body of opinion is capable of withstanding logical analysis.

The appeal to the House of Lords was dismissed because the views of both the plaintiff's and the defendant's experts could be supported in logic.

In family planning, there are a number of identifiable risks which may result in litigation or complaint:

Hormonal contraception

Poor patient selection or inadequate counselling regarding risk can result in patients with risk factors such as smoking, obesity, family or personal history of venous thromboembolism receiving the pill and suffering an ill effect. A patient who suffers a stroke in such circumstances may well need significant ongoing care and any claim for damages could be substantial.

Concomitant prescribing of some antifungals, anti-epileptic medication or antibiotics can reduce the efficacy of hormonal contraception. This should be borne in mind when prescribing contraception and enquiries made about a patient's drug history.[26] Drug interactions may not be recognized until the patient presents with an unplanned pregnancy. Similar problems may arise when a patient is changed over from one pill to another without adequate advice. In either situation, the patient may well be able to establish a claim in negligence and, if an unwanted pregnancy has arisen, claim for this or for the pain and suffering endured in undergoing a termination of pregnancy.

Box 15.7 The McFarlane case[27]

Mr and Mrs McFarlane had four children and did not wish to have any more. Mr McFarlane therefore underwent a vasectomy and the couple were told subsequently that it was safe for them to have unprotected intercourse. Less than 3 years later Mrs McFarlane gave birth to a healthy daughter.

Mr and Mrs McFarlane brought a claim for damages, on the basis that they had been inadequately counselled, for £10 000 for maternal pain and suffering and £100 000 for the cost of rearing their fifth child. The case went to the House of Lords.

The damages for pain and suffering were allowed, but not the more substantial sum for bringing up a child. It was found that the birth of a healthy child could not amount to a personal injury. This claim radically reduced the level of damages paid out in so-called 'wrongful birth' cases.

Intrauterine devices

Common problems include a failure to diagnose either pregnancy or ongoing infection at the time of insertion with predictable sequelae for the patient.

Difficult or painful insertions may also result in a claim. Patients should be made aware beforehand that, if difficulties are encountered, the procedure can be abandoned, either on their say so or on the basis of the operator's clinical judgement. Persisting with a difficult insertion can lead to litigation, as can failing to recognize and manage a perforation.

Sterilization

For both male and female sterilization procedures, failure resulting in pregnancy is a common source of complaint and claim. Thorough counselling should include discussion of the possibility of failure. Until relatively recently, a claim for 'wrongful birth' would attract significant damages and still has the potential to do so if the child is disabled and requires extra care.

The case which reformed this area is McFarlane (see Box 15.7).

Depot preparations/implants

Common complaints or claims include failing to warn of side effects such as irregular menstrual bleeding.

Care should always be taken to ensure what has been prescribed is administered – there have been cases where a patient has received the wrong type of depot preparation because of carelessness and misunderstanding.

If implants are being inserted or removed, the practitioner must have the appropriate training and follow manufacturers' or good practice guidance. Particular difficulties have arisen in respect of difficult removals, especially when the operators have failed to recognize their own limitations and seek help.

Termination of pregnancy

The common problems leading to complaints or litigation are predictably failure (i.e. ongoing pregnancy), incomplete evacuation, perforation and delay. The procedure for counselling patients prior to termination of pregnancy should be followed carefully and the operator should ensure that this has been carried out and that the patient is aware of the risks.

Any postoperative symptoms should be taken seriously.

If avoidable delays arise in referring a patient and this results in the patient enduring a more unpleasant experience than would otherwise have been necessary, legal action may follow.

THE LAW ON ABORTION

The Abortion Act 1967 substantially liberalized the law in England, Scotland and Wales.[28] Provided practitioners complied with the provisions of the Abortion Act, they had a defence against the crimes described in the Offences Against the Person Act 1861.

The grounds for lawful termination of pregnancy are now listed in the Human Fertilisation and Embryology Act 1990, which amends the 1967 Act as follows[29]:

  a. 'that the pregnancy has not exceeded its twenty-fourth week and that the continuance of the pregnancy would involve risk, greater than if the pregnancy were terminated, of injury to the physical or mental health of the pregnant woman or any existing children of her family; or
  b. that the termination is necessary to prevent grave permanent injury to the physical or mental health of the pregnant woman; or
  c. that the continuance of the pregnancy would involve risk to the life of the pregnant woman, greater than if the pregnancy were terminated; or
  d. that there is a substantial risk that if the child were born it would suffer from such physical or mental abnormalities as to be seriously handicapped.'

The Act requires the agreement of two medical practitioners that one or more of the above apply. In emergencies, a single doctor may terminate a pregnancy where it is immediately necessary to save the life or prevent grave injury to the woman.

The Abortion Act does not extend to Northern Ireland, where the law on abortion is based on The Offences Against the Person Act 1861, which makes it an offence to procure a miscarriage unlawfully.

The Bourne judgement of 1939[30] was based on an interpretation of the word 'unlawfully' in this Act and, without specific legislation, clinicians are left to interpret this with little in the way of guidance. This uncertainty means that women from Northern Ireland may have to travel to England or Scotland and pay for a private termination of pregnancy. The Family Planning Association has campaigned on behalf of women in Northern Ireland and, as a consequence, in January 2007, the Department of Health, Social Services and Public Safety finally announced that it was releasing draft guidelines to health professionals for consultation, following which these should be published along with information for the public.

• Abortion and young people

The position regarding consent and confidentiality is exactly the same as for any other treatment or procedure. Recent case law[31] has reaffirmed this and established that the parent of a competent child has no 'right to know' if their child is being advised on abortion.

• Involvement of fathers

Although women are usually encouraged to discuss the decision to terminate a pregnancy with the father, male partners have no legal rights to involvement in the decision.

• Conscientious objection to abortion

The Abortion Act has a clause that permits doctors to refuse to participate in terminations, but obliges them to provide necessary treatment in an emergency when the woman's life may be at risk.

The GMC offers the following guidance:

'If carrying out a particular procedure or giving advice about it conflicts with your religious or moral beliefs, and this conflict might affect the treatment or advice you provide, you must explain this to the patient ... If it is not practical for a patient to arrange to see another doctor, you must ensure that arrangements are made for another suitably qualified colleague to take over your role.'[1]

REFERENCES

1. General Medical Council (2006) Good Medical Practice. GMC: London.

2. Nursing and Midwifery Council (2004) The NMC Code of Professional Conduct: Standards for Conduct, Performance and Ethics. NMC: London.

3. Nursing and Midwifery Council NMC A–Z of Advice http://www.nmc-uk.org/aSection.aspx?SectionID=11

4. General Medical Council (2006) Maintaining Boundaries. GMC: London.

5. The Family Law Reform Act 1969, section 8.

6. The Age of Legal Capacity (Scotland) Act 1991, section 2(4).

7. Gillick v West Norfolk and Wisbech Area Health Authority [1985] 3 All ER 402 (HL).

8. Re M (Child: Refusal of Medical Treatment) [1999] 2 FCR 577 and Re R (a Minor) [1992] 3 Med LR.

9. FFPRHC (2004) Contraceptive choices for young people. Journal of Family Planning and Reproductive Health Care 30(4): 237–251.

10. The Mental Capacity Act 2005.

11. Department of Health (2002) Reference Guide for Consent to Examination or Treatment. DH: London, p. 4.

12. Department of Health (2002) Seeking Consent: Working with People in Prison. DH: London, p. 20.

13. Re F V West Berkshire Health Authority [1989] 2 All ER 545.

14. Sidaway v Board of Governors of the Bethlem Royal Hospital [1985] AC 871.

15. Chester (Respondent) v Afshar (Appellant) [2004] UKHL 41.

16. Re. C (Adult: Refusal of Medical Treatment) [1994]1 All ER 819.

17. General Medical Council (2004) Confidentiality: Protecting and Providing Information. GMC: London.

18. Department of Health (2003) Confidentiality: NHS Code of Practice. DH: London.

19. Kensington and Chelsea Primary Care Trust (2005) A Guide to Giving Support and Advice to Young People about Unintended Pregnancy, p. 4. http://www.rbkc.gov.uk/youthsupport/general/ysds_teenage.pdf

20. HM Government (2006) Working Together to Safeguard Children. The Stationery Office: London. http://publications.everychildmatters.gov.uk

21. HM Government (2006) Information Sharing: Practitioners' Guide, The Stationery Office: London. http://publications.everychildmatters.gov.uk

22. The Sexual Offences Act 2003, section 14(3).

23. Department of Health (2004) Best Practice Guidance for Doctors and Other Health Professionals on the Provision of Advice and Treatment to Young People Under 16 on Contraception, Sexual and Reproductive Health. DH: London.

24. Bolam v Friern Hospital Management Committee [1957] 1 WLR 582.

25. Administratrix of the Estate of Bolitho (Deceased) v City and Hackney Health Authority [1997] 4 All ER.

26. FFPRHC (2005) Drug interactions with hormonal contraception. Journal of Family Planning and Reproductive Health Care 31(2): 139–151.

27. McFarlane v Tayside HB [1999] 3 WLR 1301.

28. Abortion Act 1967, section 1(4).

29. Human Fertilisation and Embryology Act 1990, section 37.

30. R v Bourne [1939] 1 KB 687.

31. R (on the Application of Axon) v Secretary of State for Health and the Family Planning Association [2006] EWHC 372 (Admin) 2/10.

ACKNOWLEDGEMENT

The author would like to acknowledge the assistance of Sandy Anthony in the preparation of this chapter.

16 Abortion

Audrey H Brown

Chapter contents

BACKGROUND AND DEMOGRAPHICS

Worldwide, every day, there are over 100 million acts of sexual intercourse, resulting in over 900 000 pregnancies. About 50% of these pregnancies are unplanned, and about 25% actually unwanted. As a result, 150 000 pregnancies are terminated by induced abortion every day; that is over 50 million abortions worldwide every year. The World Health Organization (WHO) estimates that at least one-third of these abortions are carried out in unsafe conditions. Even in those countries where abortion is illegal, many women attempt to terminate an unwanted pregnancy illegally (e.g. in Brazil) or travel abroad to a country with more liberal laws (e.g. from the Republic of Ireland to England). Illegal abortions are often performed in unsanitary conditions by unqualified people and result in considerable morbidity and mortality. An estimated 100–200 000 women die annually from the complications of abortion.[1] In contrast, abortion performed using modern methods in optimum conditions is an extremely safe procedure,

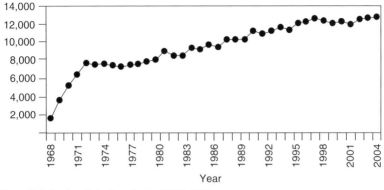

Figure 16.1 Number of abortions, Scotland 1968–2005

and legalization of abortion is always followed by a fall in maternal deaths presumed to be due to the reduction in the complications of illegal abortions.

After the Abortion Act was passed in 1967, there was a rapid rise in the number of abortions notified in England and Wales, and Scotland (Figure 16.1). Annually, over 185 000 abortions are carried out in England and Wales,[2] and 12 600 in Scotland.[3] Women of all reproductive ages undergo abortion, with peak rates in the women aged 18–24 (31.0 abortions per 1000). The majority are unmarried (77%), although around one-third are with a partner. Almost half of women have previously had a child (47%), and one-third have had at least one previous termination. Most terminations are carried out in the first trimester of pregnancy, with 87% performed before 13 weeks, and 60% before 9 weeks. Abortion forms a large part of the gynaecology workload in the UK; termination of pregnancy is one of the commonest gynaecological procedures. Although clinicians may have differing degrees of involvement in abortion services, most will come into contact with women who are currently accessing abortion, have done so in the past or indeed will do so in the future, and as such require appropriate skills and knowledge to best meet their needs. A woman may find herself with an unplanned pregnancy because of contraceptive failure, failure to use contraception and occasionally due to forced intercourse.

Of course, unplanned and unwanted and planned and wanted pregnancy may not be synonymous terms. A woman may have an unplanned pregnancy, as a result of contraceptive failure, but be happy to find herself pregnant, and continue the pregnancy. In contrast, another woman may plan to become pregnant, but experience breakdown of her relationship and feel it necessary to seek abortion. A recent study in Edinburgh showed that of women presenting for antenatal care, 66% had intended pregnancies, and 26% of women were ambivalent about the pregnancy, and the remaining 8% had actually not intended to become pregnant.[4] Today, many women outwith marriage will have a planned pregnancy, and likewise some married couples will desire no children. With the advent of widely available contraceptive methods, women and couples can choose to avoid pregnancy, and the Abortion Act allows the decision not to proceed with a pregnancy which does occur. Abortion should never be considered as a method of contraception; however, failures occur with any method and without access to abortion, the ability of women to regulate their fertility and plan their families is impaired. It is important, therefore, that anyone involved in providing contraceptive services should be aware of the legal indications and different methods of therapeutic abortion available.

LEGAL ASPECTS

Abortion on demand is not available in the United Kingdom. It is illegal to induce an abortion except under specific indications as defined by law. The conditions of the 1967 Abortion Act, as amended in 1990, state that abortion can be performed if two registered medical practitioners, acting in good faith, agree that the pregnancy should be terminated on one or more of the following grounds:

A. The continuance of the pregnancy would involve risk to the life of the pregnant woman greater than if the pregnancy were terminated.

B. The termination is necessary to prevent grave permanent injury to the physical or mental health of the pregnant woman.

C. The pregnancy has not exceeded its 24th week and that the continuance of the pregnancy would involve risk, greater than if the pregnancy were terminated, of injury to the physical or mental health of the pregnant woman.

D. The pregnancy has not exceeded its 24th week and that the continuance of the pregnancy would involve risk, greater than if the pregnancy were terminated, of injury to the physical or mental health of the existing child(ren) of the family of the pregnant woman.

E. There is a substantial risk that if the child were born it would suffer from such physical or mental abnormalities as to be seriously handicapped.

The vast majority (95%) of terminations are carried out under Clause C of the Abortion Act, and 3% because of concerns regarding wellbeing of existing children. Clauses C and D carry an upper gestational limit of 24 weeks.

Modern methods of inducing abortion are now so effective and safe that almost always it is safer for the woman to have an abortion than continue with the pregnancy. That is not to say that abortion should be recommended always, but a doctor should carefully consider the decision to refuse to recommend abortion for a woman who is convinced that her mental and/or physical health or the welfare of her children would be better preserved by ending the pregnancy.

The Abortion Act also allows abortion to be performed in an emergency, upon the single signature of the doctor carrying out the procedure. In such circumstances, the emergency grounds are:

F. To save the life of the pregnant woman.

G. To prevent grave permanent injury to the physical or mental health of the pregnant woman.

There are differences in the law between different parts of the UK. In England and Wales, it is illegal to attempt to induce abortion except under the 1967 Abortion Act even if the woman is not pregnant. The intention to induce abortion is sufficient. In Scotland, no criminal charge of inducing abortion can be sustained unless the prosecution can prove that the woman was pregnant. The 1967 Abortion Act does not apply to Northern Ireland where abortion is only legal under exceptional circumstances, e.g. to save the life of the mother.

The law concerning abortion is the subject of continuing debate within the UK. Although a vociferous lobby would wish to make abortion illegal or severely restrict its application, recent public opinion polls have shown that most people support the right to abortion. A Mori poll showed that 65% of those surveyed in 2001 agreed that if a woman wants an abortion, she should not have to continue with her pregnancy. This survey also confirmed majority approval for right to abortion in a variety of situations, ranging from carrying a pregnancy with severe abnormalities, to simply not wishing to have a child.

Women seeking abortion require the agreement of two doctors before the abortion can proceed, and women commonly rely on the support of their GP for referral. In a postal survey, 82% of a random sample of British GPs described themselves as 'broadly pro-choice', and 18% as 'broadly anti-abortion'.[5] GPs were positive regarding greater patient autonomy in the decision-making process, with almost half supporting a woman to make her own decision in the first trimester, and a further third supporting the woman to make the decision in conjunction with the doctor. Around a fifth supported the status quo, i.e. doctor-only control of the decision. A survey of trainee gynaecologists carried out in the UK in 1999, showed that around one-third had conscientious objection to abortion, with 28% being unwilling to perform abortion in the first trimester, and 38% in the second trimester. Sixteen per cent did not believe abortion should be available on the NHS, and 29% did not see abortion as part of their job. The British Medical Association guidance 'The Law and Ethics of Abortion' advises that 'Doctors with a conscientious objection to abortion should make their views known to patients seeking termination of pregnancy and should ensure that the treatment or advice they provide is not affected by their personal views'. If a doctor is consulted by a woman requesting an abortion, and that doctor is unable to make a referral, timely referral of the woman to another colleague who does not hold similar views is obligatory. At the British Medical Association annual conference in 2005, 77% of delegates rejected a proposal to reduce the gestational time limit for abortion to below 24 weeks, suggesting that senior medical staff see a need for the small number of women to continue to access late termination.

In 1990, the law was amended to reduce the upper limit from 28 to 24 weeks gestation in Clauses C and D reflecting earlier fetal viability due to advances in neonatal care. An exception was made in the case of a fetus with severe congenital abnormality, or where there is serious risk to the woman's life, when there is no upper limit (Clauses A, B and E).

REFERRAL FOR ABORTION

Most women seeking an abortion in the UK (initially) consult their GP. Others prefer to approach a family planning clinic or pregnancy advisory service directly. After confirmation of pregnancy, the woman should be referred for assessment as quickly as possible.

Provision for abortion varies throughout the UK. In Scotland and North-East England, over 90% of abortions are performed in NHS hospitals while in other areas of England, the majority are carried out in private clinics or by charities. The incidence of complications of abortion rises with increasing gestation. A guideline on the care of women requesting abortion, from the Royal College of Obstetricians and Gynaecologists (RCOG) recommends that services should be organized to minimize delay.[6] A centralized telephone booking system, with dedicated out-patient clinics results in earlier abortion. The RCOG guideline also recommends that all women should ideally be offered an assessment appointment within 5 days of referral, and as a minimum standard should be seen in no more than 2 weeks. It also recommends that once the decision to proceed to abortion has been agreed, the woman should ideally be able to undergo the termination within 7 days, or as a minimum, no longer than 2 weeks. Overall, no woman should wait longer than a total of 3 weeks from initial presentation to undergoing the abortion.

COUNSELLING BEFORE ABORTION

Faced with the news of an unintended pregnancy, some women are emotionally distraught and may have conflicting feelings about the pregnancy, e.g. to continue the pregnancy may present insoluble problems and seem quite impractical, whereas to have an abortion may seem abhorrent and contravene strongly held personal beliefs. It is important to provide sympathetic, non-directional support to all women seeking abortion, allowing the woman to explore her own feelings, and empowering her to make her own informed decision.

Although major psychological problems and rates of depression after abortion are not higher than in the background population, some women may be at a higher risk of coping with problems and distress following abortion. Pre-abortion counselling can help to identify these women, and ensure that appropriate support is offered. A history of mental health problems is an indicator of risk after abortion. Indeed, this may be one of the key factors leading the woman towards the abortion decision. Low self-esteem may also be relevant; firstly by increasing the likelihood of opting for abortion in the first place, as the woman may feel unable to cope with a child, and secondly by throwing doubt on her belief about how she will cope with the abortion. Younger women, single women and those from a cultural or religious group who do not believe in abortion are more likely to be isolated, and without a close supporting person in whom to confide. Those undergoing second trimester termination are more likely to experience psychological problems after abortion, as are those whose pregnancy was initially planned. Women who were ambivalent regarding the decision because of pressure to abort from family or partner, or indeed to economic pressures, where there is no prospect of being able to support a child will be vulnerable following the abortion. Women who blame themselves may find it difficult to come to terms with events: identifying what went wrong and agreeing a contraceptive strategy with the woman to prevent further unplanned pregnancy can help give her a more positive plan on which to move forward.

Managing a consultation with a woman seeking abortion can be daunting. There is an obligation to convey medical information, explain risks and describe the procedures, but also to give the woman the time and support to consider her options, and reach the best decision. At assessment, we may also require to scan the patient, arrange the procedure, obtain consent and prescribe medication. We are used to taking a very structured history, working our way through a series of closed questions. Of course, it is necessary to collect required factual information, such as date of last menstrual period and past obstetric and medical history, but it can help to meet the woman's emotions by utilizing some basic counselling techniques:

- Ask open-ended rather than closed questions
  e.g. 'How do you feel about the pregnancy?' rather than 'Were you upset when you found out?'
- Listen actively to the patient
  e.g. make sure you appear genuinely interested in her views, and show understanding
- Feedback empathically, which helps to reassure her that her feelings are normal
  e.g. saying 'I understand that you are finding this difficult to talk about'.

- Encourage patients to ask questions
  e.g. try asking 'What would you like to ask me about your choices?'
  rather than 'Have you got any questions?'
- Remember to be aware when someone may need more support
  e.g. young person, someone who initially planned the pregnancy,
  someone who seems ambivalent, member of religious group.

Most women make their decision within days of learning that they are pregnant. Some may require more extensive professional counselling. Women with severe medical conditions which could worsen in pregnancy, e.g. pulmonary hypertension, or with pre-existing psychiatric disorders, require particularly careful assessment of the relative risks of continuing pregnancy and expert medical or psychiatric advice should be sought. Some women may require more practical information to enable them to make a decision, for example details about maternity leave, housing rights, etc., or information about adoption. Urgent referral to a social worker should be available when necessary.

PRE-ABORTION MANAGEMENT

After it has been decided that there are grounds for abortion and the woman has been fully counselled, it is important to make a careful assessment. The RCOG guideline[6] recommends the following.

Blood tests

- Haemoglobin concentration
- Determination of ABO and Rhesus blood groups, with screening for red cell antibodies. Anti-D immunoglobulin will be required for Rhesus negative women post-abortion (250 i.u. under 20 weeks gestation, and 500 i.u. above 20 weeks). It is not cost-effective to routinely crossmatch women
- Testing for other conditions such as haemaglobinopathies or HIV infection, as clinically indicated.

Ultrasound scanning

All abortion assessment services should have easy access to ultrasound. Although not necessary in every case, it is essential if there is concern regarding ectopic pregnancy, or uncertain gestation.

Ultrasound scanning should be done sensitively and in an appropriate setting. It should not be carried out in an antenatal department alongside women with wanted pregnancies. Some women may wish to see the ultrasound image, and this should be respected. Occasionally women may request a copy of the scan, as a momento, or acknowledgement of the pregnancy.

Prevention of infective complications

Post-abortion infection complications may occur in up to 10% of cases; this risk can be reduced by about 50% with antibiotic prophylaxis. Services may choose to treat everyone, screen and only treat those who test positive or treat all but screen all since messages about safer sex may be stronger if women know that they have tested positive. As a minimum, all abortion services should offer antibiotic prophylaxis. The recommended regimens are:

- Metronidazole 1 g rectally at the time of abortion, plus doxycycline 100 mg twice daily for 7 days, *or*
- Metronidazole 1 g rectally at the time of abortion, plus azithromycin 1 g orally on the day of abortion.

Ideally, abortion services should offer STI screening, with treatment and partner notification of all positive cases. This should prevent re-infection from an untreated partner, and provides an opportunity to deliver sexual risk behaviour education.

Cervical cytology

Women who have not had a smear, or who are due a repeat smear can be offered a smear at the clinic. Women under the age of 20 should not be offered cervical cytology, in keeping with the national programme.

If a smear is taken there should be a failsafe mechanism to convey the result to the woman, referring appropriately if necessary, and notifying the smear to the local screening programme for appropriate recall. Without this mechanism, it would be inappropriate to offer cervical screening.

Provision of information for the woman

Verbal information conveyed at the time of consultation should be backed up with written information. Information may be required in alternative formats, e.g. audiotape for visually impaired women, or in a different language for non-English speakers.

Several national organizations have comprehensive information leaflets which can be downloaded from the internet and adapted for local use (see additional resources at end of chapter). An additional leaflet about the specifics of the local service can be provided.

Information should convey details about:

- Rights to abortion, including right to confidentiality
- How to access abortion services
- What abortion options are available
- Risks and sequelae of abortion
- Local contact information.

ABORTION TECHNIQUES

In the past two decades, there have been several advances in the techniques to induce abortion so that safe and effective methods are now available at all stages of gestation. Since mifepristone was licensed in 1991 use of medical methods has increased; in Scotland around two-thirds of abortions below 10 weeks gestation are now performed medically.[3] Both medical and surgical abortion can be offered at all gestations to 24 weeks, but in reality, choice may be governed by local availability. The optimum method depends on gestation, parity, medical history and of course on the woman's wishes. The RCOG guideline recommends that services should be able to offer termination by at least one of the methods at each gestation, but ideally should be able to offer a choice of techniques. Termination of pregnancy in the late second trimester requires specialist skills and training, and may not be available in every area. Service providers should ensure that referral and funding arrangements are in place for women seeking late termination. This may involve agreement with a charitable sector organization such as the British Pregnancy Advisory Service (BPAS) or Marie Stopes International.

• Medical termination

Although a number of substances are historically known to have been used to induce abortion, the discovery of the antigestogen mifepristone (RU 486) in 1980 made medical abortion a practical reality. Mifepristone (Mifegyne) is a synthetic steroid chemically similar to norethindrone (the gestogen in one of the first combined oral contraceptives) which blocks the biological action of progesterone by binding to its receptor in the uterus and other target organs. Mifepristone is administered orally under supervision of a doctor or nurse, in a premises licenced to carry out abortion, and the woman is then allowed home. She returns 24–72 hours later (most commonly 48 hours in UK practice) and is admitted for administration of a prostaglandin, to complete the termination process. Bleeding usually begins within a few hours, followed by passing of the gestational sac and fetus. The woman can usually be managed as a day case, and allowed home after around 6–8 hours. Current UK law and accepted practice dictate that both parts of medical termination are administered in the licenced place setting, although work in other countries, particularly the United States, has demonstrated the efficacy and acceptability of home administration of the prostaglandin component.[7] Most women experience period-like pains although there is great variability, with some needing no analgesia while about 10–20% require opiates. Bleeding usually continues for about 10 days although the total amount of blood lost (around 80 mL) is similar to that occurring during surgical termination.

Early medical termination – up to 9 weeks gestation

Below 7 weeks, medical abortion is the most effective option for termination of pregnancy, with a lower failure rate than early surgical abortion. It continues to be effective between 7 and 9 weeks (63 days) gestation. The licensed regimen in the UK is 600 mg mifepristone (3 tablets) orally, followed by 1 mg of vaginal gemeprost. However, 200 mg (a single tablet) of mifepristone is as effective as 600 mg.[6] In addition, an alternative prostagladin analogue, misoprostol, has been shown to be effective, and is now used conventionally in the UK. It is stable at room temperature, and is significantly cheaper than gemeprost.

The RCOG recommended regimen for early medical termination, based on efficacy, side effects and cost, is:

- Mifepristone 200 mg orally, followed by misoprostol 800 μg vaginally, 24–72 hours later.

If abortion has not occurred within 4 hours of misoprostol administration, a second dose of 400 μg can be given for women between 7 and 9 weeks

Medical termination in the late first trimester (9–13 weeks)

Conventionally, surgical termination has been the standard method offered to women in the late first trimester, as initial studies suggested a higher failure rate of medical termination at this gestation. However, a randomized trial of women at 9–13 weeks to either medical or surgical abortion, demonstrated comparable complete abortion rates.[8]

It is now recommended that medical abortion should be offered as an alternative option to surgical termination in the late first trimester, with a suggested regimen of:

- Mifepristone 200 mg orally, followed by misoprostol 800 μg vaginally 36–48 hours later. Up to a further 4 doses of misoprostol 400 μg, either vaginally or orally, can be given until abortion has occurred.

Medical termination in the second trimester (13–24 weeks)

Traditionally, midtrimester medical abortion has been carried out using prostaglandin alone, or in combination with an oxytocin infusion. However, pretreatment with mifepristone is effective, and significantly reduces the induction to abortion interval to between 6 and 8 hours. Rates of complete abortion remain high; under 10% of cases require surgical evacuation to complete the process. Like the first trimester process, the reduced dose of 200 mg of mifepristone is effective, with no difference in efficacy, time interval to abortion or side effects between misoprostol and gemeprost.

The recommended regimen in the UK for medical termination between 13–24 weeks is:

- Mifepristone 200 mg orally, followed by misoprostol 800 μg vaginally 36–48 hours later. Up to a further 4 doses of misoprostol 400 μg orally, can be given until abortion has occurred.

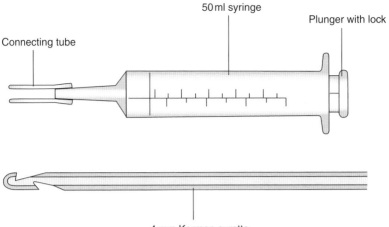

Figure 16.2 Manual vacuum aspiration equipment

• Surgical termination of pregnancy

Surgical termination below 7 weeks gestation

Surgical termination below 7 weeks gestation has a higher failure rate than that performed at higher gestations, and is less effective than medical termination at this gestation. Surgical termination is therefore usually deferred until 7 weeks gestation in the UK. However, some centres now offer manual vacuum aspiration at very early gestation. This is performed using a narrow suction curette of 4 or 5 mm diameter, inserted into the uterus under local paracervical block. Aspiration is provided by a 50 ml syringe (Figure 16.2). It is essential that a rigorous protocol is followed with this procedure, to include magnification of the aspirated material, with βhCG follow-up if products of conception are not identified.

Surgical termination between 7–15 weeks

In the UK, surgical termination at this gestation is usually performed by suction or vacuum aspiration, using a flexible suction curette, and a mechanical or electrical pump. The suction curette is inserted into the uterine cavity, after cervical dilatation, and the contents gently aspirated. Sharp curettage is not recommended. In the UK, the procedure is usually carried out under general anaesthesia, but local anaesthesia or conscious sedation are acceptable choices.

Complications increase with advancing gestation, and are inversely related to the experience of the surgeon. At all gestations, surgical termination should be performed by an appropriately experienced practitioner. In some areas surgical termination is not performed above 12 weeks gestation.

Late surgical termination (15–24 weeks)

Dilatation and evacuation, preceded by cervical preparation can be offered as a choice in the second trimester. It is the method of choice in the USA, but in the UK its use is confined largely to gynaecologists in private practice or in the charitable sector. It may be necessary to dilate the cervix up to a diameter of 20 mm before the fetal parts can be extracted using special instruments.

In skilled hands, D&E is safe, with complication rates no higher than medical abortion at the same gestation. It requires careful training if complications such as haemorrhage and perforation of the uterus are to be avoided, and the surgeon requires to carry out enough procedures to maintain his or her skills. D&E has the advantage that the woman is unaware of the procedure, which can be performed as a day case. There is evidence from the USA that women prefer D&E to medical methods although many nurses and doctors find it disturbing.

• Cervical preparation prior to surgical termination

Cervical preparation before surgical termination reduces the risk of cervical trauma and uterine perforation. RCOG recommends that cervical preparation should be considered for all surgical abortions, and should be used routinely when the woman is under 18 years of age, or gestation is above 10 weeks. The recommended regimen for both first and second trimester surgical termination is:

- Misoprostol 400 μg given vaginally, 3 hours prior to surgery.

COMPLICATIONS OF TERMINATION

When undergoing counselling about termination of pregnancy, women should be advised that the risk of complications is low. Indeed a termination is safer than continuing the pregnancy to term. Nonetheless, complications do occasionally arise, and women should be aware of the risks, and should know where to seek help or advice if concerned.

• Incomplete termination/retained products of conception

This is the commonest complication following abortion. Incomplete abortion is more common after medical abortion in the first trimester; up to 5% of women will require surgical evacuation of the uterus within the first month. However incomplete abortion also occurs after surgical termination, especially at the extremes of gestation. Ongoing pregnancy after attempted abortion is uncommon, but occurs in 2.3 per 1000 women undergoing surgical termination, and between 1 and 14 women having medical termination. All women should be advised of the importance of returning for follow-up, particularly if products of conception were not seen at the time of termination, or there are ongoing symptoms of pregnancy.

The occurrence of bleeding and presence of residual trophoblastic tissue in the uterus at 2 weeks after a medical or surgical abortion are not in themselves indications to evacuate the uterus. Although an ultrasound scan of the uterus and the measurement of hCG may help in diagnosing ongoing pregnancy, the decision to evacuate the uterus should be made on clinical grounds, i.e. continued heavy or persistent bleeding from a bulky uterus in which the cervix is still dilated.

The majority of women with an incomplete abortion will pass the residual tissue with time, without additional intervention. Minor complications such as lower abdominal pain, vaginal bleeding and passage of clots or trophoblastic tissue are relatively common and usually only require reassurance.

• Post abortion infection

Pelvic infection can occur in up to 10% of women after termination, but the incidence is significantly reduced by pre-abortion STI screening and prophylactic antibiotics. Women should be advised about signs and symptoms of infection such as pyrexia, abdominal pain and offensive vaginal discharge, and should attend for review if concerned.

• Trauma to the genital tract

The risk of perforation of the uterus is around 1 in 1000, and is greater with increasing gestation, and with limited experience of the practitioner. Cervical trauma is also rare (less than 1 in 100) and is further reduced by cervical preparation. Uterine rupture has been described with midtrimester medical abortion, but certainly occurs in less than 1 in 1000 cases.

• Haemorrhage

Haemorrhage at the time of termination is rare, occurring in around 1 in 1000 cases. Risk increases with increasing gestation.

• Future reproductive outcome

Women can be reassured that there is no proven association between previous termination of pregnancy and future infertility, ectopic pregnancy or placenta praevia. There may be a slight increase in subsequent miscarriage and preterm delivery, although the evidence is mixed.

• Breast cancer

There is no association between termination of pregnancy and future risk of breast cancer.

• Psychological sequelae

A large study carried out in the UK in the first decade after the Abortion Act compared incidence of major psychiatric sequelae in women undergoing abortion, and in women delivering after being denied abortion. The incidence of psychosis was 0.3/1000 in post abortion women, and 1.7/1000 in postpartum women.[9]

In 1990, the American Psychological Association convened an expert panel, to review the published evidence on the psychological impact of abortion. This panel found no evidence of lasting psychological harm, concluding that abortion is generally 'psychologically benign' for most women.[10]

FOLLOW-UP

A follow-up visit about 2 weeks after abortion is desirable for all women, to ensure there are no complications, and to encourage ongoing use of reliable contraception. Follow-up is essential when products of termination were not seen at the time of termination. Although the incidence of ongoing pregnancy is low (less than 1%), it may be necessary to evacuate the uterus because of incomplete abortion in about 2–5% of cases. Follow-up can be undertaken by the general practitioner, family planning clinic or abortion service. Careful co-ordination of these services is essential to ensure ongoing pregnancies are identified promptly and complications treated.

POST TERMINATION CONTRACEPTION

Over a quarter of terminations are carried out on women who have previously had a termination, and it is good practice to ensure that the woman has the opportunity to consider her contraceptive options fully before discharge following abortion.

All methods of hormonal contraception can be instituted immediately following termination either on the day of surgical termination, or on the prostaglandin treatment day of medical termination, with immediate contraceptive effect. Services should ensure that a supply of the chosen method is available to the woman. Injectable contraception can be given on the day of termination, prior to discharge, or the etonorgestrel implant can be fitted. Intrauterine contraception (copper device or levonorgestrel intrauterine system) can be fitted immediately following the end of the surgical procedure, or following expulsion of the products of conception with medical termination. Services should consider arrangements to ensure that an appropriately trained person is available to institute the use of the long-acting reversible methods. Male and female condoms can be used immediately after termination, although women are usually advised not to use a diaphragm or cap within 6 weeks of midtrimester termination, in case refitting is required.

Decision about sterilization is best deferred until at least 6 weeks after termination. Sterilization at the time of termination is associated with a higher failure rate, and an increased incidence of regret. However, as ovulation returns rapidly after abortion, alternative contraceptive precautions should be strongly advised in the interim.

CONCLUSION

Almost 200 000 women undergo termination of pregnancy each year in the UK. Women and their practitioners need to be well informed about termination options and implications, so that a truly informed choice can be made. Services should strive to provide minimal waiting times, and work to evidence-based recommendations to make termination as safe and acceptable a procedure as possible. Repeat abortion is common, and practitioners should ensure that the full range of contraceptive options is available to women at the time of termination.

REFERENCES

1. Fathalla MF (1992) Reproductive health in the world: two decades of progress and the challenge ahead. In: Khanna J, Van Look PFA, Griffin PD (eds) Reproductive health: a key to a brighter future. World Health Organization, Geneva, pp. 3–31.

2. Government Statistical Service for the Department of Health (2004) Abortion Statistics, England and Wales: 2004. Also available at http://www.dh.gov.uk/PublicationsAndStatistics

3. Scottish Health Statistics (2005) Available at http://www.isdscotland.org/isd/info

4. Lakha F, Glasier A (2006) Unintended pregnancy and use of emergency contraception among a large cohort of women attending for antenatal care or abortion in Scotland. Lancet 368(9549): 1782–1787.

5. Francome C, Freeman E (2000) British General Practitioners' Attitudes Toward Abortion. Family Planning Perspectives 32(4): 191–198.

6. Royal College of Obstetricians and Gynaecologists. Evidence-based Clinical Guideline Number 7. The Care of Women Requesting Induced Abortion. Available at http://www.rcog.org.uk/guidelines

7. Harper C, Ellertson C, Winikoff X (2002) Could American women use mifepristone-misoprostol pills safely with less medical supervision? Contraception 65: 133–142.

8. Ashok PW, Kidd A, Flett GMM, et al. (2002) A randomized comparison of medical and surgical vacuum aspiration at 10–13 weeks of gestation. Hum Reprod 17: 92–98.

9. Brewer C (1977) Incidence of post-abortion psychosis: a prospective study. BMJ 1: 476–477.

10. Adler N, David H, Major B, Roth S, Russo N, Wyatt G (1990) Psychological responses after abortion. Science 248(4951): 41–44.

USEFUL WEBSITES

Patient information leaflets can be downloaded:

www.rcog.org.uk – a nationally developed leaflet.

www.fpa.org.uk – information and support organization, with a nationally developed leaflet.

www.sandyford.org/sandyford/profpages/leaflets.html – an adaptation of national information for local use in Glasgow, presented as a series of five leaflets.

17 Screening and health promotion

Sally Hope

Chapter contents

SCREENING

Screening is, by definition, the examination of asymptomatic individuals in an attempt to identify preinvasive disease, early disease or the risk factors for a disease. The screening test must be acceptable, reliable and economically possible within the resources of the healthcare service of the country concerned. The screenable disease must be amenable to treatment and there must be an advantage in treating the disease at a stage before the patient would otherwise present. This all seems simple but screening programmes are fraught with controversy. The basic concept is well supported by the medical profession and by the general public: people want to remain well and healthy.

Many people are falsely reassured by screening, believing that if they have been checked by a health professional, nothing could possibly go wrong in the future. Evidence-based patient choice now places the responsibility on

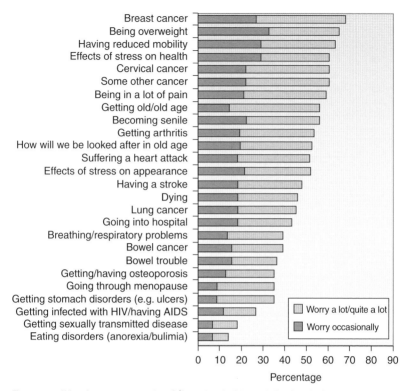

Figure 17.1 What do women worry about? (Reproduced with permission from BBC Factual & Learning, London, UK).

the individual him- or herself to decide whether or not he or she wants a particular test.

The family planning consultation offers an excellent opportunity for screening and for promoting health. Open questions in a consultation allow a woman to raise issues that particularly concern her. Women may have been coming to the same clinic for 20–30 years. During that time their health needs and the appropriate screening measures will have changed, and information or technologies related to specific diseases may have become more refined. Screening is dynamic, and not static.

A final strand of this complex tapestry of health is the woman's own health beliefs and fears. For example, most women fear they will die of breast cancer (Figure 17.1). Cardiovascular disease is still the major overall cause of death in the UK, although total cancer deaths are commoner in women at younger ages (Figure 17.2, Table 17.1). More women currently die from lung cancer than from breast cancer. Unless a woman's fears and

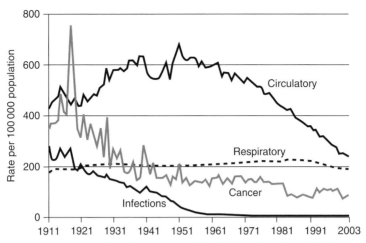

Figure 17.2 Selected causes of death by age and sex ONS 2002 England and Wales 2002. (Reproduced with permission from Mortality Statistics 2002 Office for National Statistics © Crown Copyright 2002.)

Table 17.1 Age-standardized mortality rates for selected broad disease groups, 2002–2003, England & Wales

England & Wales	Rates per 100 000 population					
	0–14	15–29	30–44	45–64	65–84	85 and over
Males						
Infectious diseases	2	1	3	6	30	142
Cancers	4	6	23	245	1403	3422
Circulatory diseases	1	4	27	232	1861	7982
Respiratory diseases	2	2	5	41	566	3610
Injury and poisoning	4	41	45	36	59	299
All causes	28	71	139	654	4427	18806
Females						
Infectious diseases	1	1	1	4	24	115
Cancers	3	5	32	218	921	1858
Circulatory diseases	1	3	11	88	1269	7016
Respiratory diseases	1	1	4	30	403	2654
Injury and poisoning	3	10	12	15	45	294
All causes	21	28	80	416	3155	15983

(Reproduced with permission from Mortality Statistics 2002 Office for National Statistics © Crown Copyright 2002.)

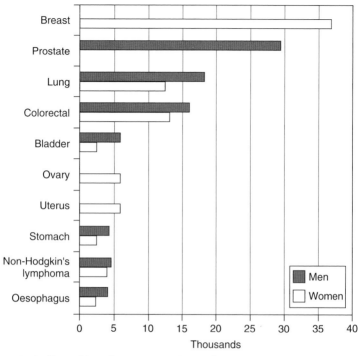

Figure 17.3 Incidence of the major cancers, 2004 England. (Reproduced with permission from Mortality Statistics 2002 Office for National Statistics © Crown Copyright 2002.)

misconceptions are addressed, very little of the value of health promotional activity will be understood by the individual.

BREAST CANCER

In the UK, 1 in every 9 women will develop breast cancer at some time in their lives. It is the most common cancer in women worldwide and in the UK (Figure 17.3). In 2004, there were 36 939 new breast cancer registrations and 12 347 women died from the disease (Figure 17.4). In the UK, almost 20% of deaths among women aged 40–50 years are due to breast cancer. More than 90% of breast cancers are detected by the woman herself.

• Breast self-examination

In the past women were encouraged to do breast self-examination (BSE), a monthly palpation performed by a woman at the same time each month in a routine manner, on the premise that the earlier the lump was found the

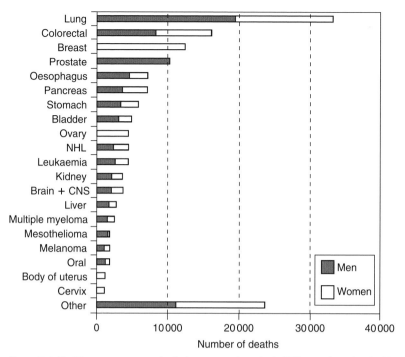

Figure 17.4 The 20 commonest cancer deaths in women and men in the UK in 2004 (reproduced with permission from Cancer Research UK 2006)

better the prognosis. Large clinical trials have however demonstrated that BSE is ineffective. It tends to increase anxiety by generating unneccessary referrals and should not therefore be recommended.

• Breast awareness

BSE was replaced by the concept of breast awareness where women are advised to be conscious of what is normal for them about the feel and look of their breasts throughout the menstrual cycle and to seek help if they notice anything different. Women should be aware of their breasts in everyday activities such as bathing and dressing. This can be easily discussed in the family planning consultation and instruction given.

• Routine breast examination

The Department of Health (DH) in the UK has stated that there is no evidence to support the efficacy of breast examination by health professionals of well women without symptoms, as it is liable to give false reassurance and discourage breast self-awareness. The DH advise that palpation of the breasts by any healthcare professionals should not be included as part of a routine health screening for women.

There is no need for breast examination of an asymptomatic woman prior prescribing to the combined oral contraceptive pill or hormone replacement therapy. However, breast awareness should always be discussed (see Chapters 3 and 22).

• Mammography

Regular mammography for women aged between 50–69 years has been demonstrated to be effective in reducing mortality from breast cancer. On the basis of this, the NHS Breast Screening Programme in the UK began inviting women for screening in 1988. The latest research shows that the NHS Breast Screening Programme is now saving 1400 lives every year in England. In England, the cost of the breast screening programme equates to around £37.50 per woman invited or £45.50 per woman screened.

The current UK guidelines are that all women between the ages of 50 and 70 years should be screened routinely every 3 years with a two-view radiographic examination. There is no routine screening for women under 50 years, and women over 70 years may continue to be screened if they wish.

It has been demonstrated that women are more likely to attend mammographic screening if there has been a brief discussion prior to the screening invitation with a healthcare professional.[1] In one study, 81% of women who had mammography claimed to experience discomfort (actual pain in 46% and severe pain in 7%). However, of the women questioned 60% said that a cervical smear or venepuncture was a more uncomfortable procedure.[2]

• Special groups

Women with a strong family history

Women with a strong family history of breast cancer affecting a first-degree relative under the age of 50 may be offered screening outwith the national guidelines. This service varies greatly from region to region. In some areas, there are specialist genetic clinics, and in other regions, breast specialists advise and screen these high-risk women. Recently, the National Institute for Clinical Excellence (NICE) recommended that women aged 30–49 years at high risk because of known genetic mutations have annual magnetic resonance imaging (MRI) breast scans.[3]

Women with symptoms

A woman with a breast lump must be examined and referred as appropriate.

Women with breast cancer

Women with breast cancer will generally be given more frequent mammograms and follow-up than the standard 3-yearly recall but this will be at the discretion of the clinician looking after that particular woman.

WEIGHT

Women are generally concerned about being overweight. In a survey for the BBC Radio 4 programme *Woman's Hour*, 33% of women in the UK over the age of 16 were concerned about being overweight.[4] The commonest reason for discontinuation of combined oral contraception (COC) is perceived weight gain.

Offering advice about healthy diet and exercise is an important health promotion issue but there is no evidence to show any efficacy on preventing obesity. Most women do not appreciate that being extremely thin puts them at higher risk of future osteoporosis and Alzheimer's disease. Conversely women who are significantly overweight (BMI > 30) double their risk of breast cancer. Obesity is also a risk factor for diabetes and cardiovascular disease in women.

DOMESTIC VIOLENCE

Domestic violence is defined as a pattern of aggressive and controlling behaviour from one adult, usually a male, to another, usually a female, within the context of an intimate relationship. The abuse can be physical, sexual, psychological or emotional. It is estimated that in England and Wales domestic violence results in more than 125 deaths a year.

Healthcare professionals rarely ask about domestic violence and, across the socio-economic classes, women are often too ashamed to talk about it. Those affected may present in the family planning consultation in urgent need of contraception or even termination of pregnancy. It may be helpful to have information posters in waiting rooms or on toilet doors which women can read and obtain information from, without making it obvious to others that they need help.

Strategies for detection and management of the problem include understanding the dynamics of the family, careful enquiry about victimization, screening for risk factors such as previous violence and high alcohol intake, and assuring patient safety. Healthcare professionals should be aware of available services locally to facilitate referral and should provide the victim with non-judgemental and confidential support.

SEXUALLY TRANSMITTED INFECTIONS

Women may confide during the family planning consultation that they are worried that they might have a sexually transmitted infection (STI) (see

Chapter 13). Within Genito-urinary Medicine Clinics (GUM), testing for STIs is well established but exact protocols will vary in different regions. General practitioners throughout the UK with an interest in sexual health are often enthusiastic about involvement in STI screening. With 2.7 million attendances at family planning clinics in England per annum and an estimated 23% of women aged 16–19 visiting a clinic per year, family planning clinics are important screening sites for STIs.

• Chlamydia screening

The National Chlamydia Screening Programme (NCSP) in England offers opportunistic screening for chlamydia to men and women under 25 years of age. Randomized trials show that systematic screening for genital *Chlamydia trachomatis* might reduce the incidence of pelvic inflammatory disease by about 50%. Nearly 100 000 NCSP chlamydia screens were undertaken in 2005/06 (the third year of the programme) with an overall positivity rate of 10.2% in women and 10.1% in men. Positivity was highest in black ethnic groups and lowest in Asian and Chinese populations. Only 18% of those screened were men. Recent roll outs of the NCSP have involved healthcare auxilliaries, GP receptionists, and Boots the Chemist chain of pharmacies. SIGN (Scottish Intercollegiate Guidelines Network) has also recently updated national guidelines for chlamydia screening and management.

In a comparison of individuals aged between 16–40 diagnosed with chlamydia in primary care with those diagnosed in GUM, women in primary care reported fewer sexual partners and were less likely to have had an HIV test in the past 5 years than their counterparts diagnosed in GUM.[5] Age, ethnicity, social class, educational attainment and urbanization of area of residence did not differ between the two groups. Too few men were diagnosed in primary care to allow for such a comparison. Women with chlamydia infections who attend primary care may perceive themselves as low risk through age or sexual behaviour, yet are likely to comprise a substantial proportion of all infections.

In a study undertaken in Bristol, 60.4% of men and 75.3% of women aged 16–24 years attended their GP at least once in a 1-year period and could be offered opportunistic screening.[6] Postal screening projects show lower responses in areas with more non-white residents, along with poorer uptake in more deprived areas and among women at higher risk of infection.

Four main themes emerged from a qualitative study describing the experience of those screened.[7] There was initial discomfort with screening arising from an unease with sexual health issues; anxiety, especially after receiving a positive test result, due to the fear of informing sexual partners, the risk of infertility and the possibility of having other undetected infections; women's concern about being stigmatized for having been infected with chlamydia, which affected how they felt about themselves and how they thought others would perceive them; and recognizing the need to balance the harms of screening with the benefits. Importantly, despite some reported adverse effects, no one regretted their decision to be screened.

Public education and discussion of sexually transmitted infections should help to increase the acceptability of chlamydia screening and destigmatize a diagnosis of chlamydia. Those working in primary care settings who opt to offer chlamydia screening must be suitably trained to inform individuals of the potential adverse effects and to deal with their consequences. They should also be aware of the need for partner notification/contact tracing and referral to GUM for this if no local facilities are available.

CHOLESTEROL

The American College of Physicians recommends that young healthy adult men aged under 35 and pre-menopausal women under 45 should not be screened for elevated cholesterol concentrations because of concerns about the costs and health risks associated with over-use of pharmacological therapy. Their recommendation was that these individuals should be given lifestyle advice. In the UK routine screening is not recommended for men or women under the age of 40 years. If a young woman is particularly worried about a strong family history of hypercholesterolaemia this can be discussed, but all women should be offered advice about a healthier lifestyle; increasing exercise, decreasing weight if obese, stopping smoking and adopting a Mediterranean-style diet.

SMOKING

The single most important health prevention measure any healthcare professional can do is to help an individual stop smoking. Around 70% of smokers would like to stop if they could. Unfortunately, young women are continuing to smoke and the decline in smoking is less among female than among male smokers. Ex-smokers can substantially restore their life expectancy to that of non-smokers, but if they do not stop, half of those who smoke will die prematurely.

The essential features of the individual smoking cessation advice are:

1. Ask (about smoking at every opportunity).
2. Advise (all smokers to stop).
3. Assist (the smoker to stop).
4. Arrange (follow-up to monitor progress and/or additional support).

In the UK, the government has set up new specialist support services to give healthcare professionals assistance in helping individuals to stop smoking. Most general practices now have a 'stopping smoking support clinic' run by a nurse or health visitor.

CERVICAL CANCER

Cervical cancer has a preinvasive phase which may last for many years and accounts for the success of screening for the disease. The abnormalities seen during the pre-invasive phase are known as 'cervical intraepithelial neoplasia' or CIN and are graded according to severity (Figure 17.5). In order that cervical screening is cost effective, at least 75% of the female population must attend for regular smears. Since the advent of the cervical screening call/recall programmes in the UK in the late 1980s, the incidence of the disease has fallen by more than 40%. Deaths from cervical cancer have also decreased (in Scotland by 50%) – partly because of increased early detection at the preinvasive phase and also because of advances in the treatment of established cervical cancer.

• Risk factors for cervical cancer

- • Human papilloma virus is the essential causative factor
- • Smoking – which reduces immunity
- • Immunosuppression – including HIV
- • High parity, use of combined oral contraception and co-infection with STIs are also factors, although less important.

• Human papilloma virus

The role of human papilloma virus (HPV) in cervical dysplasia and neoplasia has been recognized since the 1970s. Several subtypes of this virus have been implicated in the aetiology of cervical cancer. The most relevant of these are

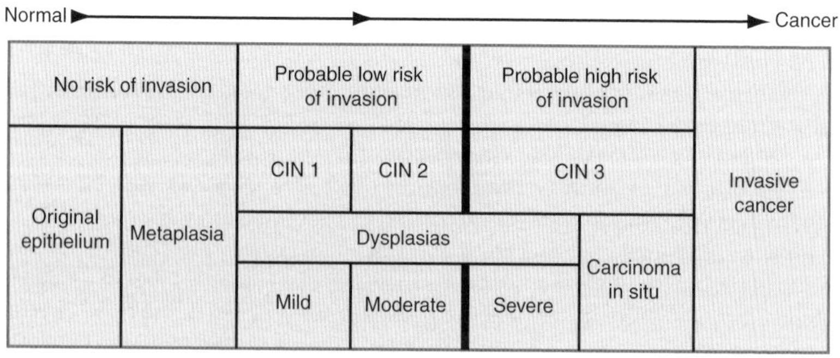

Figure 17.5 Three stages of cervical intraepithelial neoplasia (CIN).

16 and 18 which are 'highly oncogenic' and account for 70% of all cervical cancers. HPV types 6 and 11 cause genital warts but not cervical disease and there is no need therefore to screen women with warts more frequently.

Around 60% of women with mild dyskaryosis reported on cervical cytology will spontaneously clear the virus and subsequent smears will be normal. Approximately 10% of those with mild dyskaryosis will however progress to having severe dyskaryosis within 2–4 years. It is not currently possible to distinguish these two groups. Although it is possible to test for HPV types, this is neither cost effective nor widely available.

All women with abnormal smears should be strongly encouraged to stop smoking to improve their immune response. There is evidence that the combined pill more than doubles the relative risk of cervical cancer after 10 years of use. Since the overall relative risk in Western populations is low and since population screening is routine this doubling is not very clinically relevant but it is relevant in many parts of the developing world where there are no screening programmes. Women of high parity are also at increased risk of cervical cancer since the larger transformation zone during pregnancy is vulnerable to infection from HPV.

• National screening programme

Screening for cervical cancer has been in place in the UK since 1967 and, like breast cancer screening, is now under the auspices of the NHS Cancer Screening Programme. In England, the current recommendations comprise a first invitation at 25 years of age, interval screening 3-yearly from 25–49, and 5-yearly from 50–64 years. In Scotland and Wales, the recommendations differ in that all women over the age of 20 are invited every 3 years until the age of 60. By screening every 5 years, the incidence of the disease falls by 84%. Reducing the screening interval to 3-yearly leads to a further reduction in incidence of cervical cancer of 91%. Women who have never been sexually active have an extremely low chance of developing cervical cancer and, although they will be invited for cervical screening, they can choose to decline. Women who have had a subtotal hysterectomy (i.e. have the cervix retained at surgery) must continue to have routine smears.

Every woman needs to have the test explained, and arrangements made for receipt of the results. It is the responsibility of the smear-taker to instigate further investigation and follow-up all abnormal results. Computerized call and recall systems are in place in most areas.

Opportunistic screening should be offered to women who have never had a smear or who have not had a smear within the past 3–5 years. There is evidence that a woman who has always had normal smears prior to the age of 50 is highly unlikely to develop cervical dysplasia and therefore could decline further screening. If she changes partner however, she should have further smears. Teenage girls should **not** be screened. The incidence of HPV infection in young women who are becoming sexually active is very high.

Around this time many of them will have some cervical dysplastic cells but most will resolve these by their early 20s. Cervical smears in teenagers will only therefore lead to unnecessary colposcopy and treatments.

• HPV vaccines

Two vaccines against HPV have been developed. One is now licensed and the other will apply for licensing later in 2007. These vaccines induce neutralizing antibodies to the oncogenic subtypes from their virus like particles (VLPs) from the major coat or capsid protein L1. Cervarix (Sanofi Pasteur) is a bivalent vaccine against HPV 16 and 18 and Gardasil (Glaxo Smith Kline) a quadrivalent vaccine against HPV 6, 11, 16 and 18 which thus also protects against genital warts. In Phase III trials of both vaccines there was 100% efficacy against development of HPV 16/18 associated CIN 2/3. As yet, the duration of protection of these vaccines is unknown, or whether booster immunization will be required. There is some evidence of cross-protection against other HPV types which are less oncogenic.

Guidance as to who should receive which HPV vaccination is currently awaited. Ideally young people should be vaccinated prior to becoming sexually active. However, vaccination could provide protection for those who are already sexually active but have not been exposed to the specific HPV types. The debate as to which vaccine should be recommended will continue meantime. Arguments in favour of vaccinating boys with the quadrivalent vaccine to attempt to eradicate genital warts and girls with the bivalent vaccine which may provide longer protection against HPV 16 and 18 are currently being made. Cervical screening will remain necessary for many years to come as it is unlikely that all women will be vaccinated and even those who are will remain vulnerable to infection with other HPV types which may cause abnormalities.

• Taking a cervical smear

This requires adequate training and a sensitive and gentle approach. The smear-taker should be aware that many women feel anxious about having a cervical smear, particularly about the indignity and discomfort of the procedure, as well as concern about the outcome.

The woman should be welcomed, and her identity and details checked: name, date of birth, current address, NHS number. The technique of taking the smear should be explained. How the result will be communicated to her and the likely timescale for this should be discussed.

The room for taking a cervical smear needs to have a strong and comfortable couch, with adequate lighting and be at a warm, pleasant temperature. There needs to be a supply of clean specula of varying sizes to cope with different women; Cervex-Brush® and endocervical brushes (Figure 17.6); fixative vials: ThinPrep or SurePath; black ball point pen; sample forms; specimen bags and information leaflets.

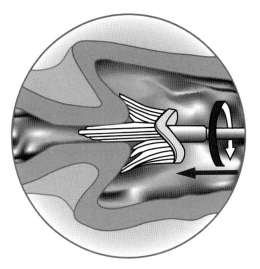

Figure 17.6 Taking a cervical smear: rotate the spatula through 360°

The commonest error in taking a smear is failing to take an adequate sample from the squamocolumnar junction, the area where neoplastic change occurs (Figure 17.7). In nulliparous women, and in women beyond the menopause, the squamocolumnar junction may be well within the cervical canal and it is not always possible to sample this area.

Technique

Offer the woman a chaperone prior to beginning the examination and ensure that there is a sheet with which she can cover her lower abdomen.

1. Ask the woman to lie on her back or on her left side.
2. With good illumination, insert the speculum, lubricated only with water, and expose the cervix.
3. If the presence of an invasive carcinoma is suspected on clinical examination, refer the woman for urgent gynaecological assessment irrespective of and prior to the smear result. Do not postpone the smear of a suspicious cervix should active bleeding be present.
4. Using the Cervex-Brush®, insert the central bristles of the brush into the endocervical canal so that the shorter, outer bristles fully contact the ectocervix.
5. Using pencil pressure, rotate the brush five times in a clockwise direction.
6. In order to ensure good contact with the ectocervix, the plastic fronds of the brush are bevelled for clockwise rotation only. A high cellular yield will be achieved with correct use of the brush.
7. Immediately fix the sample using the appropriate instructions below.

Figure 17.7 Types of sampling spatula.
Cytobroom, cytobrush and ThinPrep (R) pap
preparation. (Reproduced by courtesy of
Cytyc corporation and affiliates)

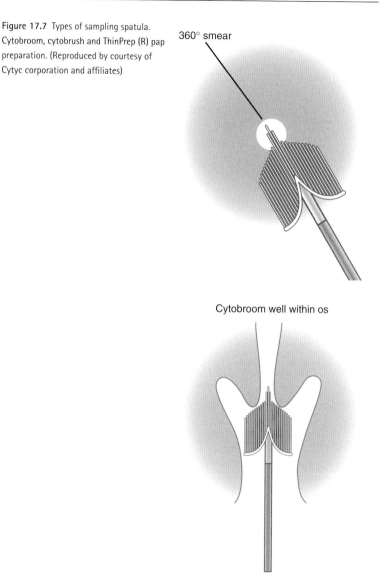

360° smear

Cytobroom well within os

ThinPrep

- Rinse the brush into the fixative vial using a vigorous swirling motion.
- Push the brush into the bottom of the vial at least 10 times, forcing the bristles apart. Firm pressure is necessary or the cells will cling to the brush.

- Inspect the brush for any residual material and remove any remaining by passing the brush over the edge of the fixative vial.
- Ensure that the material reaches the liquid or it will not be preserved.
- Tighten the cap so that the torque line passes the torque line on the vial.
- If you have placed any material on the edge of the vial give it a shake.

SurePath

- Simply remove the head of the brush from the stem and place into the vial of fixative.
- Screw the lid on and shake to ensure that the cells do not cling to the device.

N.B. For both methods, it is essential that the sample is placed in the vial at once in order to achieve immediate fixation.

8. Remove the speculum.
9. Complete the consultation:
   - ask the woman to dress and join you at the desk to finish the consultation
   - check that the woman's name and date of birth are recorded on the vial
   - check that the form is complete
   - ensure that the woman understands how and when she will receive her result
   - discuss possible results and follow-up if appropriate
   - ensure that the woman understands that if, in the future, she has any abnormal bleeding or discharge she should seek advice
   - complete notes/computer record
   - place the vial in an appropriate package for transport to the laboratory
   - dispose of equipment and waste safely
   - send the sample to the laboratory as soon as possible.

• Management of abnormal smears

The follow-up recommendations after abnormal smears should be documented by the laboratory on the written result. Swift referral to colposcopy is required for cervical carcinoma, severe dyskaryosis or moderate dyskaryosis. Women with a mild or borderline smear should have a repeat smear in 6 months time with colposcopy referral if this is again abnormal.

Doctors should be clear about the facilities for investigation and treatment available locally. Colposcopic examination and treatment services are widely available in the UK and the traditional cone biopsy will be avoided in the vast majority of women with abnormal smears. Local ablative treatments include excision by loop diathermy, cold coagulation and laser vaporization.

CARCINOMA OF THE OVARY

Carcinoma of the ovary is the fourth commonest female cancer. The lifetime risk of developing ovarian cancer in England and Wales is 1 in 48. It is uncommon in young women. Ovarian cancer is often undetected until it presents at a late stage of the disease with poor survival rates. Overall 5-year survival is only 40%, but rises to over 75% if treated early when disease is localized to the ovaries.

Women with one affected first-degree relative have a two to three times greater risk of ovarian cancer than the general population. When more than one relative is affected, the relative risk increases 11-fold. The main genetic marker is BRCA1 mutation although this is present in only 5% of women with ovarian cancers diagnosed before the age of 70 years.[8] Early menarchy, late menopause, few children and never use of combined oral contraception are all independent risk factors.

• Ovarian cancer screening

Ovarian cancer is difficult to detect in asymptomatic women, and as yet there is no evidence that this enhances survival. It would be logical to assume that screening would be more appropriate for women at higher risk, but at present there is no clear evidence to support this.

A number of combinations of screening tests for ovarian cancer are being evaluated including measurement of the tumour marker CA125, pelvic ultrasound and colour Doppler imaging. None of the signs, e.g. raised CA125, are specific for ovarian cancer. Current evidence suggests that the harm of a false positive outweighs potential screening benefits. Any screening undertaken at present should be in the context of a randomized trial and these are underway in the UK and abroad.

• Routine pelvic examination

Performing bimanual pelvic examination on asymptomatic low-risk women to 'check' for ovarian cancer is not helpful. Pelvic examination is of low specificity for detecting any ovarian enlargement when used without ultrasonography. As with breast examinations, it is hard to make a case for pelvic examinations in asymptomatic women. Again, they often lead to false-positive results causing needless anxiety and leading to further invasive investigations.

OTHER SCREENING PROCEDURES

• Blood pressure

Blood pressure should be recorded as a baseline investigation in all women when attending for the first time in a family planning consultation. It is the single most important test in women being prescribed COC or HRT and should be checked regularly (p. 61, p. 399).

• Pre-pregnancy screening

Many women attending a family planning consultation are considering stopping contraception to have a planned pregnancy. Screening for rubella immunity and discussion of any inherited conditions are important. Pre-pregnancy health advice for women such as stopping smoking, getting fit and taking adequate levels of folic acid is important.

REFERENCES

1. Austoker J, McPherson A, Clarke J, Lucassen A (1997) Breast problems. In: McPherson A, Waller D (eds) Women's Health, 4th edn. Oxford University Press, Oxford, pp. 71–127.

2. McIlwaine G (1993) Satisfaction with NHS breast screening programme: Women's views. In: Austoker J, Patnick J (eds) Breast screening acceptability: research and practice. NHS BSP Publications, Sheffield, pp. 14–16.

3. NICE (2006) Familial Breast cancer October 2006

4. McPherson A, Waller D (1997) BBC Woman's Hour survey. Women's health and its controversies – an overview. In: McPherson A, Waller D (eds) Women's Health, 4th edn. Oxford University Press, Oxford, pp. 1–21.

5. Cassell JA, Mercer CH, Fenton KA, Copas AJ, Erens B, Wellings K (2006) Implications for a national screening programme. Public Health 120(10): 984–988.

6. Salisbury C, Macleod J, Egger M, et al. (2006) Opportunistic and systematic screening for chlamydia: a study of consultations by young adults in general practice. Br J Gen Pract 56(523): 99–103.

7. Mills N, Daker-White G, Graham A, Campbell R (2006) Population screening for *Chlamydia trachomatis* infection in the UK: a qualitative study of the experiences of those screened. Fam Pract 23(5): 550–557.

8. Strutten JF, Gather SA, Russell P, et al. (1997) Contribution of all BRCA1 mutation to ovarian cancer. New England Journal of Medicine 338: 1125–1130.

FURTHER READING

Joint British Societies (2005) JBS 2: Joint British Societies' guidelines on prevention of cardiovascular disease in clinical practice. Heart 91(Suppl 5): v1–v52.

USEFUL WEBSITES

www.cancerscreening.nhs.uk/cervical/cervical-cancer

www.cancerscreening.org.uk/breastscreen

• UK National Health Service cancer screening programmes

www.hpa.org.uk/publications/2006/ncsp

• for National Chlamydia Screening Programme reports

18 Sexually transmitted infections

Christopher Wilkinson

Chapter contents

INTRODUCTION

The provision of high-quality reproductive health care requires the knowledge and skills to be alert to, diagnose and manage sexually transmitted infection (STI). Whilst some aspects of care require referral to a specialist sexual health service providing STI care, the majority of patients can be appropriately managed in community settings; this facilitates early diagnosis and treatment, which is an important component of STI management to prevent spread of infection. Whilst the main focus of this chapter is STI, lower genital tract infections such as bacterial vaginosis (BV) and candida will also be discussed.

BASIC PRINCIPLES OF MANAGING STI

Some of the key principles of managing STI are listed in **Box 18.1** and are discussed generally below or in later sections of the chapter.

Box 18.1 Key principles in managing STI

1. Confidentiality – only tell people who need to know about a diagnosis
2. Know when to test (see **Table 18.1**)
3. Sexual history taking – to help you decide when to test for STI and carry out partner notification after a positive STI diagnosis
4. Appropriate use of tests:
   a. Taking the sample correctly, don't forget storage and transport times
   b. Using the right test – e.g. HVS is not the test for gonorrhoea
   c. Using nucleic acid amplification tests (NAATs)
5. Partner notification – initiate at the time of diagnosis to help prevent the spread of infection and re-infection
6. When STI is diagnosed, advise against sex until the index patient and partner(s) are treated
7. Correct treatment and follow-up, the latter can often be done by phone
8. Epidemiologic treatment

Box 18.2 NHS Trusts and Primary Care Trusts (Sexually Transmitted Diseases) Directions 2000 (England)

'Every NHS trust and Primary Care Trust shall take all necessary steps to secure that any information capable of identifying an individual obtained by any of their members or employees with respect to persons examined or treated for any sexually transmitted disease shall not be disclosed.
Except:

a. For the purpose of communicating that information to a medical practitioner, or to a person employed under the direction of a medical practitioner in connection with the treatment of persons suffering from such disease or the prevention of the spread thereof, and

b. For the purpose of such treatment or prevention'

• Confidentiality

There is specific legislation concerning confidentiality and the management of STI. This used to apply only to GUM clinics, however in 2001 a revision of this legislation in England extended the requirements to maintain confidentiality to all sites where STI are diagnosed or managed. The principles in this guidance are a good basis for any service or practice confidentiality policy (see **Box 18.2**).

Table 18.1 When to consider testing for genital STI

On demand	Especially if identified risk or symptoms present – remember the patient may not actually disclose risk to you
Identified risk	<25 years of age
	New partner in previous 12 months
	More than one partner in previous 12 months
	High-risk partner
Symptoms	Vaginal discharge +/− odour, urethral discharge, dysuria
	Genital pruritis, soreness, ulceration, lumps
	Intermenstrual, breakthrough or post-coital bleeding
	Pain (abdominal or pelvic), dyspareunia
Iatrogenic risk	Before termination of pregnancy or before insertion of intrauterine contraception. Offer testing to all women but recommend testing in women with identified risk
Screening	Sexually active men and women under the age of 25 years as part of NHS Chlamydia Screening Programme

---

Box 18.3 Sexual history – risk assessment, a positive answer indicates an increased risk for common STI such as chlamydia, and supports the decision to test

- Has the patient had sex with a new partner in the last 12 months?
- Has the patient had sex with more than one partner in the last 12 months?
- Is the patient aged 25 or less?
- Does the patient have any concerns that their partner may have put them at risk of STI?

• When to test for STI

The principles of when to consider testing for an STI are outlined in Table 18.1.

• Taking a sexual history

Ask only what you need to know and when you need to know it. Avoid questions that are not helpful particularly if they appear judgemental. Remember not all clients are comfortable telling healthcare professionals about why they are concerned that they may have an STI.

A sexual history can help you to:

1. Decide whether to test for STI: some key questions are in Box 18.3. Notice that these questions do not include questions such as, 'are you married,' or 'how long have you been in your relationship,' which are not good discriminators of STI risk.

2. Decide which sites to take tests from. This is particularly important for men who have sex with men.

3. Initiate effective partner notification. In practice, detailed questions relating to partner notification should be asked after a positive diagnosis.

Using the right tests: nucleic acid amplification tests

These highly sensitive and specific tests are now the test of choice for chlamydia testing and screening. Similar tests are also being developed for other genital infections, including gonorrhoea and trichomonas vaginalis. In addition to being highly sensitive, NAATs allow non-invasive testing; for women using first-catch urine specimens or self-taken low vaginal swabs, and for men self-taken urethral meatal swabs. First-catch urine specimens should be taken after 1–2 hours of not passing urine. Most laboratories will carry out confirmatory tests on all positive results; this reduces the risk of giving a false-positive result. These tests have allowed a major increase in the number of tests being taken from community settings, which has consequently increased the number of diagnoses. One disadvantage of NAATs for gonorrhoea (GC) is that they cannot test for antibiotics resistance; it is therefore recommended that, where possible, patients with positive NAAT GC tests should have appropriate samples taken before treatment to allow antibiotic sensitivities to be tested.

For each infection, there are a number of different test kits available and your laboratory will be able to advise for which infections they are being used locally and for which samples they are validated for (e.g. urine or self-taken swabs) and refrigeration or transportation requirements.

• Partner notification

Partner notification, formerly known as *contact tracing*, is an important public health aspect of managing STI. It is the process by which other cases are identified, tested and treated to prevent ongoing transmission. Partner notification should be initiated at the point of diagnosis usually by the clinician managing the patient. Partner notification does not require the healthcare professional initiating this to actually *see* the partner or to be obliged to carry out testing and treatment on that partner. Partner notification involves:

- discussing with the client the implications of the diagnosis, the mode of transmission and how to prevent re-infection
- taking a sexual history to identify other potential contacts
- providing written information for the client to pass onto those contacts to enable them to be tested and treated
- If possible, the outcomes of partner notification should also be recorded to measure against auditable standards.

This written information should include information about the infection concerned, its mode of transmission and how the contact can access testing and treatment.

The question of how far historically one goes to identify partners is debatable. A man who presents with symptomatic gonorrhoea and recent partner change was probably only exposed to the infection recently, whereas someone with asymptomatic chlamydia could have had it for many months. However, as a rule of thumb, it is advisable to consider all partners in the previous 3–6 months. This practice can be individualized, bearing in mind that the aim is to identify other potentially infected people and to ensure they are tested and treated depending on the patient's sexual history.

The person initiating partner notification should ensure that follow-up, which can be by telephone, is carried out 1–2 weeks later to ensure that treatment has been taken; this would include a further discussion about partner notification to ensure that the partner(s) has been tested and treated.

• Epidemiologic treatment

It is usual to offer treatment to contacts of chlamydia, gonorrhoea, trichomonas and syphilis before the results of diagnostic tests are known. This is known as epidemiologic treatment and it aims to reduce the risk of transmission at the earliest possible opportunity. Previously this only applied to known contacts who were verifiable through the GUM network, however as more and more people are being tested in other settings it is usual to offer treatment on the basis of declared contact.

COMMON CLINICAL PRESENTATIONS

• Male urethral symptoms

Men with urethral symptoms should have a sexual history taken, as sexually transmitted urethritis is the commonest cause in sexually active men, especially the young. Urethral discharge (which may be mucopurulent or clear), dysuria, or urethral itch are the most common presenting symptoms of urethritis. Sexually transmitted urethritis is caused by gonorrhoea, chlamydia (CT) and non-specific urethritis (NSU). NSU is urethritis in the absence of GC or CT and is managed as an STI; there are a number of putative causes including TV, mycoplasmas or ureaplasma. Although GC is probably associated with more severe symptoms, it is not possible reliably to distinguish clinically between chlamydia and gonococcal infection. Referral to GUM for microscopy and treatment enables a rapid diagnosis, but if this is not possible a pragmatic approach is to take tests for GC and CT and treat empirically for CT and, if suspected, GC. Ensure partner notification and appropriate follow-up.

Table 18.2 Summary of vaginal infections

	Candida	BV	TV
Discharge	White (curdy)	White/grey homogenous	Yellow green frothy
Smell	Nil (yeasty)	Fishy or like onions	Malodorous
Pruritis	Yes	Occasionally	Yes
Vulvitis	Yes/no	No	Yes/no
Vaginitis	Yes	No	Yes
Cervicitis	Occasionally	No	Yes
PH	<4.5 *	>5	>5
Microscopy (HVS)	WC + Candida	CC + absence of normal flora	WC + TV
Culture (HVS)	Yes	No	No **

WC = Leucocytes
CC = Clue cells
TV = *Trichomonas vaginalis*
HVS = High vaginal swab
* Unless coexisting TV or BV
** NB Some labs will process special culture media

• Vulvo–vaginal symptoms

Vaginal discharge is most commonly physiological or due to the non-sexually transmitted infections, bacterial vaginosis or candida. However as TV, GC, CT and HSV occasionally lead to abnormal vaginal discharge, a sexual history should be taken to assess STI risk. Other relevant symptoms to direct management are itch, soreness and malodour. Women at low risk for STI can be managed empirically in the first instance on the basis of symptoms, discharge and itch suggesting candida, and discharge with (fishy) malodour suggesting BV. TV, which is sexually transmitted, usually causes discharge, itch or soreness and malodour and if suspected should be appropriately investigated. Table 18.2 summarizes the features of vaginal infections.

Women at risk of STI who request testing, have failed empirical treatment or vulval pain or soreness should be examined and have appropriate STI tests taken. As a minimum these would include pH of vaginal discharge, high vaginal swab (HVS) for microscopy culture and sensitivity (MC&S), a test for CT (usually NAATs) and a test for GC (endocervical swab (ECS) for MC&S or NAATs). Clinical findings suggestive of genital herpes, which can be cervical, vaginal or vulval, warrant appropriate testing. Partner notification and follow-up should be dictated by the diagnosis.

• Genital lumps

Men and women presenting with lumps in the genital region should be examined to exclude genital warts, molluscum contagiosum, and an early herpes episode.

• Female pelvic pain

Pelvic inflammatory disease should be considered in the differential diagnosis of women presenting with pelvic pain. It is a clinical diagnosis and requires pelvic bimanual examination. It cannot be diagnosed without bimanual examination. If present, tests for CT and GC should be taken and treatment with partner notification initiated. Although the clinical diagnosis has a poor specificity, positive laboratory test results are not essential to make the diagnosis, but do support the clinical diagnosis. Although PID is not always sexually transmitted it should usually be treated as such, and partner notification should be carried out irrespective of the laboratory results.

BACTERIAL INFECTIONS

• Gonorrhoea

Gonorrhoea is caused by *Neisseria gonorrhoeae*. It is almost always sexually acquired. Asymptomatic disease is common and hence represents a reservoir of infection.

Clinical features in men

1. Most patients with urethral gonorrhoea develop symptoms 2–10 days after sexual intercourse with an infected partner. Symptoms commonly are urethral discharge ($>80\%$) and/or dysuria ($>50\%$), but infection can be asymptomatic ($<10\%$).
2. Rectal infection is usually asymptomatic but may cause anal discharge (12%) or perianal/anal pain or discomfort (7%).
3. Pharyngeal infection is usually asymptomatic ($>90\%$), rarely a mild sore throat may be present.
4. Complications in men are rare. The most common complications are epididymo-orchitis, prostatic and seminal vesicle abscesses and disseminated gonococcal infections; haematological spread is rare ($<1\%$).

Clinical features in women

1. Uncomplicated genital infection: most women (about 50%) with uncomplicated gonorrhoea are asymptomatic. Some, however, complain of increased vaginal discharge (50%), dysuria (12%) or occasionally intermenstrual bleeding. The only abnormal clinical finding may be a mucopurulent exudate from the cervical os. Urethral discharge is occasionally present and is associated with para-urethral gland infection. More than 50% have a normal clinical examination.

2. Uncomplicated non-genital infection: as in the male, pharyngeal and rectal gonorrhoea are usually asymptomatic (90%). Rectal gonorrhoea is usually as a result of contamination from infected vaginal discharge and is not necessarily indicative of prior anal intercourse.

3. Complicated infection: pelvic inflammatory disease (PID) occurs as a complication in <10% of women with untreated gonorrhoea. Bartholinitis with abscess formation may develop occasionally in infected individuals, and, less commonly, disseminated gonococcal infection (presenting as a febrile illness with polyarthralgia and vasculitic skin lesions or as a septic arthritis) may result.

Diagnosis

The gold standard test is culture with antibiotic sensitivities of appropriate specimens, urethral in men, and cervical swab in women. To avoid contamination that may affect the culture results the ectocervix should be wiped to remove vaginal secretions before an endocervical swab is taken. Swabs from other potentially infected sites can be taken if gonococcal infection is thought to be likely but are not indicated routinely. Specimens should be refrigerated and sent in charcoal transport media to arrive at the laboratory as soon as possible within 24 hours of the specimen being obtained. Samples from community sites where transport to the laboratory is required do have a sensitivity about 10% lower than immediately plated samples, but have the advantage that samples can be taken at the time the need is identified as it is well recognized that there is variable attendance of clients advised to attend GUM for testing. Positive culture results are usually available between 24 and 48 hours after the laboratory receives the specimen. A high vaginal swab frequently yields negative results and is unreliable for the diagnosis of gonorrhoea.

Routine microscopy has been advocated, but this is not a diagnostic test. In patients who have gonorrhoea, microscopy enables a presumptive diagnosis of GC to be made prior to culture results being available in about 80% of men and 40% of women. Negative microscopy does not exclude gonorrhoea. Thus, whilst microscopy can speed up the diagnosis in a small number of patients, gonorrhoea is not a common infection, it is time consuming, requires laboratory space, and quality control can be difficult to maintain where practitioners carry out microscopy infrequently or in isolation. Microscopy is therefore not essential for community settings providing STI testing.

Nucleic acid amplification tests (NAATs) on first-catch urines or self-taken vaginal swabs are now available for gonorrhoea, and are more sensitive than culture but specificity is less than 100% so false-positive results occur. Their non-invasive nature makes them useful in community settings. However, whilst all positives should be treated, it is currently recommended that positive results be confirmed by culture, mainly to check sensitivities. The availability of nucleic acid tests will vary from area to area but is likely to be increasingly available either as a test for single infections or multiplex tests for multiple infections such as GC, CT and TV.

Treatment

Although the choice of antimicrobial agent should depend on the sensitivity pattern of the gonococcal isolate, treatment may be started before this is known. A suitable drug can be selected with knowledge of the drug sensitivities of the strains in the community, laboratories usually monitor this and local GUM clinics will be able to advise on current first-line treatments for your area, including for the treatment of pharyngeal infection, infection acquired abroad and pregnant women.

As up to 20% of men and 40% of female patients with gonorrhoea have a concurrent chlamydial infection, many clinicians give simultaneous treatment for this if the patient's chlamydia status is not known.

Partner notification

Partner notification should take place for all index cases of gonorrhoea. The nationally agreed standard is that 0.6 contacts should be identified and treated for each index case.

Follow-up

Routine test of cure (ToC) is not required for uncomplicated anogenital gonococcal infection provided the correct treatment was prescribed and taken, symptoms have resolved, and that re-infection is not likely to have occurred. The most common reason for failed treatment is re-infection and requires further partner notification. All treatments are less effective at treating pharyngeal infection and test of cure is recommended. Both culture and NAATs tests can be used for ToC and should be performed no earlier than 72 hours and 14 days after completing treatment respectively.

• Syphilis

Syphilis, caused by *Treponema pallidum*, is uncommon in the UK and the incidence was declining due to safer sex practices. Although the absolute numbers are small, between 1998 and 2004, rates of diagnoses of infectious syphilis in males increased by 1520%. This is largely as a result of a number of localized outbreaks. Unlike other bacterial STIs the highest rates are seen in older age groups rather than in teenagers. More than 50% of cases are in men who have sex with men (MSM). Antenatal serological screening has reduced the prevalence of congenital syphilis. The majority of syphilis diagnoses are made serologically in the absence of clinical findings. Suspicion should be raised in the presence of atypical genital ulceration or generalized rash, particularly in MSM. Serological testing should form part of a routine

STI screen. Suspected clinical syphilis and untreated syphilis diagnosed serologically should be referred to GUM to confirm the diagnosis, assess the stage of disease, plan management and carry out partner notification. Specific serological tests may remain positive for life.

Chlamydia

Chlamydia trachomatis is the most common bacterial sexually transmitted infection in the UK. It is present in 5–10% of sexually active women under 24 and men between 20–24 years. Genital chlamydial infection is frequently asymptomatic in both men and women and ongoing transmission in the community is sustained by this unrecognized infection. Spontaneous resolution can occur, but there is a high rate of progression to complicated infection.

Clinical features in men

1. After an incubation period of about 3 weeks, men develop a mucoid or mucopurulent urethral discharge and dysuria of variable severity. At least 25% of infected men, however, are asymptomatic

2. Non-genital infection: chlamydial ophthalmia is usually the result of autoinoculation of infected material from the genital tract but can exist in isolation. Proctitis, which may be asymptomatic, is sexually transmitted.

3. Epididymitis is the most common complication of untreated chlamydial infection. Chlamydiae probably play a part in the aetiology of reactive arthritis (including Reiter's disease) in both men and women.

Clinical features in women

1. Most women (70%) with a chlamydial cervical infection are asymptomatic; 30% have usually mild symptoms of intermenstrual or postcoital bleeding, mucopurulent vaginal discharge or dysuria. There may be no specific signs. The cervix may appear normal or there may be an endocervicitis with mucopus exuding from the os.

2. Non-genital infection: chlamydial ophthalmia is usually the result of autoinoculation of infected material from the genital tract but can exist in isolation. Proctitis, which may be asymptomatic, is sexually transmitted.

3. Around 10–40% of untreated women will develop PID with subsequent risk of infertility and an increased risk of ectopic pregnancy. Very rarely, perihepatitis is a complication; there is an acute onset of pain in the right hypochondrium, the pain being exacerbated by deep inspiration, nausea, anorexia and low-grade pyrexia. Chlamydiae probably play a part in the aetiology of reactive arthritis (including Reiter's disease) in both men and women.

Diagnosis

It is recommended that NAATs should be used, although some labs still use culture or Eliza Immunoassay (EIA) and the actual test kit available locally will vary from area to area. NAAT tests allow non-invasive testing using first-catch urines (FCU) after not passing urine for 1–2 hours and, some tests also enable self-taken low vaginal swabs in women and self-taken urethral meatal swabs in men. Although the sensitivities and specificities are comparable to those using specimens taken from the infected site itself, if an examination is being carried out at the potential site of infection, e.g. cervix, it should be sampled directly; FCU samples perform less well than vaginal or cervical samples with some NAATs. Results of NAATs tests can now be used for medicolegal reasons.

Treatment

Tetracyclines and the macrolides are equally effective in the treatment of adult chlamydial infections. Uncomplicated genital, rectal and pharyngeal chlamydia infection can be treated with the following agents:

Doxycycline 100 mg bd for 7 days (contraindicated in pregnancy)

or

Azithromycin 1 g orally in a single dose

If either of the above treatments is contraindicated:

Erythromycin 500 mg bd for 10–14 days

or

Ofloxacin 200 mg bd or 400 mg once a day for 7 days.

Pregnant women can be treated with erythromycin (500 mg bd, 14 days, or 500 mg qds for 7 days), amoxicillin 500 mg tds for 7 days, or azithromycin 1 g stat. The latter is unlicensed for use in pregnancy, however it is recommended by the World Health Organization (WHO) and available data, though limited, are reassuring. The manufacturer recommends use in pregnancy or breast-feeding only if other treatments are unavailable.

Partner notification

Partner notification should take place for all index cases of chlamydia. The nationally agreed standard for rates of partner notification is that 0.64 contacts (0.43 in cities) should be identified and treated for each index case.

Follow-up

A test of cure is not routinely recommended but should be performed in pregnancy or if non-compliance or re-infection is suspected. It should be deferred for 5 weeks (6 weeks if azithromycin given) after treatment is completed.

• Bacterial vaginosis

Bacterial vaginosis (BV) is the commonest cause of abnormal vaginal discharge in women of reproductive age, with up to 30% prevalence in some populations. The actual aetiology is unknown, but it results from the replacement of the normal lactobacilli with mixed organisms, including anaerobes, *Gardnerella vaginalis* and *Mycoplasma hominis* and is associated with an increased pH. BV is not sexually transmitted, but it is related to sexual activity.

Bacterial vaginosis may be associated with pelvic infection after termination of pregnancy and with post-operative wound infection. There is increasing evidence that, in pregnant women, the condition may be associated with late miscarriage, premature rupture of the membranes, premature delivery, low birth weight, and postpartum infection. Routine screening in pregnancy is not recommended but if detected in pregnancy, BV should be treated.

Clinical features

1. Increased vaginal discharge, greyish-white in colour with a fishy odour, particularly after intercourse.
2. It is not an inflammatory condition and is not associated with itch or soreness or vulvovaginitis, unlike candida and *Trichomonas*.
3. Fifty per cent of women with BV do not report symptoms.

Diagnosis

A presumptive diagnosis can be made on the basis of history, clinical findings and a raised vaginal pH. Microscopy of an HVS may demonstrate clue cells, which support the diagnosis. Not all laboratories report the presence of clue cells, so it is worth establishing if this is the case. It is of note that it is the *microscopy* of an HVS that is useful in the diagnosis of BV, not the culture result.

The pH of the vaginal discharge is measured using narrow-range (pH 4–6) pH paper (Whatman) held in a pair of forceps avoiding the alkaline cervical secretions. The pH of vaginal secretions is normally less than 4.5 but in bacterial vaginosis it is greater than 5. However, the pH of vaginal fluid can be raised in women who do not have the condition; vaginal medications and hygiene products, water, lubricant, semen, blood and the menopause are all associated with raised pH.

There are also well-defined diagnostic criteria for the microscopic diagnosis of BV, the Hay-Ison criteria and the Nugent criteria. GUM clinics usually use the Hay-Ison criteria. Detailed microscopy such as this can be useful to assess recurrent symptoms or where there is uncertainty over the diagnosis. The potassium hydroxide test is no longer recommended.

Treatment

Oral metronidazole (either 400 mg twice daily for 5 days or as a single dose of 2 g), or clindamycin cream 2% (a 5 g applicator-full inserted vaginally every night for 7 nights) are both effective. Recurrence, however, is common. Treatment of the sexual partner is not indicated.

PROTOZOAL INFESTATION

• Trichomoniasis

Trichomoniasis is caused by the protozoan flagellate *Trichomonas vaginalis* (TV) that colonizes, but only rarely invades, the mucosa of the lower urogenital tract. The organism is almost always sexually transmitted. There is increasing evidence that TV infection can have a detrimental outcome on pregnancy and is associated with preterm delivery and low birth weight. There is evidence that TV infection may enhance HIV transmission.

Clinical features in women

Up to 50% of women are asymptomatic; yellow, offensive vaginal discharge, vulval soreness, dysuria are the classic symptoms. Occasionally lower abdominal discomfort may be noted.

The vulva may be normal on inspection, but in some cases there is a vulvitis, which may be severe. The vaginal wall is reddened and a frothy, yellow discharge pools in the posterior fornix; punctate red spots on the ectocervix ('strawberry cervix') may be noted (2%). These features, however, are not present in up to 15% of infected women and are not pathognomonic of trichomoniasis.

Clinical features in men

Most men who are infected with *T. vaginalis* are asymptomatic or have minimal symptoms of discharge and dysuria and have no clinical abnormality, although discharge may be noted.

Diagnosis

Apart from the recently developed NAATs, which are not yet widely available, there are no very sensitive tests for TV readily available. Culture, which can be used in men and women, is performed in few laboratories. Direct observation by examination of a 'wet smear' or stained slide remains the predominant test and in women will detect between 40–80% of cases compared to culture. GUM clinics usually perform microscopy of a wet smear, which has the advantage that the characteristic motile flagellated protozoa are readily seen.

Sometimes, trichomonads may be found on cervical cytology, sensitivity up to 80%, but in some labs there is a high false-positive rate of up to 30%, check with your local laboratory, and if necessary consider confirmation by microscopy or culture if available.

Treatment

Metronidazole (a single oral dose of 2g stat, or 400mg bd for 7 days) is usually curative. In the event of persistent disease, re-treatment and checking that partners have been treated should be carried out in the first instance; resistance is rare and reinfection is the most likely cause. Truly persistent TV is probably best referred to GUM where the diagnosis can be confirmed and various other treatment strategies can be tried.

Partner notification

The regular sexual partners of women with trichomoniasis should be treated, even when asymptomatic and when tests for TV are negative.

FUNGAL INFECTION

• Vulvovaginal candidiasis

Vulvovaginal candidiasis (VVC) is caused by yeasts of the genus *Candida*, particularly *Candida albicans* and is not sexually transmitted. *Candida albicans* is not always pathogenic and is present in up to 20% of women without vulvovaginitis. The presence of candida on an HVS or cytology does therefore not always require treatment. It is not known precisely what leads candida to become a pathogen, and in most women there is no underlying factor. The most common condition associated with vulvovaginal candidiasis is pregnancy; occasionally other conditions, such as uncontrolled diabetes mellitus, use of broad-spectrum antibiotics, use of immunosuppressive drugs, and HIV infection are associated with recurrent vulvovaginal infection.

Clinical features in women

1. Vulval itching and abnormal non-offensive vaginal discharge are the commonest presenting symptoms. As vulvitis becomes more severe, soreness, superficial dyspareunia and external dysuria may occur, particularly in the presence of fissures.
2. Clinical examination can be normal, but a non-offensive curdy or creamy discharge may be noted together with varying degrees of vaginal and vulval erythema and occasionally vulval oedema. Erythema of the vulva sometimes extends to the perineum, perianal region, genitocrural folds and the medial aspects of the thighs.

Clinical features in men

1. Although candidiasis is not sexually transmitted, some male partners of women with candida do experience a mild macular pruritic rash on the glans penis that comes on soon after intercourse and settles within 24 hours. Treatment of the woman cures the problem.

2. Candidal balanoposthitis may be the presenting feature of diabetes mellitus in men.

Diagnosis

It is common practice to treat suspected candidal infection empirically without tests. However, examination and testing is indicated in women at risk of STI or with persistent symptoms after self-medication. Persistent symptoms after self-medication are usually due to misdiagnosis rather than treatment failure. A swab should be used to take a sample from the high vagina and lateral vaginal wall and sent for microscopy and culture. If speculum examination is not required a blind vaginal swab is also acceptable. The pH of vaginal discharge in VVC is normal (4–4.5) but in the presence of co-infection with BV, it may be raised.

Treatment

Asymptomatic infection does not require treatment.

General advice should be given about the avoidance of soaps, especially if they are perfumed, and tight-fitting synthetic clothing. Topical and oral azoles give 80–95% cure and nystatin 70–90% in non-pregnant women (Table 18.3). As topical treatments can be messy and can cause local irritation when

Table 18.3 Treatments for vaginal candidiasis

Clotrimazole*	Vaginal pessary	500 mg stat
Clotrimazole*	Vaginal pessary	200 mg × 3 nights
Clotrimazole*	Vaginal pessary	100 mg × 6 nights
Clotrimazole*	Vaginal cream	(10%) 5 g stat
Econazole**	Vaginal pessary	150 mg stat
Econazole**	Vaginal pessary	150 mg × 3 nights
Miconazole**	Vaginal ovule	1.2 g stat
Miconazole**	Vaginal pessary	100 mg × 14 nights
Nystatin	Vaginal cream	4 g × 14 nights
Nystatin	Vaginal pessary	(100 000 units) 1–2 × 14 nights
Fluconazole	Oral capsule	150 mg stat
Itraconazole	Oral capsule	200 mg bd × 1d

* Effect on latex condoms and diaphragms not known
** Known to damage latex condoms and diaphragms

applied, short courses of treatment are usually used. If using a vaginal therapy, a topical cream preparation is also recommended applied to the vulva. Fluconazole is the first-line oral preparation, with itraconazole being reserved for resistant or recurrent infections.

In pregnant women cure rates may be slightly lower and longer courses of topical treatment are recommended. Oral treatments have not been established as safe to use in pregnancy. Both oral preparations are detectable in breast milk, although no adverse effect on infants has been noted.

• Recurrent candidiasis

Recurrent candidiasis is defined as four or more episodes of VVC in any 12-month period. Always reassess the situation to ensure that the symptoms are due to VVC and consider predisposing factors, before embarking on long-term therapy. Management is empirical and not based on good evidence. There are two phases to treatment: first treat with standard regimens, repeated if necessary until the patient is asymptomatic, then give regular single-dose treatments for up to 6 months. Typical treatments are: fluconazole 100 mg weekly for 6 months or clotrimazole pessary 500 mg weekly for 6 months or itraconazole 400 mg monthly for 6 months.

VIRAL INFECTIONS

• Herpes simplex virus

Genital herpes is caused in equal proportions by HSV 1 and HSV 2 and can affect the vulva, vagina, cervix, perineum, anus, rectum and penis. Genital infection is usually sexually transmitted, but autoinoculation from a source elsewhere on the body can occur. A few patients will develop a primary infection approximately 2 weeks after exposure, after which the virus becomes latent and recurrences can occur. However, most infections are asymptomatic (80% of HSV 2), or do not become symptomatic until months or years after infection. Recurrences of clinical disease are more frequent with HSV 2 than HSV 1, in the first year after infection recurrence rates of 0.34 and 0.08 per month respectively occur. Recurrences get less frequent with time.

Herpes is most infectious during a clinical episode, but asymptomatic shedding occurs and is responsible for much transmission in discordant couples, when the risk of transmission is approximately 10% per annum.

Clinical features

Primary infections, occurring at the time of infection

1. Systemic symptoms are common and include fever, headache, malaise and myalgia.

2. Multiple small blisters containing clear fluid which progress over a few days to ulcers with grey bases and which occasionally coalesce, oedema may be present. Ulcers persist for up to 2 weeks and develop crusts before healing. Dysuria can occur either as a result of lesions at the urethral meatus or urine coming into contact with lesions. Increased watery vaginal discharge is a feature of cervical infection. Tender enlargement of the inguinal lymph nodes may be noted.

3. Aseptic meningitis or autonomic neuropathy, resulting in urinary retention may occur.

4. Systemic features usually resolve within 7–10 days and genital lesions usually heal within about 21 days.

• Recurrent genital herpes

Systemic symptoms are not a feature, but prodromal symptoms occur commonly and consist of a tingling sensation in the affected area or shooting pains in the distribution of the sciatic nerve. Lesions are usually similar to those of the primary disease but are usually much less extensive and heal more quickly. It is increasingly recognized that atypical lesions occur such as small fissures that may be confused with candidal infection.

Diagnosis

Although the diagnosis is often clinically evident it is recommended that the diagnosis is confirmed using appropriate laboratory tests. Until recently viral culture was the mainstay of diagnosis, however many laboratories are utilizing NAAT tests, which are now the test of choice. This makes accurate laboratory testing for HSV more accessible to clinicians working in the community. The role of serology is debated. It may be helpful in some cases in the following situations:

- history of recurrent genital ulceration of unknown aetiology when virus detection tests (e.g., virus culture or PCR testing of genital specimens) have repeatedly been negative
- sexual partners of persons with genital herpes, where there is a concern about transmission. Some couples may find that their HSV status is concordant. Discordant couples can identify strategies to prevent transmission.

Treatment

Basic principles of management

The aims of management are to reduce symptoms, risk of secondary infection and psychological complications. Adequate analgesia should be provided. If pain is severe oral analgesics may be supplemented by the use of topical lignocaine ointment, this should be used sparingly as sensitization may occur. Saline baths are recommended. Patients should be made aware of the risks of autoinoculation and advised not to have sex until the episode has completely healed.

Antiviral agents

Oral antiviral agents have a proven role in primary episodes when commenced within 5 days of onset of symptoms, or whilst new lesions still forming can reduce the severity and duration of the episode. Treatment has no effect on the likelihood of recurrences. There is no established role for topical antivirals. Treatments include:

- Aciclovir 200 mg 5 times per day for 5 days
- Valaciclovir 500 mg twice a day for 5 days
- Famciclovir, primary infection 250 mg 3 times daily for 5 days, recurrent infection, 125 mg twice daily for 5 days.

The use of antivirals in recurrent disease is less clear-cut. Although the clinical course of the disease is shortened somewhat, in general this is of marginal benefit to the patient. When given early, e.g. during the prodromal stage, they may reduce the duration of the recurrence. Treatment regimens may need altering in immunocompromised patients.

Suppressive treatment

Aciclovir (200 mg orally four times per day or 400 mg twice daily), or famciclovir (250 mg twice daily) reduces the frequency of recurrences and may be useful if recurrences are very frequent or disabling.

• Genital herpes in pregnancy

Neonatal infection is rare, but associated with a high morbidity and mortality; it is more common after primary maternal infection in the third trimester. Expert advice should be sought in any woman with primary genital HSV in pregnancy or clinical HSV in the third trimester. Any woman with a history of HSV should discuss this with her antenatal care provider at booking. Continuous suppressive antiviral therapy can reduce the risk of recurrence and of caesarean section, however routine suppressive therapy is not indicated and should only be given on a case-by-case basis. Primary infection in the third trimester carries the greatest risk and caesarean section should be considered in all cases, although this may not completely reduce the risk of neonatal Infection. It is usual to deliver by caesarean section when herpetic lesions are present at the time of delivery. Knowledge of local policies is essential.

• Genital warts

Warts are benign epithelial tumours caused by human papilloma virus (HPV) of which there are over 90 types. Most hyperplastic genital warts (condylomata acuminata) are caused by HPV types 6 and 11, which are not associated with cervical cancer or warts in other parts of the body. The virus is highly contagious through close physical contact leading to multifocal sub-clinical infection. Only a small proportion (1%) of those infected will develop clinical disease, which may occur several months after infection.

Clinical features

Warts may affect the vagina, cervix, urethra, anus and external genitalia, most frequently affecting areas traumatized during intercourse; in women the posterior fourchette and in men the coronal sulcus and frenulum are the commonest sites of infection. Symptoms such as discomfort or irritation are rare. Perianal lesions are not indicative of anal intercourse, unlike anal lesions which are. It is not usual to attempt to diagnose subclinical infection, which like clinical disease is usually self-limiting, albeit over several months. Secondary infection is rare.

Management

The main aims of treatment are to treat clinical disease and to prevent psychological morbidity. Other STI should be excluded, as co-infection is common. Atypical warts, especially if pigmented, should be biopsied to exclude malignancy. Although possible, it is not known whether treatment reduces the duration of infectivity. Partners should be encouraged to attend to exclude clinical disease and to be tested for other STI. Although partners without clinical disease are likely to have subclinical infection, condom use whilst the lesions are visible is recommended.

All treatments can have significant relapse rates and can cause local discomfort and blistering. No treatment is an option at any site and may apply particularly to warts in the vaginal and anal canal. Treatment choice depends on the morphology, number and distribution of warts. Soft non-keratinized warts respond well to self-applied podophyllotoxin. Use on perianal warts is unlicensed, but is commonly recommended. Keratinized lesions are better treated with physical ablative methods such as cryotherapy, excision or electrocautery. Cryotherapy using an aerosol is the simplest to provide if conventional cryotherapy is not available. Imiquimod cream is licensed for the treatment of external anogenital warts; it may be used for both keratinized and non-keratinized lesions but is more expensive and may damage latex condoms and diaphragms.

Women with genital warts should have routine cervical screening as indicated by the NHS cervical screening programme; they do not require more frequent screening than women without warts.

• Human immunodeficiency virus

The management of HIV is outside the scope of this chapter, but there are two areas of care that are relevant:

- Testing for HIV, including antenatal testing
- Post-exposure prophylaxis.

Testing for HIV

The human immunodeficiency viruses (HIV 1 and 2) can be detected in blood, semen, cervicovaginal secretions, breast milk and saliva, although there is little evidence that saliva is important in the transmission of infection. Until 2001 in the UK, men who have had unprotected anal intercourse with an infected man constituted the group at greatest risk of HIV infection, but now the majority of new diagnoses are in men and women who acquired the infection heterosexually. Heterosexual spread too is greatest in central Africa. Intravenous drug users who share contaminated syringes and needles are also at risk of HIV infection but this is relatively uncommon in the UK due to needle exchange programmes. The presence of a concurrent sexually transmitted infection, particularly an ulcerative condition, such as genital herpes, facilitates infection with HIV. It is estimated that whilst there are nearly 60 000 people known to be living with HIV infection in the UK there are nearly 20 000 people whose infection remains undiagnosed.

Although there have been reports of probable infection of neonates by breast-feeding, most infants have acquired HIV from an infected mother before or during delivery. The risk of neonatal infection varies from 22% to 51% and it is likely that there is a direct relationship between the duration of maternal infection and risk to the child. However with prenatal or antenatal diagnosis and correct management this can be reduced to as low as 1%.

Clearly anyone who is in a high-risk group or has been in sexual contact with an HIV-infected person should be advised to be tested. There is also a move to normalize HIV testing and, unless there are good reasons for not doing so, anyone requesting a test or/and STI screen should have this carried out. All women are offered antenatal screening for HIV. The concept of 'pre-test counselling' has now been replaced with 'pre-test discussion' (Box 18.4), the main purpose of which is to ensure informed verbal consent to testing and supplemented by written information. A pre-test discussion should be tailored to the needs of the patient and can be fairly brief. Having had a test alone should not affect insurance policies provided the result is negative. Patients should be given the opportunity for more in-depth discussion should they so wish.

It is helpful to have links in place to ensure that when giving an HIV-positive result an appointment with a specialist HIV service is available as soon as possible. This is to confirm the diagnosis, carry out a baseline assessment of disease and to deal with psychological or social issues the client may have.

Box 18.4 Areas that may be covered in pre test discussion

- The benefits of testing
  - The health benefits of current treatments
  - Knowing HIV status can allay anxiety
  - A positive test may motivate people to reduce risk activities
  - The opportunity to reduce the risk of transmission of the infection to others, e.g. infants, sexual partners
- A risk assessment, including date of last risk activity
- The 'window period'
- Implications of testing for mortgages, insurance, occupational risks, and confidentiality
- Details of how the result will be given
- Where appropriate to explore support and coping mechanisms
- Obtaining informed consent for the test
- Information about HIV transmission and risk reduction as necessary

---

Post–exposure prophylaxis after sexual exposure (PEPSE)

In practice PEPSE is also applicable after any potential exposure (whether sexual or not) to body fluids of someone who is known, or highly likely, to be infected with HIV. The aim of PEP is to reduce the risk of an individual becoming infected with HIV. In general the risks following an exposure are very small; the overall risk of infection after percutaneous exposure (such as injury with a needle involving infected blood) to HIV is about 1:300; for contact with mucosae, the risk is probably 1:1000. The risk of HIV infection after unprotected sex with someone known to be HIV positive varies from 3:100 to less than 1:1000 depending upon the type of sex. Evidence suggests that PEP after occupational exposure may reduce the risk of seroconversion by 80%. Individuals taking PEP frequently report side effects and completion rates are poor. Table 18.4 shows recommendations for PEP after sexual exposure and can be used as a guide, but may be varied from case to case. PEP is usually available through GUM clinics or Emergency departments.

• Molluscum contagiosum virus

Molluscum contagiosum, caused by a poxvirus, presents as hemispherical, umbilicated, pearly, flesh-coloured skin nodules 2–5mm in diameter. When acquired through sexual contact, they are found on the penis, vulva and inner aspects of the thighs. In the immunocompromised individual, including those with HIV infection, they may be extensive and recalcitrant

Table 18.4 Recommendations for PEP up to 72 hours after sexual exposure

	Source known HIV +ve	Source Unknown HIV status	
		Low risk for HIV	High risk for HIV
Receptive anal sex	Recommended	Recommended	Recommended
Insertive anal sex	Recommended	Not recommended	Considered
Receptive vaginal sex	Recommended	Not recommended	Considered
Insertive vaginal sex	Recommended	Not recommended	Considered
Fellatio with ejaculation	Considered	Not recommended	Considered
Splash of semen into eye	Considered	Not recommended	Considered
Fellatio without ejaculation	Not recommended	Not recommended	Not recommended
Cunnilingus	Not recommended	Not recommended	Not recommended
	Always check local protocols		

to treatment. The diagnosis is clinical but can be confirmed by electron microscopy of the core of a lesion that has been removed using a needle and fine forceps. Treatment is by curettage, electrocautery or piercing with a sharpened orange stick, the tip of which has been dipped in iodine solution.

ARTHROPOD INFESTATIONS

• Phthiriasis

Phthirus pubis (the crab louse) is 1.2–2 mm in length and infests the strong hairs of the pubic and perianal areas, abdomen, thighs, axillae and, rarely, the eyebrows, eyelashes and beard. The louse is transferred by sexual contact but can be acquired from clothing. Itch is the principal symptom.

Treatment
Treat with phenothrin (0.2%) or malathion (0.5%) lotions.

• Scabies

Scabies is caused by the mite *Sarcoptes scabiei* var. *hominis*. Most infestations are acquired by non-sexual contact.

1. The principal symptom is itch which is particularly noticeable at night and develops up to 6 weeks after a first infection, but earlier in second or subsequent attacks.

2. Burrows may be found on the hands and wrists, extensor surfaces of the elbows, feet and ankles, penis and scrotum, buttocks, axillae and, less frequently, elsewhere. When hygiene is good, burrows may not be apparent.
3. An erythematous rash with urticarial papules, not associated directly with the presence of the mite, is also noted in infested patients; penile and scrotal lesions are common.
4. Indurated nodules are sometimes found on the genitals and elsewhere.

Treatment

Treat with malathion (0.5% in an aqueous base) or permethrin cream (5%).

19 Sexuality and family planning

Susan V Carr

Chapter contents

Sexuality is an inherent component of the consultation when discussing family planning and reproductive health. Unfortunately, both patients and professionals may be uncomfortable about discussing sex, and it can remain a hidden part of the interaction. Usually, it is of course by having sex that conception is possible, and if the woman was not having or intending to engage in sexual intercourse, she would not need family planning advice. The vast majority of couples tend to have similar patterns of sexual activity. In a large population-based study almost 20 000 Australians aged between 16 and 59 years were asked what they did on their last sexual encounter. Around 95% included sexual intercourse, confirming that the majority of sexual encounters do carry the risk of pregnancy.[1]

SEXUALITY

Sexuality is the combination of gender identity, sexual orientation and sexual behaviour. Your sexual identity defines who you are in the biological sense, but gender identity is more about how you feel and identify in society. About half of the population are identified as female, and half are male, both emotionally and biologically. This is gender identity.

In contrast, about 8/100 000 of the population have a persisting and enduring conviction that they have been born into the wrong body, and are transsexual. These elements are believed to be well established by the age of four. Many transsexuals have children, but are unlikely to present for contraception in the transition phase. They have sexual health issues and, just as the rest of the population do, require safe sex information, and as long as they have a cervix should be aware of their need for cervical screening.

• Sexual orientation

The vast majority of the population are heterosexual, that is attracted to individuals of the opposite sex, but it is important to recognize differences in sexual orientation, as it is may have an impact on sexual health and contraceptive choices.

Bisexuality is being sexually attracted to both men and women, and accounts for 7% of the adult population. Between 5 and 10% of the male population are homosexual, or have had sexual contact with men. Although the majority of women are heterosexual, up to 2% of the population is lesbian, and sexually attracted to women.

There are some pieces of evidence suggesting a biological basis for both sexual identity and orientation. Core sexual identity and sexual orientation are believed to be fixed around the age of four.

• Lesbian and bisexual women

Many lesbian and bisexual women may use contraception as more than 80% have had sex with a man at some point in their lives. They find it difficult to disclose their sexual orientation within a clinical consultation, often due to a (probably unjustified) fear of homophobia, or lack of understanding from their clinician. Despite being shown to be at higher risk of breast and ovarian cancer than other women, they are less likely to present for breast or cervical screening[2] and should receive accurate advice about their risk. Any woman who has penetrative sex of any sort, e.g. fingers or sex toys, should have a cervical smear. These consultations also present an ideal opportunity to ask about sexual problems and refer if appropriate. It is important not to assume your female patient has a male partner. It has been shown that routinely asking a simple question, such as 'do you have a partner?' and 'is that partner male or female?' will assist the disclosure which will then ensure that an appropriate consultation can take place.

• Sexual behaviour

Sexual behaviour is dependent not only on one's sexual identity and orientation, but on many other factors and can change according to age, health, culture, beliefs, education, society and opportunity. Sexuality is inherent in everyone, but the way each individual chooses to express it or not is dependent on all these different factors and will change throughout a lifetime. Given the close link between contraception and sex, it is surprising how rarely the family planning practitioner will ask the woman during routine consultation if she is having sex, yet will happily prescribe a contraceptive if her blood pressure and menstruation are normal, even if she may not need it!

THE HUMAN SEXUAL RESPONSE

The human sexual response is dependent not only on intact neurological, vascular and endocrine systems, but also on cognition and emotions. Bancroft classically described this as the Psychosomatic Circle of Sex.[3]

A modern model, which helps clinical understanding of sexual activity, is an adaptation of the original four phase (EPOR) model of Masters and Johnson described in 1966[4]; Excitement, Plateau, Orgasm, Resolution. It is now described as Desire, Excitation, Orgasm and Resolution; the DEOR model.[5] This concept provides the framework on which some forms of therapy for sexual problems are based.

As there are both physical and psychodynamic elements to the human sexual response, both elements should be included in the treatment of any sexual disorders.

• Female sexual response

The female sexual response is a result of sensory input through the peripheral nerves of the somatic and autonomic nervous system as well as through the cranial nerves. The frontal and temporal lobes and anterior hypothalamus all have some function in mediating the sexual response, and even although imaging can show which areas of the brain are activated by incoming signals, how they are processed to cause sexual arousal is still unclear.[6] Genital responses include pelvic vasocongestion and vaginal lubrication. During coitus the vagina lengthens, the labia increase in size, the uterus draws back causing tenting of the vagina and the clitoris retracts. During orgasm there is contraction of uterine and pelvic muscles. A woman who is not sexually aroused will not respond in this way, and may complain of painful intercourse.

• Male sexual response

The male sexual response can occur within 10–30 seconds after sexual stimulation. Hormonally mediated neurovascular changes cause the erectile tissues within the corpora cavernosa to fill with blood and the intra cavernosal pressure increases. The surrounding tunica albuginea contains the pressure, and the penis becomes erect. During orgasm, the man experiences awareness that ejaculation is imminent. Smooth muscle contraction occurs, and seminal fluid builds in the prostatic urethra, and the urethral bulb dilates. The internal sphincter closes preventing the transmission of fluid into the bladder. The external bladder sphincter then relaxes, allowing the fluid into the urethral bulb. Rhythmic contractions of the bulbospongiosus and ischiocavernosus muscles, sphincter urethrae and urethral bulb propel the semen along the penile urethra and between 1 and 6 ml of ejaculate are expelled.

COMMUNICATION ABOUT SEX

Many patients find it difficult to talk about sex, even within the context of a contraceptive or sexual health consultation. It concerns the most intimate and private part of their lives, and, naturally, with most people, there are inhibitions about discussing these matters, even with trained professionals. Unfortunately many clinicians are themselves uncomfortable about talking about sex, and try to avoid facilitating disclosure of a sexual difficulty, as they are concerned at being unable to deal with the problem, and more prosaically, that it will take up too much of their clinic time. There is a growing body of evidence, however, that patients with problems of a sexual nature would like the opportunity to discuss these matters. Studies on different patient groups have highlighted lack of communication about sex. Gynaecological cancer patients felt that they would like to have had an opportunity to discuss sexual matters and they would have liked their doctor to have mentioned it.[7] The contraception consultation can be an ideal setting in which a woman can disclose problems in relation to sex, which would be difficult for her in any other setting. With a reflective, open style of consultation this helpful discussion can be facilitated.

COMMON SEXUAL PROBLEMS AND THEIR TREATMENT

For the majority of people and for most of the time, sex is a pleasurable and fulfilling activity.

It usually only comes into the domain of the family planning practitioner if there is a problem. An extensive American population-based study[8] showed that 43% of women and 37% of men have or have had a problem of a sexual nature at some point in their lives and both a proportion of family planning clinic attenders, and patients at a genitourinary medicine clinic were shown to have problems of a sexual nature.[9]

• Female sexual problems

Loss of libido

Loss of libido is essentially loss of sexual interest. It is sometimes called hypoactive sexual desire disorder. Despite the fact that various endogenous hormones, including estrogen, progesterone, testosterone and prolactin may influence female sexual function there are no physiological markers for loss of libido. Despite a recent flurry of research there is no clear evidence to date that any drug therapy improves sexual desire in women, the exception being when testosterone has been added to HRT in some post-menopausal women such as those who have had a surgical menopause and who have no other psychosexual or relationship problems. Hormonal contraception rarely can have a negative sexual effect on some women, and that is easily diagnosed by trying an alternative contraceptive, logically non-hormonal.

Loss of libido is mainly of psychogenic origin. It can have multiple underlying subconscious triggers which will differ from person to person. Loss of libido may be associated with other losses, such as bereavement, redundancy or termination of pregnancy all leading to a degree of loss of self-esteem and loss of sexual interest. Loss of libido may be partner-related, and it is unsurprising that if a woman has a core dislike of her partner she is unlikely to want to have sex with him. All of these factors may not be apparent at the outset, but after psychodynamic input the woman may be able to understand at least some of the factors underlying her libido loss. Some women have problems with any kind of contraceptive, and this may mean that they really would like to have a baby, but have not realized this themselves. In such patients it is worth exploring this idea.

The mainstay of treatment of this condition therefore is psychosexual counselling, involving the woman herself and her partner if she wishes.

Vaginismus

Vaginismus is involuntary spasm of the vaginal muscles, leading to inability to allow anything to penetrate the vagina. There is no organic abnormality, despite the frequent description of a 'blockage down below'. The treatment is ideally a combination of psychosexual therapy, and/or use of vaginal trainers. The trainers are used in order to give the woman a feeling of control over what penetrates the vagina; they are not used to dilate the vagina as it is not stenosed, and does not require dilatation.

Women with vaginismus tend to find it difficult to disclose, feeling that they are the only people in the world with this distressing problem. The alert clinician, however, should be aware that the persistent smear-avoider in the clinic may indeed have vaginismus. In all women, before taking a smear, questioning to elicit any problems with previous smear taking or with sex should avoid any distressing or painful attempts at speculum penetration in a woman with this condition. It is useful to note that women with primary vaginismus will never have used tampons. Vaginismus may also present as infertility, and again, asking about sexual activity, specifically penile penetration, will assist the diagnosis as these couples will never have had full intercourse.

Dyspareunia

Dyspareunia is painful sexual intercourse. There are multiple organic causes such as infection, dermatological reasons and rarely malignancy, which should always be excluded by appropriate investigation. One of the commonest causes however is insufficient arousal leading to lack of lubrication, which can often be helped by simple advice on foreplay techniques. If, however, the reasons for the lack of arousal are more complex, psychodynamic techniques need to be used.

Estrogen deficiency may lead to post-menopausal vaginal dryness, which can be helped by estrogen vaginal pessaries or simple lubricants. Vulvar vestibulitis is a complex condition which causes painful sexual intercourse, often through hypersensitivity of the vulval area leading to superficial dyspareunia. The multidisciplinary approach has been shown to have the best results, and a combination of gynaecological and genitourinary screening, and psychodynamic input works best.[10]

When all organic causes have been excluded and the pain persists, the woman should be referred for psychosexual therapy, as it may be of psychogenic origin.

One cause for dyspareunia in the woman can be erectile problems in her male partner. If the penis is not fully erect, any attempts at penetration can be painful.

The history-taking should address partner issues.

Anorgasmia

Orgasm is a sensation of intense pleasure which induces feelings of wellbeing and contentment. It creates an altered state of consciousness which is accompanied by contractions of the pelvic striated circumvaginal and uterine/anal muscles and myotonia which resolves sexually induced vasocongestion. Men have orgasm in around 95% of encounters and women in 70%. However, studies have suggested that up to 25% of women report orgasmic dysfunction.

Cognitive behavioural therapy lessens anxiety and promotes sexually relevant thought changes. There is no evidence to date, however, that any drugs have any proven benefit beyond that of placebo in women with anorgasmia.

• Male sexual problems

It is important to have an awareness of male sexual problems because, in a couple, the problem affects both partners, no matter who appears to have the 'primary' dysfunction.

Erectile dysfunction

Erectile dysfunction is the inability to have and maintain a penile erection. The prevalence of this condition is about 10% of the male population in their 60s rising to 40% of men in their 90s. There are many causes of this condition, which may be organic (60%), such as endocrine, vascular or drug-induced. It may be purely psychogenic (10%), or of mixed organic/ psychogenic origin (30%). It is reasonable to assume that, even if the cause of the problem is purely organic, that this is a condition which may be very distressing for the sufferer, and for his partner.

The treatment depends on the aetiology. Surgery can be performed if there is a venous shunt leading to inability to maintain erection. There are now very effective oral medications for erectile dysfunction, such as phosphodiesterase 5 inhibitors, e.g. sildenafil (Viagra®); however they will only be effective if sexual desire is present. There are alternatives of intra cavernosal injections or intraurethral pellets of alprostadil (a prostaglandin), which can also have a good local effect.

If the male with erectile dysfunction is not attracted to his partner that may be a significant part of the problem and, in that case, medication will not work.

Psychosexual assessment and counselling can help those for whom the problem is wholly or partially psychogenic and is a helpful part of the assessment of all men with this problem.

Female sexual dysfunction can be caused by male erectile problems and can be helped by treatment of the male partner's problem. A woman is more likely than a man to present at a contraception clinic, and more inclined to present a sexual problem, saying it is 'her fault', when the primary problem may lie with the male.

Ejaculatory disorders

Premature ejaculation, or ejaculation before sexual satisfaction is achieved, is the commonest male sexual problem worldwide. It is a major cause of couple sexual dissatisfaction. Behavioural techniques can be used, such as the 'squeeze' technique. This involves squeezing firmly below the glans penis at the point of orgasm; the so called 'point of no return'. This can be done by the man himself or his partner, and requires good co-ordination. It has the effect of delaying ejaculation. It is often said that the use of condoms in premature ejaculation dulls the sensation and delays ejaculation. This is anecdotal, but the use of condoms in this situation causes disruption to the act of coitus, and is more likely to worsen the problem in an already anxious man. Antidepressant medications, such as anafranil and selective serotonin reuptake inhibitors (SSRIs) used for their side effect of delaying ejaculation are now more commonly used; however the problem frequently recurs on discontinuing the medication.

Delayed ejaculation can be a side effect of some medications, such as SSRIs; the very same drugs that can be used to good effect in premature ejaculators. Ejaculation can be blocked by some adrenergic antagonists, but these men may still experience orgasm, calling this a 'dry run' experience. The majority of cases of men presenting with delayed ejaculation are psychogenic in origin, frequently related to inability to relinquish control over many areas of their life, including sexually.

With all sexual problems, especially in men, the history is important. If a problem is intermittent or situational males also suffer from loss of libido. If a man has low serum testosterone levels, then hormone supplementation can boost his sex drive. In most cases, however, as with women, the cause is psychogenic and should be treated by psychodynamic means. This can be done as an individual, or with his partner, male or female, if he chooses.

Loss of libido

Men also suffer loss of libido, and may find it even harder than women to disclose. If a man has low testosterone, replacement can help his libido. As with women, in most cases there is no disturbance of biological tests, and underlying emotional and relationship factors have to be addressed in order to improve his condition.

SEXUAL ABUSE

Trauma, such as sexual or emotional abuse, is a common underlying problem in people with sexual difficulties. Domestic violence or growing up as a child exposed to emotional abuse such as parental alcohol or drug addiction can manifest later in life as sexual or relationship difficulties. This is almost universally true of vulnerable populations such as prostitutes and the homeless. If the clinician suspects this may be the case, one key question can open up many avenues for reflection and discussion: the question is 'using one word only, how would you describe your childhood?' Anecdotally, this triggers very revealing emotions which can be used in the consultation to help the patient. Simple and direct questions about sexual violence and trauma incorporated into the routine clinic first visit can also aid disclosure.

If abuse is disclosed, then it should be acknowledged and referral for counselling offered. If refused, it may mean that the patient is not yet ready to confront the issues, or may have done so in the past, and his/her refusal should be accepted.

SEXUAL PROBLEMS IN RELATION TO CONTRACEPTION

There is no clear evidence to date that, in the vast majority of cases, use of any type of contraceptive will have any negative effect on sexual function, sexual pleasure or sexual relationships. In fact the converse seems to be true, that for most women, the comfort of being free from unwanted pregnancy will enhance her sexual experience. There are of course individual women, who may feel a particular method does cause sexual difficulties. It is essential to acknowledge this with her, take a careful and thorough general and sexual history, and allow her to discuss social and emotional issues. It may be that for her, a change of contraceptive will help.

With the exception of libido in relation to contraceptive hormones, there has been little research specifically on any link between general sexual problems and different methods of contraception. It is however worth summarizing the evidence to date in order to put the issue of sexual problems and contraceptives into context.

• The combined pill

Combined oral contraception, 'the pill', has been available in the UK since the late 1950s. Despite the immense body of excellent scientific study into this method of contraception there has been very little investigation into the sexual effects of the pill until relatively recently.

The combined pill can cause lowering of testosterone via the effect on sex hormone binding globulin (SHBG) and in some women may be associated with loss of libido. In non-pill users, androgen levels decline naturally by 50% from the mid 20s to the mid 40s,[11] so any loss of libido cannot necessarily be assumed to be caused just by the pill.

It is impossible to reach any firm conclusion from the work that has been done to date on the effects of the combined pill on libido. A classic study reported in 1995 in women from two different countries and cultures, Scotland and the Philippines, showed that the combined pill reduced sexual interest in 50% of the Scottish women but the same pill produced little change in women in the Philippines.[12] In contrast, the progestogen-only pill appeared to have had little effect in either population. Other research in different cultural settings has shown that the presence of sexual dysfunction in women had no correlation with the type of contraception used. A recent review of the published literature on the impact of the combined pill on sexual desire highlighted the mixed results, showing that some women experienced an increase in desire, some a decrease in desire and some no change whilst on the contraceptive pill.[13] Sexual enjoyment, orgasmic frequency and sexual satisfaction have all been shown to increase when on the combined pill; with no change in libido.[14]

The complexities of the human sexual response make it difficult to pinpoint the exact cause of any sexual problem in purely organic terms. Although there is some thought that any loss of libido sustained whilst on the combined pill may last beyond its use, this possibility needs to be balanced against the efficacy of the combined pill in preventing unwanted pregnancy, and the potential negative sexual effects that an abortion can trigger. Although some women may experience loss of desire on the pill, it is easy to change to another method as a therapeutic trial. Unfortunately many women come to the family planning clinic hoping that a simple contraceptive change will resolve their sexual difficulties, whereas underlying socio-emotional issues are the real cause of the problem.

• The vaginal ring

There is one study which compares oral and intra-vaginal combined contraceptives in relation to sexual function.[15] Interestingly both groups of women had improved sexual functioning compared to the placebo group. When investigating sexual fantasy however, this measure improved in both the women and the partners of the group using the ring, but not in those using the pill or in placebo groups. There was no explanation offered for this surprising finding.

• Progestogen–only contraception

Progesterone can reduce libido; this may be a potential side effect of progestogen-only methods of contraception although most deliver only a tiny dose of progestogen.

Medroxyprogesterone acetate, the hormone in the injectable contraceptive, has an anti-androgenic effect. It has been used both in male sexual offenders and male to female transsexuals to reduce androgen concentrations, in order to suppress the male sexual response. It is effective in provoking erectile failure, but its effect on libido is variable. Although a few women using an injectable method of contraception may experience loss of libido, it is a rarely mentioned side effect in the clinical setting, with weight gain being a far more troublesome complaint.

The subdermal progestogen implant and progestogen-releasing intra-uterine system (IUS) also have the theoretical risk of loss of libido listed in their patient information leaflet as a possible side effect. In the vast majority of women the benefits of these methods far outweigh the remote likelihood of any sexual problem.

• Copper intrauterine devices

There is relatively little information about the effect of an IUD on sexual well-being, but none of the published studies show a negative effect. The main problems tend to arise when there is pain or excessive bleeding with an IUD, but otherwise, as a non-hormonal method they may be a very good choice from the sexual perspective. In a comparative trial in Spain of over 1000 women, sexual desire did not vary with either pill or IUD use, and even improved in both groups between 6 and 12 months of contraceptive use.[16]

• Barrier methods

Condoms provide a useful barrier against sexually transmitted infection and pregnancy, but unfortunately to some people they can also be a barrier to sexual pleasure and satisfaction. Condom use, as the only male-controlled reversible contraceptive method, is subject to enormous cultural, religious and gender influences. To many men it reduces sexual spontaneity, and reduces their feeling of masculinity, although one study showed that men favoured its use more than women.[17]

Condom use has been widely promoted over the last 30 years, not only as a contraceptive, but to protect against sexually transmitted infections. It is unlikely to cause sexual difficulties, but latex sensitivity should be excluded before recommending condoms, as allergy can cause unpleasant dyspareunia.

Prostitutes use condoms to form an emotional, as well as contraceptive, barrier between themselves and clients which is why they often have unprotected sex with their partners.

• Sterilization

Female sterilization can lead to a significant improvement in sexual satisfaction and sexual drive, and a positive impact on sexual life.[18]

It has been shown that men who have a vasectomy do not suffer sexual problems, and in married men, vasectomy makes no difference to sexual satisfaction or frequency of sexual intercourse. In a study of 64 Brazilian men who had undergone vasectomy, there was a positive effect on sexual desire and satisfaction, and no cases of erectile dysfunction related to surgery.[19]

MODES OF TREATMENT

The majority of sexual problems have a psychosexual element to them. Even if it is organic in origin, it is deeply distressing to have a sexual problem. The sufferer who finds sex painful or unpleasant will use strategies to avoid sex, and gradually loses desire and becomes emotionally distant from the partner. Psychosexual medicine is the branch of medicine which aims to help the patient recognize and understand some of the emotional factors which are present and may be underlying the sexual problem. This type of treatment attempts to enable the patient to remove the emotional blocks and barriers to satisfactory sex and relationships.[20]

Another mode of treatment is more didactic; attempting to educate people about their sexual response, and to give them forms of behavioural therapy, including a stepwise reintroduction of sexual contact and communication, in order to improve their sex lives.

Aids to therapy such as appropriately used vaginal trainers, vibrators and vacuum devices all have their role to play, but should be accompanied by counselling sessions with a trained therapist. There are a myriad of self-help books, DVDs and websites. These can all be helpful to people who like this type of support. A carefully edited list of potentially useful materials is invaluable to any clinics that may see patients with sexual problems; this gives the patient something to do for themselves whilst awaiting specialist referral, and sometimes obviates the need for such a consultation.

All of these treatments can involve the partner if the patient wishes.

THE VAGINAL EXAMINATION IN THE CONTEXT OF SEXUAL PROBLEMS

It is frequently necessary to carry out a vaginal examination within the context of a contraceptive or sexual health consultation. If the patient appears to have a sexual problem, the examination can be carried out as part of the psychosexual assessment. Close observation of the reaction to the offer of vaginal examination, the refusal or acceptance of this offer, and the way the woman approaches the examination couch may be revealing. If any anxiety or unusual reluctance is noted, this can be reflected back to the woman and may allow discussion of matters which had otherwise been concealed in the consultation.

The vaginal examination and indeed equivalent genital examination in males can serve as a very useful and powerful psychosexual diagnostic and therapeutic tool.

Someone who is terrified of vaginal examination is unlikely to use an IUD or even a barrier method of contraception, as that would involve acknowledging her genital area. Methods such as a pill, the patch or implant are totally independent of the sexual areas of the body and that enables both the patient, and frequently the clinician, to pretend that the consultation has nothing to do with sex.

TRAINING

Many clinicians are worried about disclosure of a sexual problem during a consultation, because they are either uncomfortable about discussing sexual matters or, more commonly, are concerned because they do not know what to do about it if a problem is revealed. The important thing is to listen to the patient, acknowledge the problem and refer appropriately. With a little more training, it becomes easier to be able to conduct the consultation in a more reflective, rather than interrogative way and in many cases onward referral may not be required.

In the UK psychosexual training is offered through the organizations such as British Association of Sexual and Relationship Therapists and the Institute of Psychosexual Medicine.

REFERENCES

1. Richters J, de Visser R, Rissel C, Smith A (2006) Sexual practices at last heterosexual encounter and occurrence of orgasm in a national survey. Journal of Sex Research 43: 217–226.

2. Aaron DJ, Markovic N, Danielson ME, Honnold JA, Janosky JE, Schmidt NJ (2001) Behavioural risk factors for disease and preventive health practices amongst lesbians. American Journal of Public Health 91(6): 972–975.

3. Bancroft J (1989) Human Sexuality and its Problems. Edinburgh: Churchill Livingstone.

4. Masters WH, Johnson VE (1966) Human Sexual Response. Boston: Little, Brown.

5. Levin RJ (2005) Sexual arousal – its physiological roles in human reproduction. Annu Rev Sex Res 16: 154–189.

6. Levin RJ (2004) An orgasm is….who defines what an orgasm is? Sexual and Relationship Therapy 19: 101–107.

7. Stead ML, Brown JM, Fallowfield L, Selby P (2003) Lack of communication between healthcare professionals and women with ovarian cancer about sexual issues. Br J Cancer 10(88): 666–671.

8. Laumann EO, Paik A, Glasser DB, et al. (2006) A cross-national study of subjective sexual well-being among older women and men: findings from the Global Study of Sexual Attitudes and Behaviors. Arch Sex Behav 35: 145–161.

9. Jones AJ, Thin RN (1991) Contrasting psychosexual problems of patients attending a genitourinary medicine clinic and a community-based clinic. Int J STD AIDS 2: 124–127.

10. Bergeron S, Binik YM, Khalife S, et al. (2001) A randomized comparison of group cognitive–behavioral therapy, surface electromyographic biofeedback, and vestibulectomy in the treatment of dyspareunia resulting from vulvar vestibulitis. Pain 91: 297–306.

11. Burger H, Papalia MA (2006) A clinical update on female androgen insufficiency – testosterone testing and treatment in women presenting with low sexual desire.

12. Graham CA, Ramos R, Bancroft J, Maglaya C, Farley TM (1995) The effects of steroidal contraceptives on the well-being and sexuality of women: a double-blind, placebo-controlled, two-centre study of combined and progestogen-only methods. Contraception 52: 363–369.

13. Davis SR, Guay AT, Shifren JL, Mazer NA (2004) Endocrine aspects of female sexual dysfunction. Journal of Sexual Medicine 1: 82–86.

14. Caruso S, Agnello C, Intelisano G, et al. (2005) Prospective study on sexual behaviour of women using 30 mcg ethinylestradiol and 3 mg drospirenone oral contraceptive. Contraception 72: 19–23.

15. Guida M, Di Speiezo Sardo A, Bramante S, et al. (2005) Effects of two types of hormonal contraception – oral versus intravaginal – on the sexual life of women and their partners. Hum Reprod 20: 1100–1106.

16. Martin-Loeches M, Orti RM, Monfort M, Ortega E, Ruis J (2003) A comparative analysis of the modification of sexual desire of users of hormonal contraceptives and intrauterine contraceptive devices. European Journal of Contraception and Reproductive Healthcare 8: 129–134.

17. Grady WR, Klepinger DH, Nelson-Wally A (1999) Contraceptive characteristics: the perceptions and priorities of men and women. Fam Plann Perspect. 31: 168–175.

18. Li RH, Lo SS, The DK, et al. (2004) Impact of common contraceptive methods on quality of life and sexual function in Hong Kong Chinese women. Contraception 70(6): 474–482.

19. Bertero E, Hallak J, Gromatzky C, et al. (2005) Assessment of sexual function in patients undergoing vasectomy using the international index of erectile function. International Brazilian Journal of Urology 31: 452–458.

20. Skrine R (ed) (1989) Introduction to psychosexual medicine. Chapman Hall, London.

USEFUL WEBSITES

British Association of Sexual and Relationship Therapists (www.basrt.org.uk)

The Institute of Psychosexual Medicine (www.ipm.org.uk).

20 Gynaecological problems in the family planning consultation

Sharon Cameron

Chapter contents

Gynaecological problems are increasingly presenting in family planning (FP) consultations, particularly since a growing number of conditions are now managed medically, many using hormonal contraceptives. In this chapter the presenting features of a range of gynaecological conditions are reviewed and management options summarized. The extent to which a gynaecological problem can be managed within a family planning clinic setting will depend on the condition itself and on the expertise of the medical staff. Although the FP doctor is unlikely to be involved in any surgical gynaecological procedures, it is important to be aware of all the current options for treatment.

VULVAL, VAGINAL AND CERVICAL CONDITIONS

• Bartholin's cyst and abscess

A Bartholin's cyst is a retention cyst that results from obstruction of the duct of Bartholin's gland, which provides vaginal lubrication. It presents as a painless cystic swelling in the lower part of the labium majus. Treatment (surgical excision) is not usually necessary unless enlargement or infection occurs. Infection leads to abscess formation, presenting as a tender, red and painful swelling, which needs to be incised and drained, as an emergency gynaecological procedure. Screening for *Chlamydia trachomatis* would be advised, as for any sexually active woman presenting with vaginal infection.

• Lichen sclerosus

Lichen sclerosus is a chronic skin disorder affecting the vulva of postmenopausal women. It occurs less commonly in young women, children and men on other parts of the body. It usually presents as vulval itch (pruritis), pain or dyspareunia although it may be asymptomatic. The vulval skin looks white, thin and crinkly (because of loss of dermal support). There may be fusion of the labia minora with clitoral adhesions and narrowing of the introitus. The changes may extend around the anus in a 'figure of eight' distribution. Women with lichen sclerosus may also have autoimmune disorders. The condition may co-exist with vulval carcinoma. Five per cent of cases progress to squamous cell carcinoma. Although lichen sclerosus usually presents at the menopause, treatment with estrogen is not beneficial. The recommended treatment is topical potent steroids (e.g. clobetasol propionate 0.05% [Dermovate®]) with use of aqueous cream for washing (avoid soap as it dries skin). Referral to a specialist is advised since this condition requires long-term supervision and biopsy may be required to exclude carcinoma.

• Atrophic vaginitis

Estrogen deficiency in postmenopausal women results in thinning of the vaginal epithelium with associated dryness, irritation, pruritis and dyspareunia and occasionally postmenopausal bleeding. It responds to local vaginal estradiol (tablet or ring) or estriol (cream or pessary). Although low-potency estrogen formulations (estriol) are assumed to have few, if any, adverse effects on the endometrium, there are no long-term data to support this. Use should therefore be restricted to the smallest effective amount and need for continued treatment reviewed annually. As for all postmenopausal bleeding, any bleeding during therapy should be investigated promptly.

• Vaginal wall cysts

These can arise anywhere in the vagina but are commonest in the upper vagina and are often found by chance during cervical screening. They are usually single, thin-walled structures which are embryological remnants of the Wolffian duct. Reassurance is all that is needed, although if the cyst appears to be enlarging, the patient should be referred to a gynaecologist. They should not be confused with vaginal adenosis, a rare condition in which multiple glandular cysts occur often accompanied by profuse mucus secretion. Vaginal adenosis may be pre-malignant and can occur in women whose mothers took diethylstilboestrol (DES) during their pregnancy. Women with a history of DES exposure in utero should have regular colposcopic examinations of the vagina and cervix.

• Congenital malformations

The uterus, tubes, cervix and upper portion of the vagina are formed from fusion of the two Mullerian ducts. Disorders of embryological fusion can give rise to a range of congenital malformations. Many of these may be detected on speculum examination such as uterine agenesis (absent uterus), vaginal septum or a double cervix. Referral to a gynaecologist is indicated. In view of the high incidence of co-existent urinary tract anomalies, ultrasonography of the urinary tract is also indicated.

• Cervical ectropion ('erosion')

The lining of the cervical canal is columnar epithelium, which to the naked eye has a red, glandular appearance. In contrast, the vagina is covered with squamous epithelium, which looks pale pink and smooth. Eversion of the columnar epithelium of the cervical canal onto the vaginal surface of the cervix, leads to a rough and red ('eroded') appearance. This 'ectropion' or 'erosion' is physiological at puberty and pregnancy and is common in users of combined oral contraception (COC). A large 'erosion' may bleed if touched and can cause post-coital bleeding, or profuse vaginal discharge. If symptomatic, it may be cauterized with diathermy coagulation (if the cervical smear is normal). However, cautery often causes a prolonged watery or blood-stained discharge and women should be warned that ectropion may recur.

• Cervical polyp

These are localized growths of the endometrium which are often asymptomatic and detected at the cervical os at routine smear taking. They can cause inter-menstrual (IMB) or post-coital bleeding (PCB). If small, they can be twisted off with polypectomy forceps. Larger polyps with a thick stalk, may bleed profusely and should be referred to a gynaecologist for removal. Although polyps are usually benign, they should always be sent for histological examination. If the patient has IMB, then ultrasound investigation of the uterine cavity is indicated, since bleeding may be due to other polyps within the uterine cavity.

PELVIC MASSES

A pelvic mass may be detected on routine abdominal or vaginal examination.

Pre-menopausal women. Pregnancy must be excluded. Fibroids or an ovarian cyst are the most likely cause. History and examination may help differentiate between them. Small 'functional' ovarian cysts are not uncommon and usually disappear with menstruation. Asymptomatic cysts are known to be common in women using low-dose progestogen-only contraception (20–50% of cycles). Women with symptomatic, large or persistent cysts should always be referred for ultrasonography and for further specialist assessment.

Post-menopausal women. Ovarian cysts are common in healthy post-menopausal women and whilst most are benign, these women should always be referred for further evaluation. The prevalence of ovarian cancer is 61 per 100 000 women aged 68. A combination of vaginal ultrasonography and serum CA125 levels can predict the likelihood of malignancy. Suspicious features on ultrasound include a large size, solid areas within cyst, bilateral lesions and ascites.

• Fibroids

Fibroids are benign tumours of myometrium that vary in size from microscopic to large abdominally palpable masses. They are present in approximately 20% of women. Many are asymptomatic but they can cause heavy menstrual bleeding, infertility, miscarriage, dyspareunia or pelvic discomfort. Fibroids may also present due to compression of surrounding organs causing urinary frequency or difficulty with defecation. Growth of fibroids is hormone dependent and so they can grow during pregnancy and shrink after the menopause. Malignant change (leiomyosarcoma) is rare (0.1%).

History

Symptoms as above.

Examination

A bulky, enlarged uterus is suggestive of fibroids.

Investigation

Ultrasound examination is important to map the site and size of fibroids, since this will determine treatment.

Management

See Table 20.1.

Table 20.1 Management of fibroids

Fibroid management	Considerations
Medical	1. Medical treatments (as for heavy menstrual bleeding – see p. 348). Often poor response
	2. LNG–IUS may be considered if no significant intracavity (submucous) fibroid
	3. Gonadotrophin releasing hormone agonists (GnRH-A) cause fibroid shrinkage but result in hypo-estrogenism and bone loss. Use limited to short term (3 months) with 'add back' HRT for longer duration
Surgical	1. Hysteroscopic resection possible for small submucous fibroids
	2. Hysterectomy if childbearing complete
	3. Myomectomy (excision of each fibroid) if wish to preserve fertility
Fibroid embolization	• Interventional radiological technique
	• Interrupts blood supply to fibroid by blocking uterine arteries with tiny particles, via catheterization of femoral artery
	• Fibroid shrinkage ~50%
	• Potential complications of infection, exposure of the ovaries to radiation
	• Childbearing must be complete

ENDOMETRIOSIS

Endometriosis is the presence of functional endometrium outside the uterine cavity. It can be asymptomatic or cause dysmenorrhoea, deep dyspareunia, chronic pain and infertility, as a result of the chronic inflammation which occurs. The disease varies from a few small lesions to large ovarian endometriotic cysts (endometriomas), fibrosis of utero-sacral ligaments and adhesion formation causing marked distortion of pelvic anatomy.

Examination

Pelvic tenderness, a fixed retroverted uterus, tenderness or nodules in the pouch of Douglas or enlarged ovaries are suggestive of endometriosis. Findings may however be normal.

Investigation

1. Transvaginal ultrasound can exclude ovarian endometriomas.
2. Laparoscopy is the gold standard diagnostic test. At present there is insufficient evidence to determine if MRI is useful to diagnose or exclude endometriosis.

Management

See Table 20.2.

Table 20.2 Management of endometriosis

Endometriosis management	Considerations
Medical	1. COC (monthly or tricycling) or continuous oral or systemic progestogens (Depo-Provera®) are effective for reducing pain, and may be used long term
	2. LNG-IUS is effective at reducing pain
	3. GnRH-A is effective. HRT needs to be given to counteract bone loss, but does not affect GnRH-A effectiveness
	4. Danazol (antigonadotrophic, androgenic drug) widely used in the past, use now limited due to adverse androgenic effects
	4. Pilot studies suggest that letrozole (aromatase inhibitor) may be effective, although associated with significant bone loss
Surgical management	1. Ablation of endometriotic lesions at laparoscopy (laser, diathermy, etc.) reduces pain and improves fertility in minimal/mild endometriosis
	2. Endometriomas may be excised or drained
	3. Radical surgery involves hysterectomy and bilateral salpingo-oophorectomy

Medical therapy may be used for empirical treatment of pain (before laparoscopy), or for medical treatment following laparoscopic diagnosis. Medical treatments do not improve fertility. Pain relief may be incomplete and symptoms can recur within 6 months of stopping treatment.

MENSTRUAL DYSFUNCTION

Women in developed countries now experience ten times the number of menstrual periods (400 versus about 40) in their lifetime than their ancestors did 100 years ago, due to earlier menarche, fewer pregnancies, reduced lactation and use of hormonal contraception.

• Menstrual irregularity

Occurs commonly at menarche and peri-menopause when it is usually associated with anovulation. Irregular menses also occur in polycystic ovarian syndrome (page 353). Investigation should be as for oligo-amenorrrhoea (page 350). In most cases, good cycle control will require hormonal therapy in the form of COC, or progestogens (page 349).

• Intermenstrual (IMB) and postcoital bleeding (PCB)

This may be due to a local cervical problem including ectropion, polyp, infection with *Chlamydia trachomatis*, malignancy or an intrauterine lesion such as a polyp or submucous fibroid. Some women bleed around mid-cycle due to a fall in estrogen at ovulation. Pelvic examination and cervical smear (if due or if cervix suspicious) should be performed, with testing for *Chlamydia trachomatis* and ultrasound to detect intracavity lesions. Local causes should be treated appropriately. A trial of ovarian suppression with the COC, or progestogens should be considered if mid-cycle bleeding and/or investigations are normal.

• Heavy menstrual bleeding

The commonest menstrual complaint in the UK is that of heavy menstrual bleeding, defined as excessive menstrual blood loss that interferes with a woman's physical, emotional, social or material quality of life. In most cases, there is no underlying pathology.

History

- Take careful history to determine severity of bleeding and identify risk factors for pathology or systemic disease.
- Ask about flooding (heavy blood loss onto clothing) and use of double sanitary protection (pad and tampon) which indicate excessive loss.
- Assess effect of bleeding on quality of life – disability experienced, time lost from work, social disruption.
- Look for symptoms of anaemia.
- Ask about irregular bleeding, dyspareunia, pelvic pain, IMB or PCB, raise suspicion of underlying pathology.
- Be aware of risk factors for endometrial cancer – tamoxifen use, unopposed estrogen, family history of endometrial or colon cancer, polycystic ovarian syndrome.

Examination

Abdominal and pelvic examination should be performed.

Investigations

1. Cervical smear (if due, or suspicious appearance of cervix).
2. Full blood count. Tests of thyroid function and of coagulation are unnecessary unless indicated by the history.

Figure 20.1 outlines the further assessment of heavy menstrual bleeding (see Ref. 1 for further details).

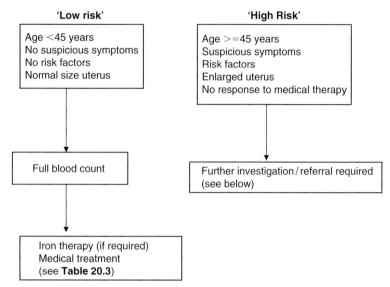

'Low risk'	'High Risk'
Age <45 years No suspicious symptoms No risk factors Normal size uterus	Age >=45 years Suspicious symptoms Risk factors Enlarged uterus No response to medical therapy

| Full blood count | Further investigation / referral required
(see below) |

Iron therapy (if required)
Medical treatment
(see **Table 20.3**)

Figure 20.1 Assessment of heavy menstrual bleeding

Further investigations

1. Ultrasound can measure endometrial thickness, determine site and size of any intracavity lesions, e.g. polyps and submucous fibroids, and assess ovaries. Saline infusion sonography (SIS) can better define questionable intrauterine pathology. SIS involves the instillation into the uterus of a few millilitres of sterile saline, through a fine catheter (such as those used in insemination techniques). Intracavity lesions are more clearly visualized against the background of saline.

2. Endometrial biopsy using a plastic sampler (e.g. Pipelle, Eurosurgical UK), is well tolerated and has similar sensitivity to D&C for detecting endometrial cancer and hyperplasia.

3. Hysteroscopy allows direct visual examination of the uterine cavity. With the advent of fine (2–3 mm) hysteroscopes, the procedure is increasingly performed as an outpatient procedure, with accuracy and patient acceptability equivalent to inpatient hysteroscopy under general anaesthetic.

Management

Management of heavy menstrual bleeding is almost always medical initially and many women will respond favourably. Hysterectomy is now less

Table 20.3 Medical management of heavy menstrual bleeding

Therapy	Mode of action	Recommended regimen	Reduction in blood loss
NSAID	Reduces endometrial prostaglandins that increase blood loss and contractions	Mefenamic acid 500 mg TDS	25%
Anti-fibrinolytic	Reduces endometrial fibrinolysis that cause increased bleeding	Tranexamic acid 1 g TDS	50%
COC	Endometrial suppression		50%
LNG-IUS	Endometrial suppression	Mirena®	90%
Progestogens	Endometrial suppression	Norethisterone 15 mg daily from day 5–day 26	80%
		Depo-Provera® every 12 weeks	Amenorrhoea (in 60% users at 12 months)

commonly performed for menstrual dysfunction unless there is significant underlying pathology.

1. For medical management see Table 20.3.
2. Surgical treatment – endometrial ablation.

With highly effective and simpler devices for destroying the endometrium, many experts view endometrial ablation as an alternative to medical therapy and not as a last option. This procedure aims to destroy the endometrium and to reduce menstrual flow (80% of women have lighter periods). Childbearing must be complete. New ablative techniques that are performed on selected patients under local anaesthesia include a thermal balloon (Thermachoice®); a microwave ablative method (Microsulis®); and an impedance device (Novasure®) that 'vaporizes' the endometrium. Hysterectomy is the final option if other treatments are unsuccessful.

POSTMENOPAUSAL BLEEDING

Postmenopausal bleeding is bleeding that occurs more than 1 year after the menopause. It should always be investigated to exclude an underlying gynaecological cancer which is present in 10% of cases. This is usually endometrial cancer but cervical, ovarian or bladder cancer can give rise to abnormal vaginal bleeding in the post-menopause. A common 'benign' cause is atrophic vaginitis (see page 384). Abnormal bleeding in association with HRT is discussed in Chapter 22.

History

1. Date of LMP.
2. History of weight loss/gain with pelvic mass may suggest ovarian/ uterine cancer.
3. Vaginal discharge may suggest infection or atrophic vaginitis.
4. Risk factors for endometrial cancer (obesity, late menopause, diabetes, PCOS, family history of endometrial or colon cancer, tamoxifen, unopposed estrogen use).
5. Drug history – use of HRT, or alternative remedies that have estrogenic properties.

Examination

Pelvic examination may reveal a vaginal or cervical cause or pelvic mass. Atrophic vaginitis is common. Its presence should <u>not</u> preclude consideration of other causes.

Investigations

1. Do a cervical smear if cervix looks suspicious or is due.
2. Pelvic ultrasound – first-line investigation (unless the woman is taking tamoxifen when hysteroscopy with endometrial sampling is the preferred investigation). If endometrium is regular and $</= 3$ mm thick then no further endometrial assessment is required. If endometrium is not clearly defined, irregular or >3 mm thick then endometrial sampling should be performed. This may be performed with a plastic disposable sampler (e.g. Pipelle). Alternatively, sampling or curettage may be performed with hysteroscopy as an outpatient or under general anaesthesia (see Figure 20.2 for investigation of PMB).

OLIGOMENORRHOEA AND AMENORRHOEA

Infrequent or absent menstruation occurs commonly. Pregnancy should always be excluded. Depending on the woman's age, need for contraception or desire to start a family, investigation may be delayed for 6 months. See Table 20.4 for causes of oligomenorrhoea or secondary amenorrhoea.

History

1. Ask about menstrual patterns since menarche. Problems which appear to have arisen after stopping the pill often predate its use and have simply been masked by the pill-induced regular withdrawal bleeds.

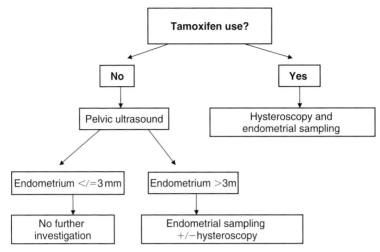

Figure 20.2 Investigation of PMB

Table 20.4 Causes of oligomenorrhoea or secondary amenorrhoea

Site	Cause
Hypothalamus	Weight loss
	Over exercise
	Chronic illness
	Idiopathic
Pituitary	Pituitary adenoma (hyperprolactinaemia)
	Hypopituitarism
Ovarian	Premature ovarian failure
	PCOS
Uterine	Asherman's syndrome
	Cervical stenosis
Endocrinopathy	Thyroid disease
	Cushing's disease

2. A history of weight loss, excess exercise, galactorrhoea or stress should be sought.
3. A drug history for medicines known to cause hyerprolactinaemia (see Table 20.6) or recreational drugs (e.g. heroin, marijuana), which can result in oligo- or amenorrhoea.

Table 20.5 Investigation of oligomenorrhoea or secondary amenorrhoea

Investigation	Interpretation	Further investigations
LH (taken during menses if oligomenorrhoea)	If <5 IU/L suggests pituitary or hypothalamic problem If >10 IU/L suggests PCOS	
FSH (taken during menses if oligomenorrhoea)	If <5 IU/L suggests pituitary or hypothalamic problem If >30 IU/L indicates ovarian failure	If premature menopause (age <40 years) blood for autoantibodies and karyotype
Testosterone	If >6 nmol/L suggests adrenal hyperplasia, neoplasia or Cushing's	Refer to specialist
Prolactin	If >1000 IU/L suggests pituitary adenoma	MRI of pituitary gland. Refer to specialist
TSH	High TSH indicates hypothyroidism	Refer to specialist
Transvaginal ultrasound	Identifies polycystic ovaries	

4. Recent use of Depo-Provera® should be excluded.
5. Uterine curettage or endometritis following miscarriage, abortion or childbirth might suggest Ashermann's syndrome (intrauterine adhesions).

Examination

General physical and pelvic examination, BMI, signs of thyroid disease, hirsutism and the presence or absence of galactorrhoea (a sign of raised prolactin – see Table 20.6 for causes).

Investigations

See Table 20.5.

Management

If investigations are abnormal, the problem persists or a pregnancy is desired, refer to a specialist.

1. If Asherman's syndrome is suspected then refer to a gynaecologist, since hysteroscopy with division of intrauterine adhesions would be indicated.
2. If investigations suggest polycystic ovarian syndrome (PCOS) and fertility is not required, COC will give regular cycles (see page 61).
3. If investigations show a pituitary microadenoma, then a dopamine agonist will suppress prolactin and lead to resumption of normal cycles.
4. If investigations give normal results, normal cycles may resume spontaneously within a few months. Review in 6 months time.

Table 20.6 Causes of hyperprolactinaemia

Stress
Drugs (e.g. phenothiazines, metoclopramide, domperidone, cimetidine, antihistamines, morphine, marijuana)
Primary hypothyroidism
Chronic renal failure
Pituitary adenoma, compression of pituitary stalk
Idiopathic

Women with amenorrhoea or oligomenorrhoea may occasionally ovulate spontaneously and so should use contraception if they wish to avoid pregnancy. COC is appropriate for women with amenorrhoea and low gonadotrophins since it will protect them from osteoporosis due to low estrogen (although COC will not protect from osteoporosis if the woman is nutritionally undernourished with anorexia nervosa). COC is best avoided in women with hyperprolactinaemia, since the estrogen component stimulates prolactin secretion (Table 20.6).

• Primary amenorrhoea

If a girl reaches the age of 16 years with primary amenorrhoea, endocrine tests as for secondary amenorrhoea should be undertaken (Table 20.5). If FSH is elevated, karyotyping should be undertaken. If this is abnormal (e.g. 45XO Turner syndrome), refer to a specialist. Otherwise, if secondary sexual characteristics are normal, then only reassurance is required.

Abdominal ultrasound may be reassuring to confirm the presence of a uterus and ovaries.

These girls should be followed-up to ensure that menses do occur and that the girl does not wish puberty to be induced.

POLYCYSTIC OVARIAN SYNDROME

Polycystic ovarian syndrome (PCOS) is a common endocrine disorder estimated to affect up to 10% of women. It is characterized by the presence of at least two out of three of the following features:

1. Oligo-menorrhoea.
2. Ultrasound appearance of large volume ovaries ($>10\,cm^3$) and/or multiple small follicles (12 or more follicles $<10\,mm$).
3. Clinical evidence of excess androgens (hirsutism, acne) or biochemical evidence (elevated free or total testosterone).

Management

This depends on which symptoms are present.

1. If overweight – weight loss improves symptoms and can correct the abnormal endocrinology.
2. Menstrual cycle control is best achieved with COC. Alternatively, cyclical progestogens (non-androgenic, e.g. medroxyprogesterone acetate or dydrogesterone) may be given cyclically to induce regular bleeding. The LNG-IUS may also be a good option to protect the endometrium against the effects of unopposed estrogen but will of course not induce regular menstruation.
3. Hirsutism and acne can be managed medically (see page 355).
4. If anovulatory infertility, ovulation may be induced with clomifene citrate, under specialist supervision and monitoring. If unsuccessful, treatment may involve metformin, gonadotrophin injections or laparoscopic ovarian diathermy.

HIRSUTISM

Excessive hair growth (androgen-dependent) in women can cause extreme distress. It is usually present on the upper lip, chin, breasts or lower abdomen. In 95% of women the cause is PCOS or idiopathic. Rare causes include Cushing's syndrome, adrenal hyperplasia and androgen-secreting tumours of the ovary and adrenal.

History

1. Severity (frequency of cosmetic hair removal and by what method, e.g. shaving, electrolysis, depilatory creams) and sites affected.
2. Signs or symptoms of virilism (deepening of voice, male pattern baldness) should raise suspicions of neoplasia.
3. Medication – any androgenic medicines (e.g. anabolic steroids, danazol – formerly used to treat endometriosis) or drugs that cause hair growth (antiepileptics, e.g. phenytoin)

Examination

1. Document sites and degrees of hirsutism.
2. Male pattern baldness or cliteromegaly (>1 cm) are signs of virilism and require specialist referral.
3. BMI.

Investigation

1. Blood for LH, FSH, and testosterone (during menses if not amenorrhoeic). If serum testosterone is >6 nmol/L, then refer

Table 20.7 Anti-androgen therapies

Anti-androgen	Action
Cyproterone acetate	Androgen receptor blockade
Spironolactone	Potassium-sparing diuretic with anti-androgenic activity
Finasteride	5 alpha reductase inhibitor (inhibits conversion of androgens to more potent forms)

to a specialist for exclusion of androgen-secreting tumours and Cushing's disease.

2. Ultrasound of uterus and ovaries for characteristic features of PCOS.

Management

1. If BMI raised – weight loss.
2. Cosmetic measures – shaving, waxing, bleaching. Permanent hair removal, such as electrolysis and laser (dark hair only).
3. Topical – for facial hirsutism, a topical preparation eflornithine (Vaniqa®) may be used which slows hair growth by inhibiting a decarboxylase enzyme (important for proliferation of hair follicles). It is applied twice daily to affected areas of face with effects noticeable after 8 weeks.

Medical therapy

1. COC – suppresses ovarian androgen production, increases sex hormone binding globulin which 'mops up' free testosterone. The preparations containing the anti-androgen cyproterone acetate (Dianette® or the generic Clairette®) is the most effective, but has increased risk of VTE compared to other COC.
2. Anti-androgens – only to be used with highly effective contraception, as risk of masculinization of a female fetus if pregnancy occurs. Contraception advised for 3 months after discontinuation. This treatment (Table 20.7) should be initiated and supervised by a specialist. Response to medical therapy is slow (>3 months) but stops progression and decreases the rate of hair growth. Success of treatment is best judged by a fall in the frequency of need for hair removal.

DYSMENORRHOEA

Dysmenorrhoea (excessive menstrual pain) is one of the most common causes of absenteeism from school and work. Primary dysmenorrhoea is present from the onset of ovulatory cycles after menarche and is thought to be a consequence of prostaglandins which increase contractility of the myometrium and cause the cramping pain.

Secondary dysmenorrhoea usually has its onset many years after the menarche and may be due to pathology such as endometriosis or fibroids. Dysmenorrhoea may be increased with the presence of an intrauterine contraceptive device (IUD) but is reduced with the LNG-IUS.

Management

A careful history with precise details of timing of pain should be taken. Pelvic examination may not be helpful in primary dysmenorrhoea, but is essential for secondary dysmenorrhoea. Women who have no abnormalities on examination may be safely treated without further investigation as below. If a pelvic mass is suspected then pelvic ultrasound should be performed. A laparoscopy may be indicated if endometriosis is suspected, or when standard medical therapy has been ineffective.

Reassurance that pain does not indicate sinister pathology may help the woman cope with her symptoms. If dysmenorrhoea is unresponsive to standard medical therapy (see below), then consideration should be given to the possibility of underlying pathology and appropriate investigation should be instituted.

Treatment

1. Prostaglandin synthesis inhibitors.
   NSAIDs reduce the production of uterine prostaglandins and dysmenorrhoea. Mefenamic acid and ibuprofen are most commonly used.
2. COC – reduces the severity of pain and can be tricycled to reduce the frequency of dysmenorrhoea.
3. Depo-Provera® – may cause amenorrhoea.
4. LNG-IUS – in addition to reducing menstrual blood loss, the LNG-IUS is highly effective at reducing dysmenorrhoea.

MENSTRUAL HEADACHE

Some women complain of severe headaches at the onset of menses. They may result from the abrupt fall in circulating steroid hormones at the end of the cycle and seem to be more common amongst pill-users than with spontaneous cycles. Tricycling the COC may help by reducing the frequency of headaches. Clearly however, women who experience focal migraine or women >=35years who suffer from any form of migraine should not take the COC.

PELVIC PAIN

• Acute pelvic pain

In women of reproductive age, the common gynaecological causes of acute pelvic pain are ovarian cysts, pelvic inflammatory disease (PID) and ectopic pregnancy. Other causes include UTI, renal colic, appendicitis and musculoskeletal conditions.

History

Take details of LMP, use of contraception, abnormal vaginal discharge, any gastrointestinal or genitourinary symptoms.

Examination

Assess the patient's general condition to see if pyrexial, or has signs of haemodynamic instability (ruptured ectopic pregnancy). In the absence of pregnancy and in women who are sexually active, cervical excitation strongly suggests PID. A palpable or tender adnexal mass in a non-pregnant woman suggests an ovarian cyst which could have undergone torsion or rupture.

Investigation

1. Do a urine pregnancy test to exclude pregnancy (for suspected ectopic pregnancy see page 363).
2. Test for chlamydia (or other STIs depending on risk factors).
3. Undertake ultrasound to look for ovarian cyst, or evidence of recent rupture (free fluid). Hydrosalpinges and tubovarian masses may also be identified.
4. Check white cell count which is likely to be raised if infection present.

Management

If a non-gynaecological cause is suspected refer to appropriate specialist. If ovarian cyst, torsion, rupture or haemorrhage suspected then refer to gynaecology as an emergency. For suspected PID, institute appropriate antibiotic therapy (see Chapter 18).

• Chronic pelvic pain

This is intermittent or constant pain in the lower abdomen or pelvis of >6 months duration, not occurring exclusively with menstruation or intercourse and not associated with pregnancy. It should be considered as a symptom with several contributory factors rather than a diagnosis. As with all chronic pain, psychological and social factors should be considered and their influence on the pain should be discussed early in the consultation.

History

Enquire about the pattern of pain, exacerbating and relieving factors, associated bowel or bladder symptoms, psychological and social factors, including domestic violence. Explore patient's fears and ideas about the cause of the pain. Cyclical pain may suggest an endocrine cause. GI symptoms may suggest irritable bowel syndrome.

Examination

Do abdominal and pelvic examination to elicit signs of infection, adnexal tenderness or tenderness at vault that might suggest endometriotic ovarian cysts or nodules of endometriosis.

Investigations

A pain diary may be helpful in tracking symptoms or activities associated with pain. Test for chlamydia (and other STIs depending on risk).

Pelvic ultrasound should be performed to exclude/assess adnexal masses.

Diagnostic laparoscopy should be carried out if examination findings suspicious of endometriosis.

Treatment

1. If the pain is cyclical and no abnormality is evident at examination, a therapeutic trial of 'ovarian suppression' using the COC for a 3–6-month period should be considered.
2. If history suggests irritable bowel syndrome then dietary modification and/or a trial of antispasmodics should be performed.
3. Diagnostic laparoscopy is the only investigation that will diagnose peritoneal deposits of endometriosis and adhesions. However, it is a surgical intervention with risks and is 'negative' in one-third to one-half of cases. Furthermore, pathology (e.g. fine adhesions or a few spots of endometriosis) may be identified that is not the actual cause of the patient's pain. When laparoscopy is negative, the doctor may be at a loss to explain the cause of the pain and the patient may feel that the doctor thinks that the pain is 'in her head'. It is best reserved as a second-line investigation, if other treatments fail.

DYSPAREUNIA

Dyspareunia is classed as 'superficial' if pain is felt near the vaginal introitus on penetration or 'deep' if it is located deeply in the pelvis upon thrusting. Superficial dyspareunia may reflect infection or a local condition (episiotomy scar, lichen sclerosis, etc.). Vaginismus ('tensing up' of vagina at attempted penetration) may account for some or all of the dyspareunia.

Deep dyspareunia is more suggestive of pelvic pathology (fibroids, cysts, endometriosis).

History

1. Ask about the site and nature of the pain – is it superficial or deep, 'burning' in nature (vulval vestibulitis).
2. Is there abnormal discharge; blisters, warts or ulcers could indicate infective cause?
3. Pruritis could indicate an infection or lichen sclerosus.
4. Menopause or breast-feeding can cause vaginal dryness.
5. Is it related to pregnancy; feelings about a recent birth, miscarriage or termination of pregnancy may impact on sexual intercourse?
6. Is there foreplay and sufficiency of arousal before penetration?
7. Ask about the relationship with the partner and their response to the woman's dyspareunia.

Examination

Do an abdominal and pelvic examination to exclude any physical causes.

Management

If physical causes are found, then treat as appropriate.

1. Vaginal dryness (menopause or breast feeding) improves with a lubricant or local estrogen therapy.

2. Vulval vestibulitis is characterized by burning pain at the introitus on attempted penetration. The cause is unknown and the evidence for treatments is poor. Local anaesthetic, steroid or estrogen cream, and ketoconazole may be tried. Patients are best referred to a specialist vulval clinic but are often reassured by the fact that it is not psychosomatic.

3. If psychological factors related to pregnancy or relationship problems are present, then referral to a counsellor is indicated.

4. If vaginismus is present then refer for psychosexual therapy. Programmes such as penetration 'desensitization' programmes can prove effective (see Chapter 19).

URINARY PROBLEMS

Urinary problems often go unreported due to embarrassment. Many women with urinary incontinence suffer depression, relationship and sexual difficulties and low self-esteem as a consequence. Prevalence increases with age, with almost half of women >80 years, suffering from urinary incontinence.

Risk factors include:

1. Pregnancy and childbirth – increasing maternal age, parity, heavy babies and difficult childbirth (e.g. forceps delivery), have detrimental effects.
2. High BMI.
3. Menopause is contributory rather than causal.

History

Determine severity of symptoms and risk factors as above. History taking should also cover medication, bowel habit, sexual dysfunction and quality of life.

Examination

Abdominal and pelvic examination should be performed to exclude a pelvic mass, atrophic vaginitis, prolapse, cystocele, demonstrable stress incontinence and neurological abnormality.

Investigation

1. Urinalysis – glycosuria (screening for diabetes), leucocytes – suggestive of UTI.
2. Mid-stream specimen of urine (MSU) – to confirm UTI.
3. Frequency–volume chart (voiding diary), to confirm frequency, volumes passed and total output of urine. Small volumes passed frequently, in absence of UTI would suggest overactive bladder (detrusor instability).
4. If symptomatic uterovaginal prolapse, pelvic mass, haematuria, recurrent UTI, or voiding dysfunction then refer to specialist services.

• Urge incontinence and overactive bladder

1. Lifestyle – reduce intake of caffeine, alcohol and weight (if overweight).
2. Review fluid intake – excessively small or large fluid intake can exacerbate incontinence. Patients should adjust their intake to produce 1–2 L urine daily.
3. Bladder retraining is effective for mild symptoms. This involves the patient gradually increasing duration between micturitions, thus slowly increasing bladder compliance.
4. Antimuscarinics – oxybutinin is effective in reducing bladder overactivity, urgency and urge incontinence. Side effects include dry mouth, blurred vision, drowsiness, nausea and dizziness. The dose can be titrated to combat these or transdermal and

slow-release oral preparations used. A trial of 6 weeks should enable assessment of benefits. Alternatives include tolterodine, tropsium and propiverine.

- ## Stress incontinence
    1. Pelvic floor muscle re-education consisting of exercise regimens tailored to individuals and often supplemented with techniques that increase muscle awareness, e.g. electrical stimulation, vaginal cones. Exercises need to be continued long term to be effective.
    2. Intravaginal devices which support the bladder neck are effective in reducing episodes of incontinence and may be suitable in the short term (e.g. ring pessary or wearing tampon to prevent leakage during exercise).
    3. If no treatment success, refer to gynaecological urologist for consideration for surgical treatment.

- ## Dysuria

Dysuria may result from:

1. UTI. Check MSSU and exclude chlamydia in young women (<25 years). Appropriate antibiotic therapy should be given if results are positive.
2. Vaginal infection. Treat as appropriate.
3. Painful bladder syndrome – describes a condition of frequency and/or urgency, dysuria, that is without an obvious cause.
4. Urogenital atrophy at the menopause may be associated with recurrent UTI, dyspareunia, urinary frequency, dysuria and incontinence. Symptoms will respond well to local or systemic estrogen replacement.
5. Urethral prolapse/caruncle – the urethral mucosa may prolapse in elderly women, becoming red and inflamed, causing dysuria. This may need to be removal surgically.
6. General measures – after visiting the toilet women should be instructed to wipe the perineum from front to back and to empty their bladder regularly. Vaginal deodorants and bath additives should be avoided. Fluid intake should be encouraged particularly when symptoms occur. Cranberry products (juice, tablets) may be of value in preventing recurrences.

PRE-PREGNANCY COUNSELLING

The general advice is to eat a good diet, take regular exercise, stop smoking and cut back on alcohol. If the woman is in good health before pregnancy then she should be in better shape to deal with the physical and emotional stresses that can occur.

1. Stopping contraception – there is no reason to switch from hormonal contraception to a barrier method before embarking on a pregnancy.
2. Weight – women who are obese should lose weight, since obesity can result in failure to ovulate. Furthermore, obese mothers are at increased risk of gestational diabetes, hypertension, large babies and VTE. Underweight women should be advised to gain weight, since they are less likely to ovulate, and there is increased risk of babies with growth restriction.
3. Alcohol, smoking, caffeine, drugs – advise to stop smoking, reduce alcohol (women limit 1–2 units/week and men 3–4 units), and avoid recreational 'drugs', since these have an adverse effect on fertility. Furthermore, smoking during pregnancy is associated with growth restriction and prematurity. Heavy alcohol intake can cause congenital fetal abnormalities (fetal alcohol syndrome). Women should also be advised to reduce caffeine intake since high intake (e.g. >4 cups coffee/day) is associated with delayed time to conception.
4. Folic acid supplements – 400 µg folic acid/day (until 12 weeks pregnancy) to protect against neural tube defects (NTDs) such as spina bifida. Women at high risk of NTD (diabetes, epilepsy, history of NTD) should be advised to take 5 mg folic acid/day.
5. Rubella status should be checked (if unknown). Non-immune women should be vaccinated and advised to avoid pregnancy for 1 month after vaccination.
6. Specialist counselling – women with diabetes may require referral to a diabetic physician to help them gain tight glucose control to reduce the likelihood of miscarriage and fetal abnormality. Women with epilepsy may wish to discuss with a neurologist whether it is appropriate for them to discontinue medication, or use a single antiepileptic agent only, as this may reduce the likelihood of fetal abnormality. Women with a family history of a genetically transmitted condition may need referral to a geneticist for counselling on risk of transmission to offspring and of diagnostic tests that may be offered during pregnancy.

BLEEDING IN EARLY PREGNANCY

Women may already know or suspect that they are pregnant, or pregnancy may be diagnosed at the consultation. Bleeding may be due to local causes such as a cervical lesion or may be a sign of miscarriage or ectopic pregnancy.

History

A detailed menstrual history with details of any accompanying abdominal pain should be elicited. Unilateral pelvic pain should raise the suspicion of ectopic pregnancy. Other suspicious symptoms include feelings of faintness and shoulder tip pain. A history of pelvic infection, subfertility or IUD use should be sought.

Examination

The patient's general condition should be assessed. Spontaneous miscarriage and ectopic pregnancy can both cause heavy bleeding and shock. If the patient is shocked, she should be transferred immediately to hospital. A urine pregnancy test should be performed, to confirm pregnancy. Most tests detect levels of hCG of at least 25 IU which corresponds to day 9 post conception. A negative result will therefore usually indicate that the patient is not, or is no longer, pregnant. If clinical suspicion persists regarding possibility of an ectopic pregnancy, then serum hCG would be indicated.

Speculum examination may reveal a local cervical cause for bleeding. Testing for *Chlamydia trachomatis* should be considered, particularly in women <25 years. Products of conception may be evident. If distending the cervical os, this can cause shock and they should be removed with sponge-holding forceps. Pain on cervical excitation, unilateral forniceal pain and a mass may suggest ectopic pregnancy.

Management

The patient should be referred to hospital as an emergency if ectopic pregnancy is suspected. In all other cases, an ultrasound should be conducted to determine whether the pregnancy is ongoing. Ideally, this should be performed in a dedicated early pregnancy unit with specialist staff to provide support and counselling. If miscarriage is confirmed then this may be managed expectantly, medically or surgically.

RECURRENT MISCARRIAGE

Recurrent miscarriage is defined as three or more consecutive miscarriages. It affects 1% of women. The causes are:

1. Genetic – in 3–5% of couples with recurrent miscarriage, one partner has a balanced chromosomal translocation. This is when sections of chromosomes change their geographical position, without any loss or gain of important genetic material.
2. Anatomical abnormalities of the uterus, e.g. uterine septum, probably account for some cases, but the extent of their contribution is uncertain. Furthermore, surgery remains controversial since the chance of live birth remains high without treatment and complications of surgery may lead to infertility.

3. Antiphospholipid syndrome – anticardiolipin antibodies and lupus anticoagulant is detectable in 15% of these women. Treatment in pregnancy with low-molecular-weight heparin and low-dose aspirin, significantly improves the likelihood of a live birth.

4. PCOS – there is a higher than expected prevalence of PCOS in these women (40%), but the exact mechanism for miscarriage is unclear and there is no effective treatment.

5. Unexplained (50%) – three-quarters of this group will go on to have a successful pregnancy if offered nothing more than reassurance and support.

Investigations

Recurrent miscarriage should be investigated and managed in a specialized clinic.

Initial investigations include:

1. Male and female chromosome analysis.
2. Pelvic ultrasound – to exclude obvious uterine abnormality or PCOS.
3. Anticardiolipin antibodies and lupus anticoagulant.
4. Endocrine investigations – LH, FSH, testosterone (PCOS).

INFERTILITY

Around 15% of couples experience difficulty in conceiving. Usually investigations are undertaken after 1 year of trying to conceive. Earlier investigation is indicated if there are predisposing factors such as amenorrhoea, oligomenorrhoea, PID, undescended testes, women's age $>/=35$ years, or prior treatment for cancer.

General measures

1. Reassure that 84% of couples achieve pregnancy by 12 months, rising to 92% by the end of 2 years. Advise also that fertility declines with female age.

2. Advise on minimal alcohol (1–2 units/per week for women and 3–4 for men) and to stop smoking if smokers. Women who are overweight or underweight should aim for a normal BMI ($19–25 \, \text{kg/m}^2$).

3. Advise against using tests to predict ovulation, since these add further stress to an already stressful situation. Instead, instruct to have sexual intercourse every 2 days during the fertile period (days 10–17 if 28-day cycle).

4. Advise about prescribed, over-the-counter and recreational drugs and occupational hazards that affect fertility. Advise on taking folic acid to protect against NTD.

Causes of infertility

The common causes of infertility are:

- Male infertility – low sperm count or motility.
- Failure of ovulation.
- Tubal disease.
- Any combination of the above.

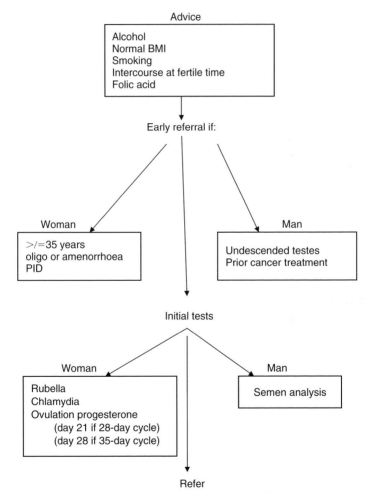

Figure 20.3 Flow chart for investigation and management of infertility (data from guidance from NICE[2])

History

1. Ask about menstrual cycle – women with irregular cycles are unlikely to be ovulating on a regular basis.
2. Any previous abdominal, gynaecological surgery or PID may suggest tubal disease.
3. In the male, a history of undescended testes, testicular torsion, hernia repair, drugs that affect sperm (anabolic steroids, some drugs used to treat ulcerative colitis), may suggest male infertility.
4. Intercourse. Occupations or lifestyles which involve one partner being away from home at the 'fertile time' will affect ability to conceive.
5. Erectile, ejaculatory and other sexual problems may be important.

Initial investigations

Initial investigations are useful while couple awaits an appointment for the infertility clinic (see flow chart – **Figure 20.3**, see previous page).

1. Assessment of ovulation – day 21 serum progesterone if 28-day cycle or later in longer cycle (day 28 if 35-day cycle). No other endocrine tests are required if ovulation confirmed. If anovulation (or if woman has amenorrhoea or oligomenorrhoea) then serum FSH, LH, testosterone, prolactin and TSH should be performed to elucidate cause of anovulation (page 352).
2. Semen analysis.
3. It is advisable to screen for chlamydia and to check rubella status of woman (and vaccinate if non-immune).

REFERENCES

1. NICE (2007) NICE Clinical Guideline no 44. Heavy Menstrual Bleeding.
2. NICE (2004) NICE Clinical Guideline. Fertility: assessment and treatment of people with fertility problems.

21 Premenstrual syndrome

P M Shaughn O'Brien

DEFINITIONS

It is important to be clear what is meant by premenstrual syndrome (PMS). Other terminology used in relation to PMS includes premenstrual tension (PMT), premenstrual tension syndromes (PMTS), menstrual distress, late luteal phase dysphoric disorder (LLPDD) and premenstrual dysphoric disorder (PMDD). PMS is the term most often used in the UK but this may change. The term PMDD is used to a large extent by psychiatrists in the US because of the tendency there to focus on psychological aspects of the disorder.

Until quite recently there has been a reluctance to accept PMS as an established condition. This has arisen because of the difficulty in distinguishing true PMS and PMDD from the milder physiological premenstrual symptoms, which occur in the normal menstrual cycle of most women in their reproductive years. They exhibit the same wide range of symptoms in the luteal phase of the cycle and they resolve by the end of menstruation but the normal physiological symptoms do not reach such a severity that they impact on normal day-to-day functioning.

Box 21.1 Patients who may present at a premenstrual syndrome clinic

- Physiological premenstrual symptoms
  - Occur only in the luteal phase
  - Resolve completely with menstruation so that there is a symptom-free week between menstruation and ovulation
  - Are not severe and do not disrupt normal functioning
- Premenstrual syndrome/premenstrual dysphoric disorder
  - Occurs only in the luteal phase of the cycle
  - Resolves completely with menstruation so that there is a symptom-free week between the end of menstruation and ovulation
  - Symptoms are severe and have a major effect on normal functioning and interpersonal relationships

(Premenstrual disphoric disorder is considered the extreme psychological end of the PMS spectrum)

- Premenstrual exacerbation of medical disorder
- Premenstrual exacerbation of psychological disease
- Co-existing PMS and underlying psychological disorder
  - Either symptoms of an underlying disorder increase premenstrually or there is PMS superimposed on an underlying problem. These are difficult to distinguish
  - Symptoms resolve with menstruation but only to the level of the background disorder
- Non-cyclical psychological disorder
  - Patients complain of symptoms which typify PMS but they do not resolve by the end of menstruation
  - Alternative diagnoses such as depression, personality disorder, drug/alcohol abuse and other psychological/psychiatric diagnoses must be considered

---

What characterizes PMS is that the symptoms are so severe that they disrupt the woman's normal functioning and her interpersonal relationships (work and family particularly). There are also women who have an underlying psychological disorder, which co-exists with PMS, and there can be premenstrual exacerbation of a pre-existing psychological disorder.

Finally, there are women who self-diagnose PMS but who actually have depression unrelated to the cycle; these women can be identified by the fact that their symptoms fail to resolve after menstruation (Box 21.1).

SYMPTOMS

An enormous range of symptoms has been described: they may be psychological/behavioural or somatic. As many as 200 have been described in the literature. Typical psychological symptoms include irritability, aggression, tension, depression, mood swings and feeling out of control. Commonly reported physical symptoms include bloatedness, breast swelling and pain. It is usually the psychological symptoms that cause the most distress and bring women to seek medical attention. The character of symptoms is less important than the timing and severity.

For a diagnosis of PMS, the symptoms must occur in the luteal phase of the cycle and resolve by the end of menstruation.

The severity must be sufficient to have a major impact on normal functioning. Women may experience symptoms for any portion of the luteal phase; some in the few days immediately prior to the period, whereas others have symptoms from ovulation right through the luteal phase to the end of menstruation.

PREVALENCE

Accurate prevalence figures cannot be given. Various papers quote 80–95% of women as having physiological symptoms, which are mild and normal. Very few women in their reproductive years appear to have absolutely no symptoms before their period. Estimates for the prevalence of true PMS are around 5%.

CONSEQUENCES

Numerous consequences have been claimed to result from PMS. Though they are based on anecdotal reports, it does seem likely that many serious problems are due to the disorder. These include psychosocial events such as poor work performance, marital problems (perhaps leading to divorce), suicide, murder, shop-lifting and child battering.

Certain medical problems also appear to relate to PMS, or at least occur in the luteal phase of the cycle; these include behavioural problems, migraine, epilepsy and asthma.

QUANTIFYING SYMPTOMS AND DIAGNOSIS

Research methods include specific charts, which may be Likert or visual analogue scales, and questionnaires such as the Moos' Menstrual Distress Questionnaire. A hand-held computer-based technique has been developed to record this information and it is under validation (Figure 21.1). This can be contrasted with a PMS diary from an asymptomatic woman (Figure 21.2).

For clinical purposes, a prospective symptom-rating diary is the most appropriate tool but in reality most clinicians rely on the history at initial consultation.

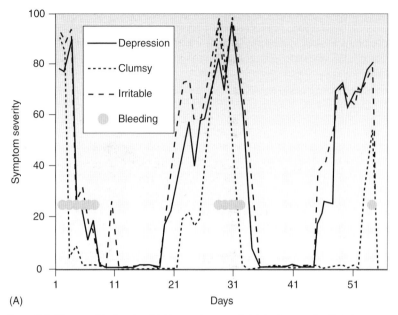

Figure 21.1 PC-screen data from hand-held computer-generated data of a severely affected woman with menorrhagia, dysmenorrhoea and severe psychological and somatic symptoms of PMS. (A) Typical psychological symptoms

The three essential clinical criteria for the diagnosis are that the symptoms:

1. occur in the luteal phase
2. have a major impact on normal functioning
3. disappear by the end of the menstrual period.

AETIOLOGY AND HYPOTHESES

The underlying cause of PMS has not yet been elucidated but some recent theories are quite convincing and an understanding of them enables the clinician to comprehend the thinking behind current treatment methods. Although the concept of a hormone imbalance has been popular, e.g. of progesterone deficiency, no evidence exists to support such theories. Indeed, the current consensus is that PMS sufferers and asymptomatic women do not differ regarding their hormonal status. Women with PMS are thought to be *more susceptible to the effects of their normal ovarian hormone cycle* than are

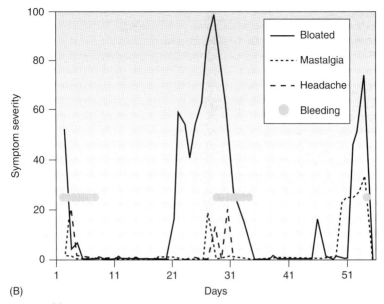

(B)

Figure 21.1 (B) Typical somatic symptoms

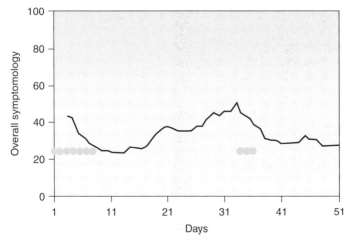

Figure 21.2 Asymptomatic woman with minimal physiological premenstrual changes

asymptomatic women. The reason for the increased sensitivity is thought to be related to neurotransmitter function. Candidates for this include abnormal function of beta-endorphins, GABA, dopamine, acetylcholine and serotonin.

All of the evidence in favour of these theories is indirect, e.g. the evidence for serotonin deficiency relies on research showing (a) that peripheral blood levels of serotonin are reduced and (b) that selective serotonin re-uptake inhibitors (SSRIs) improve symptoms.

If the broad philosophy of these theories is correct, then it appears that the *normal* ovulatory cycle provides the trigger for events in women who have an abnormal response to progesterone (or related steroids) which could result from a deficiency of serotonin function (or other neuropeptides). It is thus a psychoneuroendocrine disorder responding to an ovarian steroid trigger and so approaches to treatment fall into two broad strategies:

1. Correction of the neuroendocrine anomaly.
2. Suppression (or modulation) of the ovarian trigger.

MANAGEMENT

• Range of proposed treatment regimens

Until recently, most treatment approaches have been empirical. The wide range of therapies used probably reflects the high placebo response where almost any therapy produces an apparently favourable initial response. As a result, claims have been made for ovarian irradiation, vitamin B6, progesterone, estrogen, testosterone, dietary change, magnesium, endometrial resection, hysterectomy, oophorectomy, lithium, antidepressants, psychotherapy, hypnosis, yoga, diuretics and many other logical and illogical approaches.

• Evidence-based approach

In research into PMS therapy, symptoms must be quantified precisely and prospectively. Diagnostic inclusion and exclusion criteria must be strict. The studies must be randomized, double blind, placebo-controlled and include sufficient numbers of women to demonstrate clinically and statistically significant differences in efficacy between active therapy and control. Clinicians must be aware of these requirements in order to avoid accepting the claims of poor-quality treatment studies.

Few studies merit inclusion in good meta-analyses because they fail to meet the above standards. For this reason, few adequate meta-analyses have been published.

• Non-hormonal therapy

- **Diet**. All published dietary advice for PMS is not specific and is based on good dietary advice for health. This cannot be criticized but there are no controlled studies demonstrating a specific role for dietary modification in PMS. The advice to take frequent carbohydrate meals or exclude various foodstuffs is not supported by trials.

- **Vitamin B6**. A recent meta-analysis by Wyatt et al.[1] has demonstrated the inadequacy of all studies but the trends demonstrated in favour of vitamin B6 provide the justification for large multicentre studies. Vitamin B6 is cheap but prolonged overdosing can produce peripheral neuropathy.

- **Evening primrose oil**. This contains gammalinolenic acid. One systematic literature review demonstrated possible beneficial effects but, at present, adequate evidence exists only for the positive treatment effect in premenstrual breast symptoms.[2]

- **Minerals**. *Calcium and magnesium*. Research studies are of insufficient quality to recommend magnesium or calcium treatment though limited studies suggest a possible benefit for both.

- **Alternative therapies**. Many alternative therapies have been suggested but they have not been subject to appropriate trials. St John's Wort is a fashionable non-medical remedy and has many effects including serotonergic activity. It may therefore be acting as a weak SSRI. Conventional SSRIs should not be taken at the same time as St John's Wort because serious interactions have been reported and it can also reduce efficacy of the combined oral contraceptive pill.

- **Exercise and relaxation therapy**. There are controlled studies which suggest benefit.

- **Psychotherapy**. Cognitive behavioural therapy has gained widespread acceptance, particularly amongst clinical psychologists. There are some well-controlled studies which demonstrate efficacy over and above that of control therapy though others do not. Access to clinical psychology services is very limited in the UK.

- **Psychotropic drugs**. Benzodiazepines, lithium, monoamine oxidase inhibitors and tricyclic antidepressants have been used and assessed in a limited number of trials. SSRIs appear to be the most effective agents and there are many well-conducted studies of fluoxetine (at least seven) and sertraline (at least three) which fulfil criteria for meta-analysis.[3] Dimmock et al.[4] have produced a meta-analysis of all RCTs of the SSRIs; this includes some of the best conducted trials with the most convincing results in PMS research. Somatic as well as psychological symptoms appear to improve with these drugs. It appears that when SSRIs are given in the luteal phases only, they are effective for all symptoms. This is true particularly for irritability but less so for depression – possibly indicating the mechanism of action is different for the two symptoms. Although fluoxetine used to be specifically licensed for the treatment of PMS in the UK, this indication was withdrawn when there was harmonization of European licensing requirements and <u>not</u> because of lack of efficacy or safety concerns. There are recognized side effects of SSRIs but dependence is not a problem.

- **Diuretics**. There is convincing evidence that fluid retention is *not* an essential prerequisite of PMS even where bloatedness is a major symptom. Therefore there is little logic in giving diuretics. Despite this, diuretics have been prescribed for many years. In trials, only spironolactone demonstrates efficacy in PMS, particularly for somatic symptoms.

- **Prostaglandin inhibitors**. Mefenamic acid and naproxen sodium have been assessed in five RCTs. All reported significant improvement in symptoms. Many PMS sufferers report co-existing menstrual dysfunction, with pain and heavy bleeding, and therefore treatment of the latter may well improve general well-being.

- ## Hormonal therapy

  - **Progesterone/progestogens**. Despite the popularity of progesterone and progestogens (and the fact that they remain licensed in the UK for treating PMS) there are surprisingly few supportive data to justify this. Systematic reviews of progesterone and progestogen treatments have been published.[5] Of 12 RCTs available, two with micronized progesterone and two using progesterone suppositories suggest benefit, whilst eight (seven with suppositories and one with an intramuscular injection) show no benefit over placebo.[6] Three studies of dydrogesterone show benefit whereas four do not. Two of oral medroxyprogesterone acetate showed benefit whilst a third did not. There are no studies of the depot preparations. There are no trials of sufficient quality to demonstrate the value of norethisterone. Paradoxically, it should be remembered that norethisterone and indeed all progestogens are capable of *causing* PMS when given with estrogen in hormone replacement therapy (HRT) for menopausal symptoms.

  - **Estrogen**. Suppression of ovulation with relatively high-dose estradiol patches and implants has been shown to be effective. Trials of estradiol implants and estradiol patches (100 μg and 200 μg) demonstrate significant benefit when the dose is sufficient to suppress ovulation.[7] In order to prevent endometrial hyperplasia, progestogen must be given with any estrogen therapy and this can lead to a return of symptoms. Strategies to avoid this are outlined later.

  - **Danazol**. Danazol is no longer licensed for PMS because of concerns of potential masculinizing and lipid-altering side effects.

Consequently danazol is now used less often. It is, however, very effective as evidenced by five good RCTs. When given only in the luteal phase of the cycle, it is effective for premenstrual breast symptoms with no more side effects than placebo. It is thus an effective drug but with long-term risks.

- **Gonadotrophin-releasing hormone (GnRH) agonist analogues**. GnRH alone has been demonstrated to be highly effective in seven separate trials. Menopausal side effects, including loss of bone mineral density, limit its use in the long term. These can be countered by administering add-back estrogen/progesterone or possibly tibolone.[8]
- **Bromocriptine**. There are many trials which provide good evidence that bromocriptine is *not* effective for PMS except in the management of premenstrual breast symptoms.
- **Combined oral contraception**. Four trials have failed to demonstrate superiority over placebo. In theory, continuous pill therapy should be effective but this has not yet been researched. As many younger women will request the pill for contraception, it may seem worthwhile trying this empirically. Drospirenone is a relatively new progestogen which is contained in some oral contraceptives. This progestogen has anti-mineralocorticoid actions and may well counteract the physical symptoms of PMS in a similar way to spironolactone.

• Surgical approach

Hysterectomy and bilateral oophorectomy should be and is, as shown in good studies, curative.[9] Hysterectomy alone reduces but does not eliminate symptoms. Trials are limited because of the difficulty in providing true controls. Bilateral oophorectomy alone (e.g. laparoscopically) should be effective, but the need for estrogen (and thus progestogen) limits its potential. The consequences of major surgery, surgical menopause and the need for long-term estrogen replacement virtually preclude this approach for all but a few severely affected patients and usually those who are to undergo hysterectomy for another indication.

There is no logical reason why endometrial ablation (EA) should be effective, as no 'menotoxin' has been demonstrated. There are no adequate trials of EA in PMS, merely reports of incidental findings in women who have been randomized to treat menorrhagia.

CLINICAL MANAGEMENT

Broadly speaking, treatment aims either to suppress the ovarian cycle trigger by abolishing ovulation, or to correct the neurotransmitter factors that render women hypersensitive to their endogenous hormones.

When assessing the treatment for an individual patient, it is necessary to take into account several important factors:

A. The age of the woman, her desire for pregnancy in the near or distant future and current contraceptive needs. This will influence whether approaches that are also contraceptive or that require contraception can be used, or if hysterectomy would ever be acceptable.

B. Severity of the symptoms; impact on the quality of her life and that of her family. This will allow the clinician to use a hierarchical approach to therapy and determine if the more invasive means of treatment are justifiable.

C. A woman's preconceptions of the potential method available. She may be convinced that a certain approach is the only acceptable method. She may only accept non-hormonal methods, will not accept psychotropics or only wish to use non-medical techniques. The woman must always be involved in the decision-making process.

GUIDE TO TREATMENT

1. Women will almost always have explored the simpler approaches including diet, evening primrose oil and vitamin B6. The next stage will involve both doctor and patient.

2. Early resort to the use of SSRIs is increasingly considered acceptable and, when there is co-morbid depression, this is a particularly justifiable approach. Experience in both the management of depression and prescribing SSRIs is desirable. Women should be made aware that using an SSRI for the treatment of PMS is an unlicensed indication.

3. The use of danazol and GnRH analogues is usually limited by the inadvisability of long-term therapy; with GnRH analogues this can be prolonged by means of add-back HRT but they are also very expensive.

4. Estrogen is an important approach as it can suppress ovulation without inducing the risks of the menopause; it is effective as both implants and patches. If it proves ineffective in a particular patient, it is possible that a higher dose will be required to achieve suppression of ovulation. If PMS symptoms return in the progestogen phase, then a change of progestogen, reduced dose, reduced duration or intrauterine progestogen should be tried.

5. Some treatments may be more effective for particular symptoms than others. A symptom-directed approach can be tried such as:

   a. SSRIs are highly effective for psychological symptoms (but also somatic symptoms). They are of lesser efficacy for 'atypical' premenstrual symptoms.

   b. Breast symptoms are particularly responsive to bromocriptine but may also respond to evening primrose oil and luteal phase danazol.

   c. Dysmenorrhoea responds to non-steroidal anti-inflammatory drugs.

   d. Somatic symptoms (particularly bloatedness) respond to spironolactone and possibly drospirenone (as part of combined oral contraceptive preparation).

6. COC, particularly those containing drospirenone, are increasingly considered useful. Transdermal combined patches or depot medroxyprogesterone acetate (DMPA) may be useful if contraception is required. The intrauterine system (IUS) will give contraception and treat co-existing menstrual problems. It can be used as an adjunct to estrogen therapy to provide endometrial protection.

7. Progesterone and progestogens are probably not effective but will be required to protect the endometrium when estrogen is used. We have seen that these are associated, in many cases, with the recurrence of PMS symptoms. Alternative progestogens may then be tried resorting at an early or late stage to an IUS.

PREMENSTRUAL SYNDROME IN THE CONTEXT OF FAMILY PLANNING

No single medical speciality has ever accepted the responsibility for managing PMS. General gynaecologists rarely have sufficient expertise in the use of psychological interventions and psychotropic drugs. Psychiatrists have very limited knowledge of endocrinology, gynaecology and sexual health. General practitioners' breadth of knowledge makes them ideally placed to manage most aspects of the problem. Doctors working in family planning and sexual health services will have much of this broad expertise and are in an ideal position to run a specialist PMS service.

As PMS appears only in women in their reproductive years, it will inevitably mean that PMS will, on many occasions, influence the choice of contraception:

- *Barrier methods* will not affect PMS symptoms but will be required during several treatment regimens such as danazol, GnRH analogues and estrogen therapy.

- *Copper intrauterine devices* will not affect PMS per se but may exacerbate heavy or painful periods, thereby worsening the overall situation.

- *Intrauterine systems* may suppress ovulation in the initial months of use and this is thought to explain a temporary improvement in symptoms. Thereafter, despite the amenorrhoea associated with an IUS, PMS symptoms often will continue much as before. An IUS can be used for endometrial protection in conjunction with *estrogen* for ovulation suppression. This combination appears to be highly effective though research evidence for this does not exist.

- *Combined oral contraception* (COC) has not been proven to be of value but some women do find it helpful and there is anecdotal experience that continuous pill use is most effective. An empirical approach is suggested, particularly for young women. Recently, initial studies of COC containing the progestogen, drospirenone have suggested benefit. Its mineralocorticoid effect has the potential to reduce or eliminate physical symptoms but this is yet to be tested.

- *Progestogen-only pills.* There is no evidence or rationale for an effect on symptoms with conventional progestogen-only pills. The newest progestogen-only pill which contains desogestrel (Cerazette®) consistently suppresses ovulation and anecdotally can be helpful in the management of mild–moderate PMS and menstrual migraine. Women find it a highly acceptable treatment option.

- *DMPA.* Ovulation is often suppressed and there is anecdotal evidence to suggest a beneficial effect. This would be a fruitful avenue for research.

- *Fertility awareness methods, coitus interruptus.* These will presumably have no effect on a woman's PMS.

- *Sterilization* should have no influence on symptoms. It may, however, be difficult to convince a woman that, having been sterilized, she should then take hormones or receive an IUS.

A large multicentre study is required, probably in a family planning setting, to determine the relative efficacy of continuous COC, Cerazette®, DMPA and estrogen plus IUS.

PMS INDUCED BY HORMONE REPLACEMENT THERAPY

Women with PMS may also have an inappropriate response when given conventional sequential HRT. This is due to the progestogen phase of therapy that is essential to protect the endometrium. Typically, women complain of mood disorders, irritability, aggression, bloatedness and breast tenderness during the 12 days of progestogen; this mimics PMS.

There are many possible strategies that can be used to avoid this. Women vary enormously in their response. The approach must be empirical. There are no substantial trials to support the suggestions but the potential techniques include:

1. Change the progestogen – women appear to have individual responses to the different progestogens; this can be a disappointing venture but norethisterone is a particular progestogen to avoid.

2. Less frequent progestogen such as 3-monthly – bleeding problems are common when this regimen is used in perimenopausal women.

3. Shorter duration or a lower dose of progestogen in each cycle – this has to be balanced against the potential higher risk of endometrial hyperplasia and malignancy.

4. Give unopposed estrogen without progestogen with regular endometrial assessment (by scan and outpatient endometrial biopsy) – a calculated risk requiring careful discussion and documented consent.

5. An IUS administers low-dose, continuous progestogen thereby avoiding cyclical fluctuations. Its potent local effect protects the endometrium without causing significant systemic side effects; irregular bleeding is a common initial problem.

6. Removal of the endometrium by hysterectomy. Hysterectomy may occasionally be the only acceptable treatment for a particular woman. Usually this means simultaneous removal of the ovaries. Endometrial ablation is not appropriate as pockets of endometrial tissue are likely to persist.

7. Continuous combined HRT regimens; there is some evidence that continuous progestogen is tolerated better than sequential preparations when administered systemically.

8. Tibolone – limited evidence though one study reported an improvement in PMS. It is highly effective as an add-back agent during GnRH therapy and does not counteract its beneficial effect.

9. Conventional HRT with SSRI – this is theoretical, although there appears to be a proven synergistic effect on mood.

As with the treatment of true PMS, the choice of regimen will depend on many factors including the severity of symptoms, previous PMS, the presence of co-morbid depression, time since menopause and whatever previous therapy the woman has received.

REFERENCES

1. Wyatt KM, Dimmock PW, Jones PW, O'Brien PMS (1999) Efficacy of vitamin B6 in the treatment of premenstrual syndrome: systematic review. British Medical Journal 318: 1375–1381.

2. Budieri D, Li WP, Dornan JC (1996) Is evening primrose oil of value in the treatment of premenstrual syndrome? Controlled Clinical Trials 17: 60–68.

3. Steiner M, Steinberg S, Stewart D, et al. (1995) Fluoxetine in the treatment of premenstrual dysphoria. New England Journal of Medicine 332: 1529–1534.

4. Dimmock PW, Wyatt KM, O'Brien PMS (1998) Selective serotonin re-uptake inhibitors: An interim systematic review of efficacy in treatment of premenstrual syndrome. British Journal of Obstetrics and Gynaecology 105: 104.

5. Wyatt K, Dimmock P, Jones P, O'Brien PMS (2001) A systematic review to assess the efficacy of progesterone and progestogens in the treatment of premenstrual syndrome. BMJ 323: 776–780.

6. Freeman E, Rickells K, Sondheimer SJ, Polansky M (1990) Ineffectiveness of progesterone suppository treatment for premenstrual syndrome. Journal of the American Medical Association 264: 349–353.

7. Watson NR, Studd JWW, Savvas M, Garnett T, Baber RJ (1989) Treatment of severe premenstrual syndrome with oestradiol patches and cyclical oral norethisterone. Lancet 2: 730–732.

8. Mortola JF, Girton L, Fischer U (1991) Successful treatment of severe premenstrual syndrome by combined use of gonadotrophin releasing hormone agonist and estrogen/progestin. Journal of Clinical Endocrinology 72: 252A–252F.

9. Casson P, Hahn PM, Van Vugt DA, Reid RL (1990) Lasting response to ovariectomy in severe intractable premenstrual syndrome. American Journal of Obstetrics and Gynecology 162: 99–105.

FURTHER READING

Wyatt K, Dimmock P, O'Brien PMS (1999) Premenstrual syndrome, Clinical Evidence 2. BMJ Publishing Group 748–759.

ACKNOWLEDGEMENT

Figures 21.1 and 21.2 are reproduced by kind permission of Wyatt KS, Dimmock PW and O'Brien PMS (1999) Unpublished data.

22 Menopause

Ailsa E Gebbie

Chapter contents

By definition, the menopause is a woman's last spontaneous menstrual period and is a diagnosis made in retrospect following amenorrhoea for 12 months. It occurs on average at the age of 51 years. The majority of women in the Western world can anticipate spending at least one-third of their lives in a postmenopausal state as average life expectancy of women is now around 81 years. The transitional phase of fluctuating ovarian function around the time of a woman's last menstrual bleed is known as the 'perimenopause' or 'climacteric' and lasts around 2–3 years.

The last few decades have seen considerable scientific interest and research in the area of the menopause. In addition, widespread media coverage has made hormone replacement therapy (HRT) a household name. HRT is not a panacea for every ailment of middle-aged women and cannot be universally recommended. Prescribing of HRT in the UK reached a peak around 2002 but has declined since then following the publication of large randomized trials and studies which clarified the risks and benefits of HRT.

ENDOCRINE CHANGES

The menopause signals the end of reproductive potential with the onset of irreversible ovarian failure. The exhaustion of the ovaries' store of oocytes leads to the cessation of follicular development and ovulation. This results in:

1. Very low levels of circulating estrogens once ovarian activity has ceased. The predominant estrogen after the menopause is estrone.
2. A rise in circulating gonadotrophins, follicle stimulating hormone (FSH) and luteinizing hormone (LH), as a result of the removal of the negative feedback effects of estrogen.
3. Menstrual bleeding patterns reflect the changing hormonal milieu during the perimenopause. Regular menstruation becomes gradually interspersed with spells of amenorrhoea until the final period occurs.

DIAGNOSIS

In practice, the diagnosis of the menopause is made clinically and it is only occasionally necessary to resort to biochemical investigation.

If measurement of FSH is required for diagnostic purposes, a concentration of >30 IU/L indicates menopause. A detectable rise of FSH may be found in the first 7 days of cycles early in the perimenopause.

FSH measurement may sometimes be helpful to diagnose menopausal status if:

1. A premature/early menopause is suspected, i.e. in a woman less than 45 years.
2. A woman has had a hysterectomy.
3. Very occasionally when an older woman wishes to stop using hormonal contraception.

CONSEQUENCES OF THE MENOPAUSE

• Immediate symptoms

These symptoms are common, distressing, and cause many previously healthy women to seek medical advice. They are often insidious in onset and, although very unpleasant, are generally self-limiting and are not life-threatening. Quality of life may be severely compromised in some women with menopausal symptoms and should not be ignored in any discussion on the risks and benefits of HRT.

Vasomotor symptoms

1. Hot flushes.
2. Sweats.

3. Faintness.
4. Palpitations.

Hot flushes and sweats are the commonest menopausal symptoms affecting around 80% of women. They tend to begin before the cessation of menstruation and may cluster in the premenstrual week. They persist on average for 2–5 years and are universally perceived as unpleasant and embarrassing.

Night sweats disrupt normal sleep pattern and can cause chronic sleep deprivation. Subsequent lethargy and irritability are common.

Flushes can be triggered by stress, hot weather, alcohol and spicy food, although most occur without an obvious precipitating factor.

The aetiology and exact physiological mechanism remain unclear. In response to fluctuating declines in estradiol concentrations, the thermoregulatory centre within the hypothalamus triggers cutaneous vasodilatation and sweating with a rise in skin temperature of up to 5°C.

Psychological symptoms

Many women report psychological symptoms as a problem in the climacteric years but there is little evidence to support an association between the menopause and frank psychiatric disease. Minor psychological disturbances are listed in Box 22.1. Chronic sleep disturbance from night sweats exacerbates many of these symptoms.

Personality, cultural factors and attitudes to the menopause undoubtedly affect the incidence of psychological symptoms during the climacteric.

Social stresses can also affect the well-being of a woman around the time of the menopause and may be associated with events such as:

1. Death or illness of an elderly parent.
2. Marital separation or disharmony.

Box 22.1 Psychological symptoms of the menopause

Depressed mood
Mood swings
Irritability
Anxiety
Emotional lability
Lack of confidence
Inability to cope
Loss of libido
Indecision
Poor memory
Poor concentration
Feelings of worthlessness

---

3. Poor job satisfaction.
4. Weight gain and obesity.
5. Difficult teenage children. The 'empty nest syndrome' is frequently quoted in this context but grown-up children who remain in the family home are often more of a problem than those who have 'flown the nest'.

• Medium-term symptoms

Urogenital atrophy

The tissues of the lower urogenital tract are highly estrogen-dependent and undergo atrophy as a result of estrogen deficiency. Older women frequently suffer the symptoms of atrophy in silence through ignorance and embarrassment. These symptoms may first occur several years following the last menstrual period and gradually worsen thereafter.

1. Dryness of the vagina causes dyspareunia, which in turn may result in loss of libido.
2. The vaginal pH increases and the vagina becomes more prone to infection with commensal bacterial organisms, as there is loss of the normal colonization with lactobacilli.
3. Frequency of micturition, urgency and urge incontinence all increase in incidence with advancing age, and arise from atrophic change and loss of collagen support around the bladder neck.

Skin, joint and muscle changes

1. There is a generalized loss of collagen from the dermal layer of skin.
2. Women frequently complain of thin, dry skin accompanied by hair loss and brittle nails.
3. Widespread stiffness with joint and muscle aches are common symptoms and the exact aetiology of these symptoms is unknown.

• Long-term symptoms

Osteoporosis

Osteoporosis is a progressive systemic skeletal disease characterized by low bone mass, micro-architectural deterioration of bone tissue and skeletal fragility. It is a silent condition and its clinical significance lies in the occurrence of fractures. It is estimated that there are at least three million women in the UK suffering from osteoporosis.

Estrogen is a physiological regulator of bone metabolism. Bone density peaks in women in their mid-30s and, thereafter, declines slowly until a rapid acceleration in loss of bone mass occurs following the menopause. Whether

---

Box 22.2 Risk factors for osteoporosis

Premature menopause
Steroid therapy
Small, slim build
Caucasian racial origin
Family history
Immobilization
Inactive lifestyle
Cigarette smoking
Chronic diseases such as diabetes, liver disease, rheumatoid arthritis

---

or not a woman develops osteoporosis is determined by her peak bone mass and her rate of bone loss. Women are naturally endowed with a less dense skeleton than men and their lifetime risk of osteoporotic fractures is more than double that of men.

Postmenopausal osteoporotic fractures classically affect three main sites:

1. Neck of femur.
2. Distal radius – the Colles' fracture.
3. Thoracic vertebrae – wedge compression fractures cause the typical 'dowager's hump'.

Risk factors for osteoporosis (**Box 22.2**) are only, at best, a crude guide to a woman's risk of sustaining osteoporotic fractures. The major risk factor is being a postmenopausal female!

Bone mineral density measurement

Assessment of bone mineral density (BMD) can be performed by highly accurate machines, e.g. dual X-ray absorptiometry (DXA). Measurement of BMD is recommended as a case-finding strategy in individuals with risk factors and to assess response to treatment. Population screening is not thought to be cost-effective.

Preventing and treating osteoporosis

This has been a changing therapeutic area as new agents have been developed recently and the risks and benefits of long-term treatment with HRT have been reassessed.

1. Although HRT is of proven value, it is no longer recommended as a first-line agent for the long-term prevention or treatment of osteoporosis because of its risk–benefit profile.
2. Raloxifene is currently the only selective estrogen receptor modulator (SERM) licensed for the prevention and treatment of

osteoporosis and exerts an estrogen-like effect on bone. It decreases risk of vertebral fractures but has no obvious effect on risk of hip fracture (p. 391).

3. Bisphosphonates, strontium ranelate and parathyroid hormone are potent non-hormonal drug treatments now licensed for the treatment of osteoporosis.

4. Prevention of falls in elderly individuals is clearly important and hip protectors may decrease risk of fracture although their usefulness is limited as elderly individuals tolerate them poorly.

5. Population-based strategies to prevent osteoporosis include reducing the prevalence of smoking and excess alcohol consumption, increasing levels of physical activity and ensuring an adequate dietary intake of calcium and vitamin D. Calcium supplements with vitamin D reduce risk of fracture in very elderly institutionalized women although there is no evidence that supplements are of value in perimenopausal women or in childhood.

Cardiovascular disease

Cardiovascular disease is the single most common cause of death in both men and women in the Western world. Prior to the menopause, deaths in women from cardiovascular disease are uncommon, particularly when compared to men of similar age. There is a marked increase in the incidence of cardiovascular disease in women following the menopause although it is of scientific debate whether or not this is due to loss of ovarian function per se.

Other potential long-term effects

Recent epidemiological data suggest that HRT may offer significant protection against colon cancer. There is no conclusive evidence that it is protective against Alzheimer's disease or other dementias; indeed there is some evidence that the risk of dementia increases with HRT, possibly due to increased risk of microvascular infarcts in the brain.

TREATMENT

As the symptoms and long-term sequelae of the menopause are caused by estrogen deficiency, the logical treatment would be estrogen replacement. Despite this obvious statement, prescribing of HRT in the early 21st century has become a very controversial area of modern medicine. Following the publication of long-awaited randomized trials and large observational studies on HRT, the indications for using HRT for the treatment of menopausal women have changed. Women with severe menopausal symptoms should continue to be offered HRT if their symptoms significantly affect quality of life and they have no contraindications to it. It is now generally accepted

Table 22.1 Estrogen delivery systems and dosages licensed for use in standard systemic HRT regimens

Estrogen	Delivery system	Dosage
Estradiol	Oral	0.5, 1, 2 mg
	Transdermal patch	25, 40, 50, 75, 80, 100 μg
	Gel	0.06%, 0.1%
	Nasal spray	150 μg per spray
	Vaginal ring	50 μg/24 hours
	Implant	25, 50, 100 mg
Conjugated equine estrogens	Oral	0.3, 0.625, 1.25 mg
Estriol	Oral	1 mg
Estropipate	Oral	1.5 mg

that HRT is a second-line treatment for the prevention and treatment of osteoporosis and it is not indicated at all for the long-term prevention of other chronic diseases.

A large selection of HRT preparations is available, in many different combinations and dosages of estrogens plus progestogens. A detailed list is available in the British National Formulary.

• Estrogen therapy

The estrogens used in conventional HRT are described as 'natural' because they give rise to circulating estrogens identical or very similar to those produced by the premenopausal ovary. Their pharmacological effect is achieved with plasma levels of estradiol well within the physiological range. Natural estrogens in the dosages within HRT are less potent than synthetic estrogens contained in combined oral contraception.

Estrogen therapy is effective when administered by a variety of routes (Table 22.1) and generally causes few side effects. Choice of how to take systemic HRT is largely a matter of patient preference, although for the majority of women, the cheaper, oral preparations will be acceptable.

Oral estrogens

Oral estrogen preparations consist primarily of either estradiol formulations or conjugated equine estrogens (CEE). Most of the long-term epidemiological HRT data are based on women who took CEE although some women nowadays have ethical objections to taking a preparation derived from animal sources. CEE preparations are widely used in North America and estradiol preparations are more popular in Europe.

Advantages

1. Cheap.
2. Convenient.
3. Well tolerated.
4. Easy to stop or change.

Disadvantages

1. 'First pass' through the liver – when estrogen is taken orally, it passes through the portal circulation to the liver before reaching the systemic circulation and achieving the desired effect. During this 'first pass' through the liver, at least one-third is immediately metabolized to the weak estrogen, estrone, which is rapidly excreted. A higher dose of oral estrogen has to be given compared to transdermal estrogens to achieve the same therapeutic effect.
2. Occasional nausea and gastrointestinal upset.
3. Having to remember to take a daily pill.

Transdermal estrogens

Transdermal delivery systems allow estrogen to be absorbed directly into the systemic circulation. Patches are designed to be changed once or twice weekly and are placed on smooth, dry skin anywhere below the waist. Estrogen gels are administered once per day in an exact dose and, although widely used on the continent, do not have a large market share in the UK.

Advantages

1. Highly acceptable to women.
2. Convenient to use.
3. Avoid 'first-pass' effect through the liver; therefore, more 'physiological' and can be given in lower dosage. Less effect on hepatic synthesis of other products, e.g. clotting factors and lipoproteins. May be associated with lower risk of venous thrombo-embolism than oral estrogens.
4. Combination patches with progestogen are also available.

Disadvantages

1. More expensive than oral preparations.
2. Allergic reactions occasionally occur with patches but are much less common with the current single-layered matrix patches than with the older reservoir patches.

Subcutaneous estrogen implants

These consist of crystalline pellets of estrogen, which are inserted subcutaneously under local anaesthesia as a minor surgical procedure.

The most common sites of insertion are the anterior abdominal wall or buttock. The usual dose of estrogen implant is 50 mg, which is effective for at least 6 months. Implants are now less widely used because of the increasing popularity of other non-oral routes. They are most likely to be used by younger women who have had a hysterectomy and bilateral oophorectomy.

Advantages

1. Convenience.
2. Compliance is guaranteed.
3. Relatively higher serum estradiol concentrations can be achieved with implants compared to other methods and this can be particularly beneficial in the treatment of severe vasomotor symptoms not relieved by standard dosages of estrogen.
4. Can be given simultaneously with testosterone implants when loss of libido is a particular problem.

Disadvantages

1. Insertion involves a surgical procedure and a very small risk of bruising and infection.
2. Implants may occasionally extrude spontaneously through the skin.
3. Some women experience the return of many of their menopausal symptoms while their circulating concentrations of estradiol are very high (tachyphylaxis). These women have to be 'weaned off' estrogen implants in order to try to reduce their serum estradiol levels and are a very difficult group to manage clinically.

Vaginal estrogens

Vaginal preparations can be given at a dose to achieve either a systemic effect to help menopausal symptoms or an effect only on the local vaginal and bladder neck tissues. Local vaginal treatment is an effective way of improving atrophic change within the lower genital tract and is prescribed as creams, pessaries, tablets or rings. The old highly potent estrogen creams have all been withdrawn from the market in the UK now.

Advantages

1. Can be used by women who do not wish to take systemic HRT or where contraindications exist to its use.
2. Can be used in conjunction with systemic HRT if local symptoms persist despite standard doses of the latter being used.

Disadvantages

1. Elderly women often find difficulty in using vaginal creams and for some women they are unacceptably messy.

2. Most vaginal estrogen preparations are only licensed for use over periods of 3–6 months because of the theoretical risk of endometrial cancer thereafter. Most women will require treatment for significantly longer and the addition of intermittent oral progestogen is recommended for endometrial protection.

Other routes of estrogen administration

Estrogen is also rapidly absorbed by the intranasal and sublingual route and a nasal spray product is available in the UK. An injectable depot estrogen preparation is available in some countries.

• Combined estrogen–progestogen therapy

It is well established that use of estrogen-only replacement substantially increases risk of endometrial cancer in women who still have a uterus. The addition of progestogen to estrogen replacement regimens negates this excess risk of endometrial cancer.

In order to protect the endometrium, progestogen must be given:

1. In adequate dosage.
2. For an adequate number of days each cycle.

The recommended daily dosages of different progestogens to oppose the effects of estrogen are listed in Table 22.2.

Women who have had a hysterectomy (with a few exceptions such as those with severe endometriosis) should not be prescribed HRT regimens containing progestogen. Estrogen-only HRT has fewer side effects and less effect on risk of breast cancer than combined preparations (p. 395). Calendar packs of combined estrogen and progestogen regimens assist the woman to keep to the correct sequence. Separate prescriptions for estrogen and progestogen can also be given if a particular combination is not marketed.

Table 22.2 Progestogens and dosages licensed for use in standard oral combined HRT preparations

Progestogen	Dosage
Norethisterone	0.5, 0.7 or 1 mg
Norgestrel	150 μg
Medroxyprogesterone acetate	1.5, 2.5, 5 or 10 mg
Dydrogesterone	5, 10 or 20 mg
Drospirenone	2 mg

Sequential HRT

In the standard cyclical regimens, progestogens are added sequentially for around 12–14 days each month. A regular withdrawal bleed normally follows at the end of the cycle. A 'long cyclic preparation', with a larger dose of progestogen but only administered every 3 months, is also available and will give four withdrawal bleeds per year.

Continuous combined hormone replacement therapy

Continuous daily administration of both estrogen and progestogen causes endometrial atrophy and amenorrhoea. This regimen is suitable for women who are at least 1 year postmenopausal.

1. Spotting in the early months is very common before complete amenorrhoea is achieved.
2. Women get the same beneficial effects on menopausal symptoms and prevention of osteoporosis as with estrogen only and sequential HRT.
3. When given to pre- or perimenopausal women, erratic bleeding frequently occurs because of endogenous ovarian activity.
4. It is protective against risk of endometrial cancer due to the overall higher total dose of progestogen administered, compared with a sequential regimen.
5. As there is no cyclical effect with this regimen, women appear to tolerate the progestogen better with fewer PMS-type side effects.
6. Long-term adherence with HRT is improved as most women prefer to avoid the return of menstrual bleeding following the menopause.

Tibolone

The synthetic steroid tibolone is a derivative of nortestosterone and has weak estrogenic, progestogenic and androgenic properties. It mimics the effects of a low-dose continuous combined HRT and its use should be restricted to women who are at least 1 year postmenopausal because of risk of unscheduled bleeding. As it has a weak androgen-like effect, it may have a beneficial effect in women with loss of libido and low mood. It appears to have less effect on risk of breast cancer than combined preparations but more effect than estrogen only. It is more expensive than conventional HRT preparations.

• Selective estrogen receptor modulators

Several estrogen-like compounds exist which exhibit differential effects on estrogen receptors in the body by selective agonist and antagonist actions. When first developed, they were hailed as the possible solution to avoiding the undesirable effects of estrogen on tissues like breast and endometrium but still having beneficial effects on symptoms and bone. Unfortunately, to date they have not fulfilled their early promise and development of the perfect selective estrogen-like preparation still remains elusive.

Raloxifene is licensed for the prevention of vertebral osteoporosis. It does not stimulate the endometrium and therefore does not cause problems associated with return of uterine bleeding. Recent data suggest that it reduces risk of breast cancer and has no effect on coronary heart disease risk but increases risk of venous thromboembolism and fatal stroke.[1] In absolute terms the actual gains and losses of taking raloxifene overall are incredibly small.

Tamoxifen is widely prescribed to prevent recurrence of breast cancer and is also protective against osteoporosis in postmenopausal women. In contrast to raloxifene, it causes endometrial stimulation and increases risk of endometrial cancer. Vasomotor symptoms may also be particularly troublesome with tamoxifen.

Both raloxifene and tamoxifen increase risk of venous thromboembolism to a similar extent as estrogen.

• Contraindications to hormone replacement therapy

Absolute

The few absolute contraindications to estrogen therapy are listed in Box 22.3. The summary of product characteristics and patient information leaflets for HRT preparations are updated regularly to reflect new information and advice from the regulatory authorities.

Relative

Among those commonly encountered are:

1. Hypertension – women with controlled hypertension can be prescribed HRT but must be monitored carefully. If a woman is found to be hypertensive, her blood pressure should be controlled before HRT is commenced. Transdermal estrogen is generally preferred to oral therapy in women with risk factors for cardiovascular disease because of the theoretical reduction in risk of thromboembolism.

Box 22.3 Absolute contraindications to HRT

Unexplained vaginal bleeding
Pregnancy
Active or recent diagnosis of breast cancer (see p. 395)
Active thromboembolic disease
Established ischaemic heart disease or stroke
Severe, active liver disease

---

2. Previous episode of deep vein thrombosis or pulmonary embolism – this will require full evaluation and most women should be referred for a thrombophilia screen and specialist advice prior to considering HRT. The majority of women are advised to avoid taking HRT although each woman should be considered individually. In exceptional circumstances HRT can be prescribed in conjunction with low-dose warfarin for women with severe symptoms who are at particularly high risk of further venous thromboembolism, e.g. have an inherited thrombophilia.

3. Fibroids – these may enlarge with HRT and cause bleeding problems. Use of a hormone-releasing intrauterine system can be helpful (Chapter 8) but withdrawal of HRT or even hysterectomy may have to be considered depending on the woman's individual circumstances.

4. Endometriosis – this may be reactivated by estrogen replacement but depends on the amount of residual disease present. Prescribing higher than normal dosages of progestogen or using a hormone-releasing intrauterine system (Chapter 8) may reduce the risk of recurrence.

5. Cancer – HRT has no effect on the majority of cancers.

Endometrial cancer was previously considered an absolute contraindication. Women who have early-stage disease and are disease-free after treatment may take low-dose HRT following specialist advice.

Breast cancer is still considered a complete contraindication for most women. Each woman should, however, be assessed individually and, for some with severe menopausal symptoms, improving quality of life with HRT may outweigh a theoretical risk of reactivation of breast cancer. Small studies have shown conflicting results on risk of recurrence or death when HRT is prescribed for women with pre-existing breast cancer.

Neither previous cervical nor ovarian cancer represents a contraindication. Malignant melanoma is not a contraindication.

• Side effects of hormone replacement therapy

Estrogen causes few side effects. Unfortunately, the addition of progestogen may cause troublesome side effects. These are common and lead to many women discontinuing HRT after only a few months of therapy.

Side effects of estrogen

1. Nausea.
2. Breast tenderness and bloatedness.
3. Leg cramps.
4. Headaches.

Management

1. Reduce dose of estrogen.
2. Change route of administration.

Side effects of progestogen

1. Sequential regimens induce a regular monthly withdrawal bleed which may be heavy, prolonged or painful.
2. Premenstrual syndrome-type symptoms of irritability, depression, breast pain, fluid retention and bloating.

Management

1. Reduce dose and duration of progestogen to minimum recommended for endometrial protection. Long cyclic HRT may be helpful.
2. Change progestogen to C-21 progestogen derivatives (dydrogesterone or medroxyprogesterone acetate) which are less androgenic and often tolerated better than a nortestosterone derivative (norethisterone or norgestrel).
3. Change from oral progestogen to a transdermal progestogen or a progestogen-releasing intrauterine system.
4. Stopping progestogen completely is not recommended, but some women opt to do this. Regular endometrial biopsies and transvaginal scans are mandatory. The increased risk of endometrial cancer persists for many years after estrogen treatment has been stopped and informed consent from the woman should be documented.
5. Use of the continuous–combined regimen or tibolone may be better than a sequential regimen.
6. Hysterectomy. This then allows the woman to be prescribed estrogen-only therapy.

PREMATURE MENOPAUSE

Premature menopause is generally defined as ovarian failure before the age of 40 years; ovarian failure between the ages of 40–45 years is often described as early menopause. The causes of premature menopause are listed in Table 22.3; often the cause is unexplained.

Women are often devastated to be told they are prematurely menopausal and require very sensitive counselling and management. They particularly grieve the loss of fertility if they had not started or completed their family. Pregnancies can occasionally occur in some women with premature menopause; fertility rates are very low but not zero. Assisted conception

Table 22.3 Causes of premature menopause

Cause	Specific details
Unknown	May be family history of premature menopause
Auto-immune disorders	Thyroid disease is the commonest but Addison's disease, diabetes, rheumatoid arthritis are also associated with an increased risk
Surgery	Bilateral oophorectomy Hysterectomy can sometimes be associated with ovarian failure despite conservation of the ovaries
Infection	Mumps, varicella, malaria or tuberculosis can in rare situations cause premature menopause
Chemotherapy and radiotherapy	Women undergoing cancer treatment
Abnormalities of the X chromosome	Fragile X carriers, Turner syndrome (may be mosaics)
Metabolic conditions	Galactosaemia

with egg donation has now made future pregnancy a real possibility for many women with premature ovarian failure.

Most women with premature menopause opt to take HRT for symptom relief but also, importantly, to maintain bone health until the age of normal menopause. It is widely accepted that using HRT in women with premature menopause is extremely safe and, in particular, is not associated with an increased risk of breast cancer when compared to women who continue menstruation until the age of normal menopause. Combined hormonal contraception can be used as an alternative to HRT and allows young women to feel a degree of normality about their hormonal status. It offers the same relief of menopausal symptoms and bone protection as HRT.

SPECIAL CONSIDERATIONS WITH HRT

• Breast cancer

The relationship between breast cancer and HRT is complex and the magnitude of the effect of HRT on risk of breast cancer varies considerably between studies. Although the overall effect of HRT on breast cancer risk has important public health implications, the absolute risk is probably of less concern to individual women who are using HRT.

A large re-analysis of 90% of the epidemiological data on the effect of HRT on breast cancer risk which included more than 50000 women with breast cancer was undertaken.[2] Their major findings were that:

- Amongst current users of HRT, there was a small increase in the risk of breast cancer which rose with increasing duration of usage

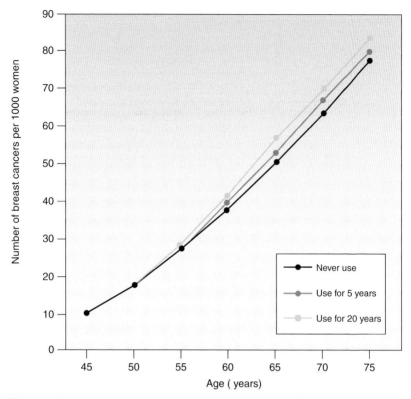

Figure 22.1 Estimated cumulative number of breast cancers diagnosed in 1000 never-users of HRT, 1000 users of HRT for 5 years, and 1000 users of HRT for 10 years (with assumption that HRT use began at age 50 years). (Reproduced from Collaborative Group on Hormonal Factors in Breast Cancer 1997 Breast cancer and hormone replacement therapy: collaborative reanalysis of data from 51 studies of 52 705 women with breast cancer and 108 411 women without breast cancer. Lancet 350: 1047–1059, with permission from Elsevier.)

(Figure 22.1). In women who had used HRT for 5 years or longer (average duration of use 11 years), the relative risk was 1.35 (95% CI 1.21–1.49) compared with never-users.

- Five years after stopping HRT, the excess risk of breast cancer was lost.

Recent data have largely confirmed the same trends. The Women's Health Initiative (WHI) trial failed to demonstrate any increased risk of breast cancer in women using estrogen-only HRT compared to placebo after 6.8 years of follow-up.[3] But in the combined estrogen and progestogen arm of the

Table 22.4 Summary of main data from Women's Health Initiative (WHI) Trial and Million Women Study

Clinical event	WHI estrogen + progestogen	WHI estrogen alone	Million Women Study estrogen + progestogen	Million Women Study estrogen alone
	Hazard ratio (95% CI)	Hazard ratio (95% CI)	Relative risk (95% CI)	Relative risk (95% CI)
Breast cancer	1.26 (1.00–1.59)	0.77 (0.59–1.01)	2.0 (1.88–2.12)	1.3 (1.21–1.4)
Coronary heart disease events	1.29 (1.02–1.63)	0.91 (0.75–1.12)	–	–
Stroke	1.41 (1.07–1.85)	1.39 (1.10–1.77)	–	–
Pulmonary embolism	2.13 (1.39–3.25)	1.34 (0.87–2.06)	–	–
Colon cancer	0.63 (0.43–0.92)	1.08 (0.75–1.55)	–	–
Hip fracture	0.66 (0.45–0.98)	0.61 (0.41–0.91)	–	–
Death	0.98 (0.82–1.18)	1.04 (0.88–1.22)	–	–
Global index	1.15 (1.03–1.28)	1.01 (0.91–1.12)	–	–

study after 5.6 years of follow-up, risk of breast cancer was significantly increased by 24% (Table 22.4).[4] This correlates to eight extra cases of breast cancer per 10 000 woman-years in the treatment group compared to placebo. The UK Million Women Study found an even greater increase in current users of combined HRT preparations and to a lesser extent with estrogen-only preparations (Table 22.4).[5]

In summary, the relevant points on risk of breast cancer associated with HRT are:

1. Combined HRT is associated with a small but signicant increase in risk of breast cancer, comparable to the range of risk conferred by late natural menopause or moderate alcohol consumption.
2. Estrogen-only HRT has less, if any, increased risk of breast cancer compared to combined HRT.
3. Risk of breast cancer relates to duration of HRT use and appears to be independent of dose.
4. Women should be routinely counselled about the effect of HRT on risk of breast cancer but in a balanced and sensitive way.

• Venous thromboembolism

Although it was originally thought that the natural estrogens contained within HRT did not increase risk of venous thromboembolism (VTE), epidemiological studies have now confirmed that there is a two- to four-fold increase in risk of VTE in women taking HRT. In the Women's Health Initiative (WHI) randomized trial, the combined estrogen and progestogen regimen doubled risk of VTE; the absolute risk equates to about two extra cases per 1000 women per year (Table 22.4). There is no indication to stop HRT routinely prior to surgery provided appropriate thromboprophylaxis, such as heparin, is used.[6]

• Arterial disease

Many observational studies have suggested that use of HRT following the menopause exerted a significant protective effect against cardiovascular disease. Estrogen was thought to induce this beneficial effect by both favourable effects on lipid profile and a direct effect on the vascular system. Recent data from randomized trials have not confirmed that HRT has a significant beneficial effect for either the primary or secondary prevention of cardiovascular disease. It should not now be recommended for these indications. Whilst it is possible that the effects of HRT on the cardiovascular system vary depending on dose and type of hormone used or the delivery system, there is still inadequate evidence to justify recommending any HRT regimen for cardiovascular protection.

Coronary artery disease

The WHI study showed little effect of estrogen-only therapy on risk of coronary events but the combined estrogen and progestogen arm of the study suggested a significant increase in risk after 5.6 years of follow-up (Table 22.4). This latter finding may well be related to the fact that the WHI study included relatively older women who may already have a degree of established atherosclerosis. In a meta-analysis of 30 trials, HRT seemed to reduce mortality from coronary artery disease in women aged under 60 years but there are so few coronary artery deaths in this younger age group that this finding is unlikely to have a significant impact on overall prevention of coronary artery prevention.[7]

In respect of HRT and women with established coronary artery disease, the best evidence comes from the HERS study which showed an overall 'null effect' after 4 years of HRT use in women with established ischaemic heart disease.[8]

Stroke

The recent trials on risk of stroke with HRT have all consistently shown slightly increased risk. The WHI trial showed a 41% increase in risk with combined HRT compared with placebo which equates to an absolute excess risk of eight more strokes per 10000 women. The estrogen-only arm of the trial showed a similar magnitude of increased risk of stroke (Table 22.4).

CLINICAL MANAGEMENT

• Assessment of a woman prior to hormone replacement therapy

Use of menopause clinic proforma sheets can be helpful and a trained menopause counselling nurse can be an invaluable resource in spending time discussing the pros and cons of HRT with each individual woman.

History

1. Current symptoms attributable to the menopause; a self-administered symptom-rating questionnaire can be used.
2. Menstrual and gynaecological history.
3. Past medical history, noting any contraindication to HRT use, and any current drug therapy.
4. Family history, particularly breast cancer, ischaemic heart disease and stroke at a young age, and osteoporosis.
5. Social history: employment, smoking, current relationship and any sexual problems.
6. Check if women are in date with both cervical and breast screening if appropriate; this is an opportunity to reinforce the health promotion importance of these procedures.

Examination

1. BP.
2. Weight may be helpful.
3. Teach breast awareness and self-examination.
4. Routine breast and pelvic examinations are not mandatory, but should always be performed if there are any symptoms or significant past medical history. It must be remembered that women seeking HRT are generally in the age range for increasing risk of breast and ovarian cancer.

Investigations

In practice, investigations are usually not necessary but may be indicated by the history or examination.

If a woman has significant menstrual problems, a full blood count and thyroid function should be checked and a gynaecological examination should be undertaken. She may also require a pelvic ultrasound scan, endometrial biopsy or hysteroscopy prior to prescribing HRT.

• Monitoring

There is no absolute agreement as to how often women should be followed-up or what exactly should be monitored. By convention, however, the first follow-up visit is usually after 3 months and, thereafter, review can be 6-monthly or more frequently if problems arise.

History

1. Assess degree of symptom relief; estrogen dose can be altered if necessary.
2. Note bleeding pattern.
3. Assess any side effects.

Examination

1. BP.
2. Weight. Weight gain is a major issue with almost all women regardless of age and is frequently attributed to HRT use. It is a feature of increasing age and studies show that women who take HRT actually put on the same or less weight overall than the non-users. Advice and support on dieting and exercise should always be offered.
3. Confirm that women are 'breast aware'. Routine breast examination by a health professional is not recommended and may be falsely reassuring. Over 90% of breast cancers are detected by women themselves.
4. Routine 3-yearly cervical smear and mammogram if within the age limits for screening. Breast and pelvic examination should always be performed in the presence of any abnormal symptoms but are not mandatory at follow-up visits.

• Adherence to therapy

Less than 60% of women who start HRT are still taking it after 1 year. Fear of breast cancer tends to discourage women from starting treatment and the withdrawal bleeds and cyclical progestogenic side effects often cause women to stop treatment after only a brief trial. Tolerance of 'no period' preparations is generally better than of those that cause withdrawal bleeding. Women also need to be given realistic expectations of what HRT will and will not help. Many women are disappointed when they take HRT and find that it is not the 'elixir of life'. Women taking HRT need good back-up support from health professionals and may have to try several different preparations before they find one that suits them.

• Duration of use

There is no rule as to how long HRT can be continued. The general advice is that the lowest dose should be used for the shortest period of time necessary. For relief of acute menopausal symptoms in the perimenopause, most women will take HRT for around 3–5 years. The decision when to stop is an individual one and many women discontinue HRT without recourse to medical advice while others are extremely reluctant ever to stop. Some women experience menopausal symptoms until well into old age.

Menopausal symptoms will often recur when HRT is stopped and it can be helpful to try to wind down the dosage gradually over many months rather than stop abruptly.

• HRT and contraception

Conventional HRT is not a method of contraception and if HRT is prescribed to a woman who is still menstruating, contraception should be recommended as well.

Barrier methods, an intrauterine device (IUD) and the progestogen-only pill (POP) can all be used in conjunction with conventional HRT. A hormone-releasing intrauterine system can administer the progestogen component of HRT (see Chapter 8).

For simplicity, the POP should be added to a sequential HRT preparation as a separate prescription. It appears to be effective and is quite widely prescribed with HRT although no scientific data exist on the efficacy of this combination. The continuous combined 'no period' HRT formulations give a daily administration of progestogen which is contraceptive although women taking these preparations are almost certainly postmenopausal anyway.

Once HRT has been started, it becomes impossible to give an accurate indication of when contraception can safely be discontinued. Two possible strategies exist:

1. For most women, contraception can arbitrarily be continued until the age of 55 years which is assumed to be the upper limit of fertility. For example, an IUD which is not causing any problems can remain in situ until this time.

2. HRT can be stopped briefly for around 6 weeks. If the woman is amenorrhoeic and has vasomotor symptoms, an FSH concentration can be measured. If this is raised, then contraception can be discontinued after 1 further year (or 2 further years if she is under the age of 50). If there is spontaneous menstruation or a low FSH concentration, then contraception should be continued and the exercise repeated 1 year later.

• Alternatives to HRT

Treatment of menopausal symptoms with agents other than estrogen frequently give largely disappointing results. Most studies on alternative therapies for menopausal symptoms demonstrate a marked placebo response or they fail to include a placebo group which makes their results hard to assess. There are few data relating to either efficacy or safety. Occasional reports of serious side effects particularly relating to liver toxicity have been reported with several herbal preparations. Whilst healthcare professionals are often sceptical about the use of herbal preparations for menopausal symptoms, women expect them to be knowledgeable about the different preparations and the value of the placebo response should not be underestimated.

1. **Anti-depressants**. Small, short studies have shown a beneficial effect of several anti-depressant therapies on vasomotor symptoms compared to placebo. Most data relate to venlafaxine but fluoxetine may also be helpful in this respect. Many women experience side effects with anti-depressant therapy and dislike the idea of taking these drugs. These agents undoubtedly improve mood and this may well be a significant benefit for symptomatic women who are struggling with their menopausal symptoms.

2. **Progestogens**. Progestogen-only therapy has been shown to have a mild to moderate beneficial effect on hot flushes but side effects are frequently troublesome. Norethisterone 5–15 mg daily and megestrol acetate 20 mg twice per day can reduce vasomotor symptoms. There are no data relating to risk of breast cancer with these agents but the general assumption is that they are safer than estrogen-only and combined preparations.

3. **Clonidine**. This anti-hypertensive agent (50 mg twice daily) is mildly effective in the short-term management of vasomotor symptoms but most women find that the beneficial effect wears off rapidly.

4. **Herbal preparations**. An enormous range of over-the-counter preparations is available. Any real benefit of these agents probably reflects a placebo response. Black Cohosh (derived from the roots of the plant *Cimicifuga racemosa*) is the most popular herbal preparation for menopausal symptoms but the data on efficacy are very mixed. Phytoestrogens are naturally occurring plant estrogens that are found within particular foodstuffs or can be taken as supplements. As these agents exert a weak estrogen-like effect, it is not possible to reassure women with conditions such as breast cancer that they are significantly safer than conventional HRT.

5. **Other complementary therapies**. Some women find relaxation techniques, specific exercise regimens or aromatherapy beneficial. Self-help groups or nurse-counselling sessions may assist women to cope better with their symptoms.

REFERENCES

1. Barrett-Connor E, Mosca L, Collins P et al. (2006) Raloxifene Use for The Heart (RUTH) Trial Investigators. Effects of raloxifene on cardiovascular events and breast cancer in postmenopausal women. NEJM 355: 125–137.

2. Collaborative Group on Hormonal Factors in Breast Cancer (1997) Breast cancer and hormone replacement therapy: collaborative reanalysis of data from 51 studies of 52705 women with breast cancer and 108411 women without breast cancer. Lancet 350: 1047–1059.

3. Writing Group for the Women's Health Initiative Investigators (2004) Effect of conjugated equine oestrogen in postmenopausal women with hysterectomy. JAMA 291: 1701–1712.

4. Writing Group for the Women's Health Initiative Investigators (2002) Risks and benefits of estrogen plus progestogen in healthy postmenopausal women: principal results from the Women's Health Initiative randomized controlled trial. JAMA 288: 321–333.

5. Million Women Study Collaborators (2003) Breast Cancer and hormone replacement in the Million Women Study. Lancet 362: 419–427.

6. Royal College of Obstetricians and Gynaecologists (RCOG) (2004) Hormone replacement therapy and venous thromboembolism. Guideline No. 19. RCOG: London.

7. Salpeter SR, Walsh JME, Greyber E et al. (2004) Mortality associated with hormone replacement therapy in younger and older women. J Gen Int Med 19: 791–803.

8. Hulley SB, Grady D, Bush T et al. for the HERS Research Group (1998) Randomized trial of estrogen plus progestin for secondary prevention of coronary heart disease in postmenopausal women. Journal of the American Medical Association 230: 605–613.

Michael J K Harper

It is evident from a study of reviews on contraceptive development that many of the purported new methods are, in fact, not new but rather represent incremental changes in formulation, composition or delivery of existing hormones, like those used in oral contraceptives. This is also true for hormonal male contraception. This is not to say that such improvements are inconsequential, since newer combinations may be more convenient, have reduced side effects or other health benefits, and thus be more acceptable. New barrier methods are also mainly modifications of existing devices. In contrast, radically new methods of contraception are still far back in the translational process from laboratory to clinical practice. Enthusiasm by industry for investment in these potential new methods, with a few exceptions, is tempered by the cost of many years of preclinical and then clinical studies, with no certainty of a successful outcome. Indeed the regulatory hurdles that must be overcome are higher for a contraceptive than for many other drug categories, since contraceptives are used by healthy people over potentially many years, unlike drugs for therapeutic indications where there is already an underlying pathology.

Although it is tempting to forecast the development of new contraceptives, past experience has often shown that interest generated by new leads or new technology is overly optimistic about both the chances of success and the time to introduction.

During the last 20 years of the 20th century a number of experts independently predicted that by the year 2000 there would be safer oral contraceptives; improved drug releasing IUDs; improved barrier contraceptives for women; improved long-acting and monthly steroid injections; and steroid implants and vaginal rings. Although a little later than 2000, products in all these categories are now available (Table 23.1).

In contrast, other potentially promising new methods did not reach fruition. These included gonadotrophin-releasing hormone (GnRH) analogues for contraception and induction of menses; prostaglandin analogues for menses induction; immuno-contraceptives; hormonal and non-hormonal methods for men, and simplified methods of sterilization. Apart from work on hormonal male contraception, little is now being done in these other areas. One discovery that post-dated these original possibilities was a progesterone-receptor blocker, mifepristone (see below).

A recent issue of *Population Reports* considers the availability of contraceptive methods, and stresses that family planners and users need more new methods that are highly effective, have less side effects, are inexpensive and are easier to use.[1]

POTENTIAL NEW METHODS FOR WOMEN

• Methods which inhibit implantation

Implantation is fundamental to reproductive success. In recent years the World Health Organization (WHO) and the Rockefeller Foundation jointly funded a basic research programme aiming to identify key factors in the implantation process which might be susceptible to disruption and provide a contraceptive opportunity. Although much knowledge was gained, only a few targets were identified. Other investigators have used knock-out mice to validate targets. Certain target molecules are under development that might provide the basis for new methods which interfere with implantation. These include molecules important in implantation, for example leukaemia inhibitory factor, interleukin-11, proprotein convertase 6 and leptin. Inhibitors of some of these might provide the next generation of female contraceptives, but for now none of these methods is likely to be available in the foreseeable future.

There are, however, other more advanced developments which hold promise.

• Combined oral contraception

It is 50 years since Pincus and his collaborators published the results of the first human studies using 19-norsteroid-based compounds, which became the initial ingredients in the first oral contraceptive pill. This area has continued to attract attention with new formulations and new combinations of steroids exhibiting different spectra of activity and with the theoretical potential to reduce side effects, e.g. more progestogenic (chlormadinone

Table 23.1 Contraceptive products by category introduced in the last 15 years

Oral contraceptives	Numerous – only recent introductions noted	Yasmin®	Drospirenone and EE
		Seasonale®	LNG and EE continuous for 84 days
		Seasonique™	LNG + EE for 84 days followed by EE alone for 6 days
IUDs	Two main types	ParaGard®	Copper T380A
		Mirena®	LNG releasing
Barrier contraceptives	For women and men: many latex-based male condoms and latex diaphragms available – only newer developments noted	Lea's shield®	Cervical cap
		FemCap™	Cervical cap
		FC1	Female condom
		Tactylon™	Non-latex male condom
		Trojan®	Non-latex male condom
Long-acting and monthly steroid injections	Monthly (women)	Cyclofem®	DMPA and E cypionate
		Mesigyna®	NET-EN and E valerate
		Deladroxate™	DPA and E EN
	Long-acting (men)	Nebido®	TU bi-monthly
Steroid implants	3 year life – single rod	Implanon™	Etonorgestrel
	5 year life – two rods	Jadelle®	LNG
Steroid vaginal rings	Insert once a month for 3 weeks	NuvaRing®	Etonorgestrel and EE
Transdermal patch	Apply a patch weekly for 3 weeks per month	Ortho EVRA®	Norelgestromin and EE

DMPA, depot medroxyprogesterone acetate;
DPA, dihydroxy-progesterone acetophenide;
E, estradiol;
EE, ethinylestradiol;
EN, enanthate;
LNG, levonorgestrel;
NET, norethisterone;
TU, testosterone undecanoate.

acetate), more androgenic (levonorgestrel and its esters), anti-androgenic (nomegestrel acetate), or anti-mineralocorticoid and anti-androgenic (drospirenone).

Among the various oral contraceptive combinations, it could be argued that each woman should be able to find one that suits her best. However, as each succeeding generation of combinations reduces levels of administered hormones to increase safety and decrease side effects, the possibility of pregnancy occurring due to missed pills increases, and patient compliance becomes more important. On the same theme, a new formulation of an oral contraceptive pill which is mint-flavoured and chewable is designed to increase patient compliance.

Nomegestrel acetate

There have been recent preliminary trials with a new oral contraceptive combination containing nomegestrel acetate and estradiol taken for 24 days, followed by a 4-day pill-free interval. This regimen gave adequate cycle control and would be the first oral contraceptive that uses the natural hormone estradiol instead of the synthetic analogue ethinylestradiol (EE) – the selling point being that a 'natural estrogen' is better.

• Emergency contraception

It has been known for many years from animal experiments that inhibition of follicular rupture can be achieved by inhibition of prostaglandin synthetase. This enzyme complex is comprised of cyclo-oxygenase-1 and -2 (cox-1 and cox-2). Non-specific inhibition of both cox-1 and -2 by indometacin increases the incidence of unruptured follicles in women. Selective inhibition of cox-2 by rofecoxib (Vioxx®) appears to achieve the same result.

Meloxicam

Meloxicam, another cox-2 inhibitor, can also delay rupture of the dominant follicle.[2] A non-steroidal anti-inflammatory drug (NSAID), meloxicam, is available in a generic version in many countries and is cheap. It does not seem to be associated with the cardiac problems seen with newer cox-2 inhibitors (rofecoxib and celecoxib). Daily administration for 5 days, or as a single dose in combination with LNG 1.5 mg, both started in the presence of a pre-ovulatory follicle, significantly delays follicular rupture. The significant advantage of meloxicam which acts to prevent follicular rupture but permits luteinization and normal progesterone secretion, is that it ensures normal cyclicity.

Once an effective and safe dose of meloxicam has been identified, an efficacy study in women coming for emergency contraception should be done.

There is also interest in using meloxicam for regular contraception, but it is difficult to envisage how the woman would know when to start it and for how long to take it. It should be noted that since meloxicam is already an approved drug, off-label use is possible, and it may not be necessary to wait for the results of the efficacy study to use the combination of LNG and meloxicam.

• Injectables

Long-acting hormonal contraceptives are highly effective, reduce the need for compliance, and avoid the first pass through the liver. There are only two progestogen-only injectables widely available in the market, depot medroxyprogesterone acetate (DMPA) and NET-EN (see Chapter 5).

Levonorgestrel butanoate

In the early 1980s there was a great demand in developing countries for improved long-acting injectable steroid contraceptives. Pharmaceutical companies had little interest in developing new injectable agents, and so WHO supported a chemical synthesis programme which identified a new levonorgestrel (LNG) ester, levonorgestrel butanoate, with desirable characteristics. This new ester has been under development for many years and work is underway to bring it to clinical evaluation. It is anticipated that it will have a 3-month period of efficacy, will not affect bone density and will not exhibit a large initial spike of LNG. It is hoped that bleeding disturbances will be less than with DMPA.

Realistically, it will be at least 5 years before levonorgestrel butanoate can reach the market. As it is anticipated that each injection will last 3 months, it could also be used as the progestogen in the hormonal combination used for male contraception.

• Progesterone receptor modulators (PRM)

Mifepristone

The first progesterone receptor antagonist to reach clinical application was mifepristone. It is highly effective in inducing abortion when combined with a prostaglandin analogue (misoprostol). Owing to the strong feelings engendered by abortion, other potentially valuable uses of mifepristone have not been pursued.

WHO conducted a large-scale trial of mifepristone 10 mg for emergency contraception.[3] Mifepristone was as effective as levonorgestrel, preventing a high proportion of pregnancies if taken within 5 days of unprotected intercourse. Mifepristone is known to have an effect on the endometrium and part of its action may be due to this. It can also delay ovulation, prolong the cycle, delay menses and expose women to the risk of pregnancy if further acts of unprotected intercourse take place in the same cycle. In contrast, it is thought that LNG acts to inhibit, rather than delay, ovulation, thus reducing the risk of pregnancy later in the same cycle. Both compounds, however, often result in delayed menses.

Mifepristone has also been tested as a daily, weekly and monthly contraceptive. Daily doses of 2 or 5 mg inhibit ovulation and menstruation in 90% of cycles while maintaining follicular development and normal estradiol levels.[4] In 200 months of exposure in 59 women no pregnancies occurred. The antiproliferative action of mifepristone diminished the risk of atypical endometrial hyperplasia which might be caused by unopposed estrogen (if ovulation is inhibited). Mifepristone appears a very viable novel method of contraception.

Higher doses given weekly (25 or 50 mg orally) also appear to provide effective contraception with a tendency for decreased bleeding and amenorrhoea in the 50-mg dose group. A once-a-month pill using mifepristone taken just before ovulation is effective in preventing pregnancy but the timing of administration is tricky. Moreover, the resulting disruption of cycle length makes administration in the next cycle even more difficult to time, rendering this method impractical.

Clearly, either daily or weekly dosing regimens of mifepristone have promise as non-estrogenic contraceptives. The problem is that the toxicology testing done in licensing mifepristone as a medical abortifacient is insufficient for the long-term use required for contraception. Given the association with abortion and the emotive feelings aroused, funding to conduct the required toxicology has not been forthcoming.

Other progesterone receptor modulators

A number of other progesterone receptor modulators have been studied. CDB-2914 has a somewhat similar mode of action to mifepristone and single mid-luteal doses of 200 mg or more caused luteolysis and shortened cycles without apparent toxicity. The clinical role of this compound has yet to be determined.

Despite their promise for contraception and treating gynaecological conditions, it seems likely that at a high enough dose all the PRM will be capable of inducing abortion with the attendant bad public image, and therefore not of interest to industry.

• Spermicides

Nonoxynol-9

Nonoxynol-9 is the most widely used spermicide. Surprisingly, it was never subjected to modern standards of toxicology testing, but was approved by the FDA by monograph in 1978. N-9 causes significant inflammation of the vagina when tested in rabbits (the standard test for vaginal compounds). This pro-inflammatory potential may be why over-frequent use of COL-1492, a low-dose N-9 vaginal gel, resulted in an increase in HIV infection in female sex workers instead of the desired reduction.[5] These results, although probably not clinically relevant to monogamous couples in parts of the world where the risk of HIV is low, spurred the research community to develop alternative vaginal gels that would prevent pregnancy. If they were also effective in preventing transmission of HIV or other sexually transmitted diseases, this dual protection would be an added advantage. Two such preparations have reached the stage of clinical trials for prevention of pregnancy.

SAVVY (C31G)

SAVVY (C31G) is an antimicrobial and spermicidal agent that contains two surface-active agents, cetyl betaine and myristamine oxide. One study compared three concentrations of SAVVY against a 3% N-9 marketed spermicidal gel.[6] The percentage of women experiencing genital irritation was lower for the 0.5 and 1% SAVVY than for the 1.7% or the N-9 preparation. SAVVY was not detected in plasma of any volunteers. In men, both circumcised and uncircumcised, SAVVY appeared to be as safe on penile exposure as Extra Strength N-9. Post-coital tests have confirmed the spermicidal effect of SAVVY. Efficacy studies are ongoing.

Cellulose sulfate

The gel cellulose sulfate (CS) (Ushercell™) is being developed for prevention of HIV and other sexually transmitted infections. In preclinical studies CS 6% vaginal gel was effective in preventing fertilization in rabbits.[7] Unlike SAVVY and N-9 which immobilize sperm, CS acts by some other mechanism. It has been shown to inhibit hyaluronidase, induce acrosomal loss and inhibit cervical mucus penetration. So strictly speaking CS is not a spermicide since it does not kill sperm, but only disables their ability to fertilize an oocyte. In vitro, CS inhibits HIV, herpes viruses, gonococci and chlamydia, but does not inhibit beneficial lactobacilli. Two HIV-prevention trials using CS, were underway. However, initial data found that not only did CS not protect women, it seemed to increase seroconversions compared to placebo gel. Consequently, both HIV-prevention trials were stopped. At this time there is no explanation for these unexpected findings. Although CS appears to be more effective than N-9 in preventing pregnancy and appears to be non-irritating and well liked by couples in whom it has been tested, it is now very unlikely that the required studies to get an approved label for contraception will be done.

• Female barrier methods

Various latex diaphragms have been available for many years, but they come in different sizes and this necessitates a gynaecological examination to select the correct size. Used with a spermicide, diaphragms provide reasonable contraception. However, there is great interest in developing a new diaphragm in which one size fits most women.

SILCS diaphragm

The so-called SILCS (SILCS, Inc.) diaphragm is being developed by PATH (Program for Appropriate Technology in Health). The novel approach taken in the development process was to conduct a needs assessment by users and clinicians. Each variation was tested by users and their feedback was used for the next modification. As a result the present device fits most women, who would otherwise need a conventional diaphragm of 65–85 mm. SILCS is non-latex and has a polymer spring. It can be fitted by the woman without help from a health professional and is more comfortable than currently available diaphragms. Various acceptability studies have been conducted in several countries. A recent US study compared the effectiveness of the SILCS diaphragm used with either 2% N-9 or lubricant gel in a post-coital test. It was concluded that the SILCS worked well and is suitable for contraceptive testing.[8] A multicentre study will commence in the US in 2007 and FDA approval is expected in 2009.

• Female sterilization

Quinacrine

The intrauterine placement of quinacrine tablets or suspension was suggested many years ago as a way to induce sclerosis of the fallopian tubes with consequent sterilization. Follow-up studies of women who were sterilized with quinacrine show no evidence of an increased incidence of reproductive cancers but there were still concerns regarding the potential safety of quinacrine.[9] The toxicological studies that had been done were not sufficient for present-day regulatory approval. Recent toxicology studies have demonstrated increased cancer risk in rats. Given these findings and the fact that pregnancy rates 5 years after treatment are as high as 12.6/100 women, work on this approach to female sterilization has ceased and it is unlikely to be resurrected.

Essure

A more sophisticated approach to non-surgical sterilization involves placement of spring-like devices, called Essure, in the fallopian tubes using hysteroscopy. During a 3-year period after its placement, scar tissue develops and permanently blocks the tubes so that sperm cannot pass.[10] The microcoil can usually be placed in 95% of women, and is almost 100% effective. This device is available in many countries but because it requires hysteroscopy will not be suitable for resource-poor countries (Chapter 12).

• Female condoms

A non-latex female condom, Reality® or FC1, has been available for several years, but has aesthetic drawbacks and is expensive. A newer latex version (FC2) has been made and tested against the FC1 in a trial in South Africa.[11] Breakage was similar for both condoms (0.7 and 0.9% for FC1 and FC2, respectively). Outer ring displacement was similar at about 3% and slippage was negligible. The biggest complaint was discomfort during insertion and this was similar for both condoms. The acceptability of both condoms appears comparable. The newer version may be available in 2007/08.

A second new female condom is the Reddy condom developed by Medtech, Inc. It is a one-size device made of latex and uses a soft polyurethane sponge to aid insertion and a firm, flexible outer ring intended to hold it in place during intercourse. A comparative trial of the Reddy version 4 and the FC1 has been conducted in India.[12] The Reddy female condom had significantly higher acceptability. It is marketed as V Amour in

Africa and as L'amour in South America. It is also approved for distribution in Brazil, Europe and India.

The third female condom is being developed by PATH. A small short-term acceptability study done in Mexico, South Africa and Thailand demonstrated that this condom is easy to use and acceptable to the users.[13] As with the development of the SILCS diaphragm, the development process is an iterative one, with feedback from users dictating modifications for the next version. It is likely that one or more of these female condoms will be available in the near future.

POTENTIAL NEW METHODS FOR MEN

Male contraception has always depended on three methods, withdrawal, condoms or sterilization. For men who have completed their desired family size, sterilization, although permanent, has been widely accepted. Its almost complete irreversibility, except by use of in vitro fertilization techniques, has restricted its appeal to older men. For many years, advocates for women's reproductive health have called for other reversible methods for men so that they could share the burden of family planning. Surveys show that both men and women are in favour of such alternatives. However, the physiology of the male reproductive system has been more difficult to alter than has been the case for the female. Nevertheless, research carried out over many years indicates that a hormonal method may be feasible and available in the medium term and that there are prospects for other non-hormonal methods in the longer term.

• Hormonal methods

Testosterone

In 1990, the World Health Organization Task Force on methods for the regulation of male fertility reported a study in which healthy men received 200 mg testosterone enanthate (T-EN) weekly for contraception.[14] Sixty-five percent of the men had azoospermia by 6 months of starting treatment. There was one pregnancy in 1486 months of use during the efficacy phase of the study. Median time from the cessation of treatment to recovery to >20 million sperm/ml was 3.7 months. One of the major reasons for discontinuation was the injection schedule.

A second study by the same group[15] then examined whether complete azoospermia was necessary for effective contraception. In this study, there were four pregnancies in 49.5 person-years among men who were oligospermic (up to 3 million sperm/ml), and none in 230.4 person-years for azoospermic men. Again, dislike of the injection schedule resulted in 5% of men discontinuing. The regimen had significant effects on skin, muscle, liver, lipid metabolism, and haemopoietic function, with variations between Chinese and non-Chinese men. These changes were felt to reflect the high peak levels and fluctuations of testosterone (T) induced by weekly injections. To develop a practical hormonal method it was concluded that a more stable level of T supplementation was necessary. However, this study conclusively proved that exogenous T supplementation can provide effective contraception in men.

Testosterone combined with progestogens

Many small studies have been done with various combinations of testosterone and progestogens or GnRH analogues using sperm numbers as a surrogate for contraceptive efficacy. One of the problems has been the development of a formulation of testosterone that would require injections no more frequently than every 2 months. This was solved when a formulation of testosterone undecanoate (TU) in oil was developed. A small study showed that 1000 mg of TU plus 200 mg NET-EN at 8-weekly intervals effectively suppressed spermatogenesis.[16] This regimen was found to be acceptable; 66% of 50 men saying at the end of the trial that they would use such a method. An efficacy trial using this regimen in 400 men in nine sites in eight countries starts in 2007, and is scheduled for completion in 2010. One disadvantage of the present regimen is that two separate injections are needed. However, if the trial is successful a single formulation containing both hormones can be made reducing the regimen to one injection every 8 weeks.

An industry-sponsored study using a combination of Implanon® (a 1-year progestogen implant) and TU injected at 3-month intervals was recently completed. This particular combination is not going to be pursued, not because of lack of efficacy, but for reasons of acceptability. A survey of over 9000 men in nine countries in four continents showed that overall acceptance of the concept of hormonal male contraception was greater than 55%, but there was wide variation between nationalities (29–71% acceptance), indicating that such a method will not be suitable for all men.[17]

With long-acting delivery routes (implant, pellet or injection), the issue of whether women would trust men to take a male contraceptive pill is not a factor. However, a survey of 1894 women in three countries showed that only 13% thought that a hormonal male contraceptive was a bad idea and only 2% would not trust their partner to take the pills.[18]

In summary, a hormonal contraceptive method for men may be available in 2012. It is likely to be effective and suitable for some men. Whether this regimen will have positive or negative health consequences in the longer term is uncertain. Concerns about the TU-NET-EN combination include the reduction of high-density lipoprotein (HDL) levels by the androgenic progestogen and effects of TU on the prostate.

• Non–hormonal methods

In 2007 no non-hormonal methods for men are likely to be available in the next 5 years. There are potential target molecules in the development pipeline which may be a reality within 15 years. Examples are Eppin, an epididymal protease inhibitor; glyceraldehyde 3-phosphate dehydrogenase-S, a sperm-specific glycolytic enzyme; hormone sensitive lipase; retinoic acid receptor antagonists; testis-specific spermatid thioredoxin system (Sptrx-1, -2 and -3), and the c-ros oncogene. Although promising, there is no guarantee that any of these targets will result in success. There are other possibilities further along the preclinical developmental pathway.

Lonidamine, Adjudin and gamendazole

In 1975, interesting antifertility activity was described for lonidamine, an anticancer drug. Unfortunately, this compound was too toxic for use as a male contraceptive.

A search for less toxic analogues with the same properties came up with Adjudin (AF2364), which causes reversible inhibition of fertility in male rats when given orally. It works by damaging the cell adhesion function between elongating spermatids and Sertoli cells in the testis, and causing premature exfoliation of immature sperm from the seminiferous epithelium. This novel mode of action gave rise to the hope that a monthly treatment regimen could be envisaged, as regeneration of mature sperm would take more than 30 days. High doses were needed because of poor bioavailability. Initial toxicity tests with a single high oral dose or five weekly doses showed no adverse effects.[19] However, significant toxicity was seen following 28 days continuous administration and work with this compound was abandoned.

Another group following the lonidamine lead, identified another analogue, gamendazole, that had better bioavailability and increased potency compared to AF2364. However, not all rats returned to complete fertility, and work is continuing to look for other analogues that permit reversal.

FSH mutant–Adjudin complex

If there was a way of targeting the activity of compounds specifically to the testis, systemic toxicity might be avoided. A recent report provides a strategy to accomplish this. It entails inducing mutations in both alpha and beta subunits of FSH so that it no longer has hormonal activity, but still binds to FSH receptors localized to the Sertoli cells in the testis. Administration of Adjudin alone (50 mg/kg/day orally) caused infertility but also led to liver inflammation and muscle atrophy. In contrast, Adjudin conjugated to the FSH mutant at a dose of 0.05 mg/kg given once intraperitoneally to male rats induced complete infertility at 4 weeks continuing up to 12 weeks with complete restoration of fertility at 20 weeks.[20] Conjugation with the mutant reduced the amount of Adjudin that reached the liver and reduced the amount needed to induce infertility by more than 1000-fold. Whether this strategy will reduce the liver and muscle toxicity seen with longer-term dosing of Adjudin remains to be seen. In addition, the present proof of principle suffers from the need to deliver the mutant–Adjudin complex by intraperitoneal injection. Even if intramuscular injection would work, we know from the studies on hormonal male methods that monthly injections are marginally acceptable. Thus, this is a work in progress but one which holds promise.

Occludin

Occludin is a peptide that plays a key role in maintaining tight junctions which are an essential component of the blood–testis barrier. Inhibition of occludin breaches this barrier, and causes infertility.[21] Peptide antagonists of occludin are being developed. Here again, the success of this approach hinges on developing a practical delivery route.

One of the problems with such peptide approaches is that they cannot be given orally due to rapid metabolism. Systemic administration, even at infrequent intervals, raises issues of acceptability and also the possibility of systemic toxicity. Again, if there was a way of targeting the activity of such compounds to the testis, similar to the FSH mutant–Adjudin complex described above, systemic toxicity could be minimized.

Miglustat

Another promising lead concerns an imino sugar, miglustat, which is already in clinical use for treatment of Gaucher's disease. Long-term low-dose treatment causes fully reversible infertility in male mice.[22] Since the drug is already in clinical use the road to regulatory approval for this second indication might be shorter than usual. In addition, miglustat also inhibits HIV replication and syncytium formation, and thus could theoretically provide dual protection against pregnancy and HIV infection. However, it does not appear to cause infertility in men. Until the discrepancy between species in response to this drug is understood, development of new analogues will be at a halt.

CatSper

A well-advanced approach to non-hormonal male contraception is CatSper, which stands for a cation channel of sperm. The cation, calcium, plays a crucial role in mammalian fertilization. CatSper is located in the principal piece of the sperm tail, and in mice with CatSper knocked out, sperm motility is decreased and the mice are infertile. Subfertile men with poor sperm motility also have low levels of CatSper.[23]

Idenopyridine compounds

A second approach which is also well advanced involves certain idenopyridine compounds. One of them, CDB-4022 (RTI-4587-073), causes disruption of spermatogenesis and infertility in male rats. Toxicology studies in rats with a related compound showed only minor side effects, but the oral doses used caused testicular atrophy. Lower doses could still produce infertility, but without testicular atrophy. Treatment of male cynomolgus monkeys with 12.5 mg/kg/day CDB-4022 by naso-gastric tube for 7 days decreased sperm concentrations to <1 million/ml by day 17 and they remained suppressed through week six. Sperm motility was also completely inhibited. By week 16 sperm concentrations had returned to normal.[24] Men with sperm concentrations reduced to this level are infertile. Although only one treatment regimen was studied, this is a most promising result for development of a non-hormonal male contraceptive. Additional dose-finding and length of treatment studies are needed to move this lead forward.

• Male barrier methods

Vasectomy is a widely used method of male fertility control, but is not easily reversible. Where cost is no option, intra-cytoplasmic sperm injection (ICSI) can be used to achieve a pregnancy. However, a more practical solution would be the development of a reversible method of male sterilization. It seems possible that at least one of the novel vas-blocking approaches could be approved within the next 5 years depending on the degree of pregnancy prevention, side effects and reversibility.

Intra Vas Device (IVD)

The SHUG, now known as the Intra Vas Device has been under development for more than 20 years. It consists of two 1 inch long flexible silicone plugs joined by a thread which remains outside the vas and is used to remove the device. The device does not completely block sperm transit through the epididymis, failing in three out of 30 men.[25] However, the numbers of sperm escaping were well below those usually needed for fertility. The device now comes in three sizes, thus ensuring a better fit and less sperm leakage. Further trials are ongoing.

A Chinese group completed a randomized trial of a different IVD comparing it to the no-scalpel vasectomy widely used in China.[26] During 1 year of follow-up no method failures were reported in either group. The degree of azoospermia was lower with the IVD than with the no-scalpel technique. Contraceptive success was similar for both groups, 94.3% for the IVD group and 98.6% for the no-scalpel group. Whether this degree of protection will be acceptable, and whether when the device is removed fertility will be restored remains to be determined.

RISUG (Reversible Inhibition of Sperm Under Guidance)

Another approach to reversible vasectomy has been the development of RISUG. A styrene maleic anhydride gel is injected into the vas, percutaneously or using the no-scalpel vasectomy technique, and then solidifies to plug the vas. Sperm coming in contact with the plug are damaged and lose motility. The polymer can be flushed out of the vas to restore fertility. A small trial resulted in azoospermia within 5 days and no pregnancies were reported during 12 months of use.[27] In another small study azoospermia took up to 4 months to appear but again no pregnancies were reported during the study period.[28] Theoretically this procedure should cause less back-pressure, and hence less irreversible damage to the epithelium of the vas, than the IVD. Some evidence has been gathered from monkeys which had vas occlusion by RISUG for 540 days. Sperm parameters returned to normal by 90–120 days after removal of the RISUG. Worryingly, during the period of occlusion focal damage to the testes was observed, but testis morphology returned to normal within 190 days.[29] There have been extensive safety studies conducted and the experience of over 25 years in animals and men shows this to be a safe and effective procedure.

Since all the work on RISUG has been done in India, the initial approval will likely be achieved there. Although some of the clinical studies have run for many years, the total number of men exposed is small and a large trial conducted to GCP standards is needed. These requirements suggest that this technique will not be available outside India in the medium term. The advantage of RISUG over vasectomy is the rapid onset of infertility. However, there is a downside in the long period required to return to normal fertility. The consequences of a pregnancy occurring during the period of sperm reversion to normality are unknown, and could potentially be a major problem.

Chemical barriers

A different way of blocking sperm from being ejaculated is a chemical, as opposed to, a mechanical barrier. For 50 years it has been known that men treated with alpha-adrenergic blocking agents, such as phenoxybenzamine, experience a dry orgasm, i.e. there is no ejaculation. Recently this notion has been resurrected and a possible mode of action identified. It seems that phenoxybenzamine blocks contractions of the vas deferens induced by norepinephrine in the longitudinal, but not in the circular muscle. Various compounds have been tested on human vas deferens in vitro and some of them can discriminate between the circular and longitudinal adrenoceptor subtypes in vas deferens muscles. Further testing has identified a promising lead, but as yet no clinical trials have been started. Provided these are successful and side effects are not an issue, this new method might be available in less than 10 years. The attraction of this approach is that the pill could be taken a few hours before need and the effect would only last for about 12 hours.

REFERENCES

1. Upadhyay U (2005) New contraceptive choices. Population Reports Special Topics 2005; Series M. no. 19, Johns Hopkins Bloomberg School of Public Health, The INFO Project; Baltimore 23pp (also available at: http://www.infoforhealth.org/pr/m19/index.shtml)

2. Bata MS, Al-Ramahi M, Salhab AS et al. (2006) Delay of ovulation by meloxicam in healthy cycling volunteers: A placebo-controlled, double-blind, crossover study. Journal of Clinical Pharmacology 46: 925–932.

3. Von Hertzen H, Piaggio G, Ding J et al. (2002) Low dose mifepristone and two regimens of levonorgestrel for emergency contraception: a WHO multicentre randomized trial. Lancet 360: 1803–1810.

4. Baird DT, Brown A, Cheng L et al. (2003) Mifepristone: a novel estrogen-free daily contraceptive pill. Steroids 68: 1099–1115.

5. Van Damme L, Ramjee G, Alary M et al. (2002) Effectiveness of COL-1492, a nonoxynol-9 vaginal gel, on HIV-transmission among female sex workers. Lancet 360: 971–977 (erratum in Lancet 360:1892).

6. Mauck CK, Weiner DH, Creinin MD et al. (2004) A randomized Phase I vaginal safety study of three concentrations of C31G vs. Extra Strength Gynol II. Contraception 70: 233–240.

7. Anderson RA, Feathergill K, Diao X-H et al. (2004) Contraception by Ushercell™ (cellulose sulfate) in formulation: duration of effect and dose effectiveness. Contraception 70: 415–422.

8. Schwartz JL, Mauck CK, Rountree RW et al. (2006) SILCS diaphragm: Postcoital testing of a new single-size contraceptive diaphragm. Obstetrics & Gynecology 107: 125.

9. Benagiano G (2001) Non-surgical female sterilization with quinacrine: An update. Contraception 63: 239–245.

10. Valle RF, Carignan CS, Wright TC (2001) Tissue response to the STOP microcoil transcervical permanent contraceptive device. Results from a prehysterectomy study. Fertility and Sterility 76: 974–980.

11. Beksinska M, Smit J, Mabude Z et al. (2006) Performance of the Reality® polyurethane female condom and a synthetic latex prototype: a randomized crossover trial among South African women. Contraception 73: 386–393.

12. Smita J, Neelam J, Rochelle DY et al. (2005) Comparative acceptability study of the Reality female condom and the version 4 of modified Reddy female condom in India. Contraception 72: 366–371.

13. Coffey PS, Kilbourne-Brook M, Austin G et al. (2006) Short-term acceptability of the PATH woman's condom among couples at three sites. Contraception 73: 588–593.

14. World Health Organization Task Force on Methods for the Regulation of Male Fertility (1990) Contraceptive efficacy of testosterone-induced azoospermia in normal men. Lancet 336: 955–959.

15. World Health Organization Task Force on Methods for the Regulation of Male Fertility (1996) Contraceptive efficacy of testosterone-induced azoospermia and oligospermia in normal men. Fertility and Sterility 65: 821–829.

16. Merriggiola MC, Constantino A, Saad F et al. (2005) Norethisterone enanthate plus testosterone undecanoate for male contraception: effects of various injection intervals on spermatogenesis, reproductive hormones, testis, and prostate. Journal of Clinical Endocrinology and Metabolism 90: 2005–2014.

17. Heinemann K, Saad F, Wiesemes M et al. (2005) Attitudes toward male fertility control: results of a multinational survey on four continents. Human Reproduction 20: 549–556.

18. Glasier A, Anakwe R, Everington D et al. (2000) Would women trust their partners to use a male pill? Human Reproduction 15: 646–649.

19. Cheng CY, Mruk D, Silvestrini B et al. (2005) AF2364 [1-(2,4-dichlorobenzyl)-1H-indazole-3-carbohydrazide] is a potential male contraceptive: a review of recent data. Contraception 72: 251–261.

20. Mruk DD, Wong CH, Silvestrini B et al. (2006) A male contraceptive targeting germ cell adhesion. Nature Medicine 12: 1323–1328.

21. Wong CH, Mruk DD, Lui WY et al. (2004) Regulation of blood–testis barrier dynamics: an in vivo study. Journal of Cell Science 117: 783–798.

22. Walden CM, Butters TD, Dwek RA et al. (2006) Long-term non-hormonal male contraception in mice using N-butyldeoxynojirimycin. Human Reproduction 21: 1309–1315.

23. Nikpoor P, Mowla SJ, Movahedin M et al. (2004) CatSper gene expression in postnatal development of mouse testis and in subfertile men with deficient sperm motility. Human Reproduction 19: 124–128.

24. Hild SA, Marshall GR, Attardi BJ et al. (2007) Development of l-CDB-4022 as a nonsteroidal male oral contraceptive: Induction and recovery from severe oligospermia in the adult male cynomolgus monkey (Macaca fascicularlis). Endocrinology 148: 1784–1796.

25. Zaneveld LJ, De Castro MP, Faria G et al. (1998) The soft hollow plug ('SHUG'): a potentially reversible vas deferens blocking device. In: Griffin PD, Rajalakshmi M, eds. Male contraception: present and future. New Delhi: New Age International, pp. 293.

26. Song L, Gu Y, Lu W et al. (2006) A phase II randomized controlled trial of a novel male contraception, an intra-vas device. International Journal of Andrology 29: 489–495.

27. Guha SK, Singh G, Ansari S et al. (1997) Phase II clinical trial of a vas deferens injectable contraceptive for the male. Contraception 56: 245–250.

28. Chaki SP, Das HC, Misro MM (2003) A short-term evaluation of semen and accessory gland function in phase III trial subjects receiving intravasal contraceptive RISUG. Contraception 67: 73–78.

29. Lohiya NK, Manivannan B, Mishra PK et al. (2005) Preclinical evaluation for non-invasive reversal following long-term vas occlusion with styrene maleic anhydride in langur monkeys. Contraception 71: 214–226.

Index

Page numbers for figures in **bold**; page numbers for tables in *italics*

Q

R

S

Y